D1563315

Crisis Intervention and Trauma

New Approaches to Evidence-Based Practice

Issues in the Practice of Psychology

SERIES EDITOR:

George Stricker, *Derner Institute of Advanced Psychological Studies,
Adelphi University, Garden City, New York*

A Continuation Order Plan is available for this series. A continuation order will bring
delivery of each new volume immediately upon publication. Volumes are billed only upon
actual shipment. For further information please contact the publisher.

Crisis Intervention and Trauma

New Approaches to Evidence-Based Practice

Jennifer L. Hillman

Pennsylvania State University
Berks-Lehigh Valley College
Reading, Pennsylvania

KLUWER ACADEMIC/PLENUM PUBLISHERS
NEW YORK, BOSTON, DORDRECHT, LONDON, MOSCOW

ISBN: 0-306-47341-0

©2002 Kluwer Academic / Plenum Publishers, New York
233 Spring Street, New York, N.Y. 10013

http://www.wkap.nl/

10 9 8 7 6 5 4 3 2 1

A C.I.P. record for this book is available from the Library of Congress

Printed in the United States of America

In honor of
those affected by the events of September 11, 2001
and in memory of
Roland Kandle

Preface

This book would not be possible without the courage of my patients. I remain in awe of their resiliency, courage, and grace. I am honored to bear witness as they share their most private experiences of trauma and survival. I also would like to send a special thank-you to the Maple Shade, NJ, United States Search and Rescue Task Force members.

A number of experienced, skilled, intelligent, open-minded, and generous clinicians and researchers have helped shape my work in crisis and trauma. These individuals include: George Stricker, Rick Zweig, Eileen Rosendahl, Michael Bibbo, Donna Chimera, Andrea Rae, Patrick Ross, Greg Hinrichsen, Jonathan Jackson, Denise Hien, Adrienne DeSimonne, Nina Yentzer, Christine Li, Elissa Lesser, Buckley Miller, Suzanne Weaver, Steven Silver, Edward Moon, and Tom Skoloda. My undergraduate research assistants, Katie Traczuk, Jason Briggs, Renee Waage, and Vanessa Milan, have been a terrific help and a constant source of encouragement. I wish them all of the best in their future endeavors.

I also would like to thank the following individuals, in addition to my family members, for their tremendous emotional support: Molly Dallmeyer, Jeffrey Kurtz, Rowena Fantasia-Davis, Francine Scoboria, Ike Shibley, Lisa Shibley, Candace Spiegelman, Danielle Richards, Henry Patterson, Willis Frankhouser, Peter Behrens, Carl Lovitt, Sandy Feinstien, Deb Guy, Ken Fifer, and, once again, George Stricker.

The Berks County, Pennsylvania, Community Foundation, Berks County AIDSNet (of the Pennsylvania Department of Health), the Berks County Area on Aging, the Berks and Lehigh Valley County Red Cross, Berks Women in Crisis, and the National Association of HIV over Fifty also provided me with a significant amount of formal and informal research support. Barbara Waller, Kathleen Kinney, Nadine Miller, Richard Mappin, Kevin Murphy, Andrea Rae, Nathan Linsk, Jayne Fowler, and Ann Barlet, among others, provide invaluable leadership in those aforementioned organizations. I thank them for allowing me to be associated with them and the valuable work that they do.

Contents

ix

1

Introductory Aspects of Crisis Intervention and Trauma Counseling

Although the ancient Chinese developed a character for the word "crisis" by combining pictographs of both "danger" and "opportunity," clearly demonstrating their understanding of its potential for both negative and positive outcomes, the formal recognition of crisis intervention as a clinical specialty by the American Psychological Association did not occur until 1989.

This text is designed to serve three broad purposes. First, it is designed to alert mental health professionals to many of the newer, and sometimes controversial, theoretical and practice issues in crisis intervention and trauma counseling. In response to increasing concerns about the effectiveness of various approaches to treatment (e.g., third party payers; managed care organizations), significant emphasis has been placed upon the integration of empirical research findings. Earnest effort also has been made to present relate clinical case reports in order to provide a balanced perspective.

Second, this text is intended to serve as a resource for both novice and experienced professionals. Consistent with recent trends in which therapists are learning to recognize the critical need for appropriate self-care, a vital feature of this text is an exploration of the personal impact that such challenging work can have upon therapists themselves. Because the vast majority of clinical case studies available in the literature tend to focus upon treatment "successes" (Stricker, 1995a) preventing clinicians from discussing various treatment challenges openly and honestly, the current text offers a variety of case studies and clinical anecdotes in which clinicians struggle with certain patients and crisis situations. Such examples of steps and mis-steps in therapy are designed to offer a more realistic view of crisis intervention, and to aid therapists engaged in both training and supervision (e.g., Stricker, 1995b).

Third, this book is intended to bear witness to the wide-ranging experience of individuals in crisis, including those affected by the recent, tragic events of September 11, 2001. Honest, unflinching appraisals of trauma are needed to help make professionals, as well as laypersons, more comfortable with necessary discussions of trauma (c.f., Herman, 1997). As evidenced by general social psychological principles highlighted in the next chapter (e.g., Lerner's Just World Theory; 1980), the social stigma typically associated with crisis and trauma can help prevent individuals from receiving necessary social support and treatment.

DEMOGRAPHICS AND TRAUMA

The prevalence of trauma and crisis in our society, which cuts across age, race, gender, ethnicity, religion, intelligence, and socio-economic status, cannot be underestimated. Various experts suggest that nearly 40% of men and 70% of women in the United States will experience at least one traumatic event in their lifetime, with more than 75% of those individuals experiencing at least symptoms of Posttraumatic Stress Disorder (Herman, 1997). Approximately one out of three female patients in a hospital emergency room is a victim of domestic abuse (Guth & Pachter, 2000), and more than two in five Americans citizens may experience some form of sexual or physical abuse throughout their lives (e.g., Avery-Leaf, Cascardi, O'Leary, & Cano, 1997). The presence of recent terrorist attacks upon the United States, including the tragic events of September 11, 2001 in which more than 6,000 people were killed when two hijacked jumbo jets felled the World Trade Center's twin towers, makes previous estimates regarding the prevalence of trauma in our society appear conservative, at best.

A significant amount of governmental legislation and funding is devoted to trauma related initiatives. International disaster relief supplied by the U.S. surpasses over one trillion dollars per year. Even before the terrorist attacks on September 11, 2001, the American

Federal Emergency Management Agency (FEMA) was appropriated an annual budget of more than 1.37 billion dollars (White, 2001). Despite this outpouring of governmental attention and resources, however, millions of dollars in U.S. revenue are lost every year due to problems in coping with a variety of traumatic events. Worker inefficiency, turnover, absenteeism, and even sabotage and theft are often linked with the presence of domestic abuse, workplace violence, substance abuse, depression, anxiety disorders, and other forms of mental illness.

In response, a number of independent professional and government related organizations have made significant efforts to acknowledge the impact of unmitigated crises upon individuals, families, cultures, and societies. The American Psychological Association officially sanctioned "Emergencies and Crises" as a member (i.e., section VII) of their Clinical Psychology Division in 1989. Two years later, the American Red Cross introduced the APA's Disaster Response Network as a professional service branch of their organization. The vast majority of state and local agencies currently work with FEMA to develop up to date emergency response plans for everything from natural disasters to biological warfare, including the utilization of mental health professionals. Although controversial (Dineen, 2000), various governmental agencies, including the FBI, have adopted specific, mandatory psychological interventions for use with their own employees in times of crisis.

Despite the increased demand for psychological services in response to traumatic incidents, practitioners and trainees in academic and clinical settings have few resources available to provide step-by-step, detailed information about how to engage in crisis intervention. Limited information also exists regarding the ability of these interventions to ameliorate suffering and prevent the development of chronic mental illness. The American Psychological Association's Task Force on Education and Training in Behavioral Emergencies (of Section VII, Division 12; 2000) itself describes current graduate training in behavioral emergencies as woefully inadequate, and calls for improved curricula and coursework in crisis intervention. Thus, this text also attempts to address a variety of issues in crisis intervention and trauma counseling, including the integration of clinical theory and practice with evidence based research findings.

HISTORICAL PERSPECTIVES

Understanding the development of professional interest in crisis intervention itself can be instructive. The first community crisis center was established in the 1940's by Eric Lindemann and Gerald Caplan. Despite the extent to which many survivors of trauma experienced severe psychological distress, including participation in suicidal acts, these two clinicians believed that with appropriate, and sometimes necessary, psychiatric intervention patients could be allowed to undergo a "normal grief reaction (1944)." Patients were encouraged to identify and work through any related feelings of anger, grief, loss, and relief, and to elicit instrumental as well as emotional assistance from various individuals and community based organizations (e.g., churches). Although Lindemann (1944) endorsed the use of shock treatment for individuals who became suicidal after traumatic events, his general approaches to crisis intervention appear quite insightful in relation to a zeitgeist that instructed an individual to "bite the bullet," "keep a stiff upper lip," and "pull yourself up by your bootstraps."

Lindemann (1944) also made the following critical assertions, which provided the foundation for future work in crisis intervention and trauma counseling:

- People in crisis can be receptive to major life changes.
- Crisis intervention can be accomplished in a relatively brief period of time (e.g., 10 sessions).
- People in crisis can be helped significantly through supportive networks with friends, paraprofessionals, and religious leaders.
- An adaptive resolution to a crisis situation can result in enduring, positive change.

POINTS OF CONSENSUS

In the more than half a century after Caplan and Lindemann opened their first community crisis clinic, many principles of crisis intervention evoke little debate or controversy among practitioners. Some of these generally accepted tenets are articulated here:

1. Crisis intervention is brief and time limited. It is not intended to foster a long-term therapeutic relationship or long-term personality change. This central feature of time as a fixed factor in crisis intervention is based upon the early work of a work efficiency expert, C. N Parkinson. Parkinson recognized that whether he had a few weeks or a few months to finish a job, he was able to complete the short-term jobs just as well as the long-term jobs, which often seemed to drag out. He also discovered that many employees with long-term deadlines tended to procrastinate, and got much of the work done in the last possible

moments. Thus, he advanced the formal supposition that "work expands or contracts to meet the time available for its completion," which became widely known in the business community as Parkinson's Law.

In the late 1970's two therapists, Appelbaum (1975) and Baldwin (1979), adapted Parkinson's Law for application in psychotherapy. Appelbaum posited that both conscious and unconscious patient motivation increases when a time limit is introduced early in treatment, and that such time limits similarly increase therapists' sense of accountability and motivation. Baldwin applied Parkinson's Law specifically to crisis intervention and reasoned that reasonable time limits imposed in crisis counseling will force the "work" of crisis resolution to fit the prescribed length of treatment. For better or worse, managed care plans' limitation in the number of individual treatment sessions is consistent with this time-limited approach.

2. Patient and therapist safety must be ensured before effective crisis intervention can take place. Tenets from even the most diverse theoretical orientations (e.g., behavioral, feminist, and analytical approaches) stipulate that patient safety must receive initial and focused attention.

3. Crisis intervention is more active than passive. Therapists must act quickly to engage a patient in the therapeutic process within their first meeting. Unlike other theoretical orientations, including Rogerian, analytic, and many dynamic approaches, therapists who provide crisis intervention are sometimes encouraged to provide direct suggestions and advice to patients in a state of extreme distress and confusion. Therapists also cannot afford to allow patients to skirt the immediate issues involving their crisis, and interpret and revisit their patient's "resistance" during a later session. Although paradoxical, crisis therapists often must provide the most active (but not necessarily directive) therapy with their most passive and disoriented patients in order to assess and ensure patient safety, and to help patients regain a sense of control over their own situation.

4. Clinical material unrelated to the patient's present crisis has limited value in crisis intervention. In other words, even though psychological testing, a detailed social history, and family map or genogram would provide valuable clinical information, the need for immediate action does not allow for such time intensive processes. Rapid assessment of the patient's problem is essential, and must often be accomplished with incomplete information. In some cases, a patient's resistance to coping with a current crisis may, in fact, be exacerbated by a therapist's unintentional emphasis upon childhood and other early life

antecedents. Similar to Yalom's seminal tenets of group work (Yalom, 1995), crisis intervention is intended to focus on the here-and-now.

5. Effective crisis intervention demands therapeutic flexibility. Effective crisis intervention borrows techniques for assessment and intervention form a variety of theoretical orientations, including cognitive, behavioral, family systems, group, existential, humanistic, person-centered, dynamic, reality based, and others. Thus, therapists must be skilled in a range of therapeutic techniques and familiar with a variety of orientations. Therapists are encouraged to select from a variety of clinical interventions, but only if an intervention is tailored to "fit" a patient, and not the patient to "fit" the intervention. Although such an eclectic (or integrative) approach can be anxiety provoking for some therapists, at times, increased opportunities for professional and personal growth are also likely.

6. Therapists must be prepared to work with diverse patient populations. Crises occur irrespective of an individual's age, sex, gender, ethnicity, cultural background, disability, intelligence, religious affiliation, or socio-economic status. A willingness to be open to different cultural, religious, and other beliefs becomes requisite. Although therapists should be familiar with general norms, expectations, and traditions for different patient groups (e.g., older adults; Chinese immigrants; Catholics), care also must be taken to avoid making assumptions about a *specific* patient's ethnicity, sexual orientation, and beliefs (also see Chapter 11). The best way for therapists to address such concerns is to simply and respectfully ask questions.

7. Effective work in crisis intervention demands constant ethical evaluation and consideration. If treatment proceeds as intended, an active approach allows patients to make significant gains in only a few sessions, and fosters immediate, effective responses to a critical event. However, therapists can inadvertently use their powerful position (i.e., the vast majority of patients who seek crisis intervention present with some kind of cognitive disequilibrium and a significant amount of distress) to lead patients to make important decisions and treatment goals, based upon the therapists underlying values and beliefs rather than their own. For example, a therapist who provides crisis intervention to an anxious, confused 16 year-old girl who just learned about an unwanted pregnancy must carefully acknowledge and process his own attitudes toward adoption and abortion in order to avoid any inappropriate, authoritarian influence.

8. Crisis intervention may take place in a variety of settings. With the primary exception of in-vivo treatment for phobias and other anxiety disorders, the majority of traditional psychotherapies takes place in

a private office or controlled, hospital setting. In contrast, many forms of crisis intervention take place, quite literally, outside of such a traditional, controlled environment. For example, mobile crisis intervention teams and wrap-around service programs send therapists into the very settings that patients themselves tend to experience as unsupportive, stressful, and even dangerous. (Such immersion in a patient's environment also often reveals a wealth of vital information about a patient's critical situation and environment.) Phone contact via hot line programs allows patients to seek crisis intervention without revealing their identity, scheduling a formal appointment, or traveling to a distant clinic, but such limited, relatively anonymous contact does not afford the professional support and structure to which most therapists have become accustomed. Without face-to-face contact, clinical assessment becomes increasingly difficult and complex.

9. Patients require crisis intervention in a variety of clinical scenarios. For example, someone may seek therapeutic support for the first time after experiencing a critical incident. Or, a patient already may be in psychotherapy when they experience a crisis. Or, a patient already in therapy may represent the focus of a crisis (e.g., a patient experiences a psychotic break or a suicide attempt). Each of these clinical scenarios is uniquely different, and will require an equally unique approach to treatment.

10. The goal of crisis intervention is to return individuals to their previous level of functioning; no assumption of previous psychopathology is made. This general assumption can translate into high expectations of adjustment and normality after a crisis among those who seek treatment. These perceived therapist expectations may foster a self-fulfilling prophesy among patients, and offer an increased sense of hope for recovery. However, it also may be detrimental to ignore the number of people with serious Axis I (e.g., schizophrenia; bipolar disorder) and Axis II disorders (e.g., borderline, narcissistic, and antisocial personality disorder) who seek help in response to crisis. Thus, despite initial considerations of normal levels of functioning before the traumatic event, the accurate and appropriate assessment of serious, chronic psychological illness remains essential in work with any patient.

POINTS OF CONTENTION

Since the introduction of Lindemann and Caplan's groundbreaking work, in which crisis intervention and trauma counseling was portrayed as a relatively straightforward yet highly beneficial undertaking, important questions have been raised regarding *when* treatment should take place (e.g., as soon as possible after traumatic incident or when the survivors seek it), *how* it should be regulated (e.g., by individual practitioners or organizational units), and *who* should offer it (e.g., licensed mental health professionals, paraprofessionals, or peers). Additional concerns regarding evidence-based treatment also have begun to influence the manner in which mental health practitioners, government agencies, and private organizations and businesses engage in crisis intervention. An examination of these opposing views (i.e., dialectics) can prove invaluable in order to address some of these aforementioned issues. A number of these dialectics will be addressed throughout the text, with some of the more central themes highlighted here:

Empirical vs. Anecdotal

Due in part to mandates from managed care, increasing emphasis has been placed upon empirical evidence or "proof" that a practitioner can provide effective, and often time-limited, treatment. At the extreme, practitioners may employ only empirically validated, rigidly structured, manualized treatments in their practice or employ only anecdotally based treatments with no regard for systematic study or review of that approach. Perhaps the more appropriate approach is to use empirically validated treatments as a benchmark or starting point in treatment, but also to encourage practitioners to use their clinical training, acumen, experience, and intuition to vary, expand, modify, and deviate from those standardized treatments. The number one priority for practitioners, however, remains reflected in the Hippocratic oath, to "do no harm." Because a number of empirical investigations suggest that some approaches to crisis intervention and trauma counseling actually may harm patients (e.g., Critical Incident Stress Debriefing, CISD; Dineen, 2000; see Chapter 10, practitioners are entreated to integrate findings from clinical research and practice into their own work.

Profit vs. Non-Profit

Another pivotal issue that emerges in work with crisis and trauma is that of profit versus non-profit (e.g., pro bono) work among both practitioners and researchers. Current APA ethical guidelines (1992) do not require but only encourage therapists to provide pro bono services. Some practitioners regard crisis intervention and trauma counseling as a socially requisite function, and conclude that such services should be offered at no charge to those in need, or that they should at least be subsidized by government agencies. Other practitioners note that individuals in any helping profession, including that of mental health, deserve to charge fees that allow them to pay off increasingly high student loans, enjoy a decent standard of living, and seek appropriate compensation for their level of professional training and skill. Some clinicians suggest that by offering inexpensive services, the field of mental health will garner a second-rate reputation in comparison to other health care fields.

From a market-based perspective, practitioners (and researchers) should be entitled to market their products and services in response to general conditions of supply and demand. Critics of this approach argue that the "psychology industry" has purposefully identified all survivors of trauma and crisis as potential victims in need of specific services (Dineen, 2000) in order to artificially generate increased demand for service. The emergence of specialized training centers, for profit organizations, and required certifications in various aspects of treatment related to crisis intervention and trauma counseling (e.g., Critical Incident Stress Management; Eye Movement Desensitization and Reprocessing) may force practitioners to examine the positive and negative aspects of personal and professional gain.

Peer vs. Professional

Important questions can be raised regarding the specific training, skills, and background required for individuals to perform effective crisis intervention and trauma counseling. Many crisis hot lines employ individuals without a bachelors degree in psychology, social work, or mental health, and require only a few sessions of in-house or on-the-job training. In response to personnel shortages, certain states now hire individuals with 60 college credit hours in psychology to serve as therapeutic support staff (TSS) in state-funded home based treatment and crisis intervention programs (also see Chapter 12). Similarly, paraprofessionals (e.g., grief counselors; Steven's ministers; 12 step group leaders) often engage in crisis intervention and trauma counseling. In contrast, only licensed mental health professionals such as psychologists and social workers can perform certain interventions, such as EMDR (see Chapter 4). Unlike paraprofessionals, licensed psychologists and other mental health care providers may have hospital privileges and immediate access to inpatient treatment options and facilities in various states.

In a frequently cited and often criticized (e.g., Brock, Green, & Reich, 1998) study published in *Consumer Reports*, Seligman (1995) found that licensed mental health practitioners and paraprofessionals had similar, favorable treatment outcomes, particularly in response to substance abuse. Various experts assert that crisis intervention with emergency service workers (e.g., fire fighters; police officers; paramedics) is likely to be effective only if those services are provided by an appropriately trained, identified peer (Mitchell & Everly, 1998). Other mental health practitioners describe situations in which paraprofessionals overlooked, were unaware of, or were unable to assess a patient's chronic mental illness until significant alterations in mental status created or led to a serious state of crisis. Until additional, empirical information is available, the critical issue of *who* provides the most effective crisis intervention *under what conditions, and why* remains to be fully addressed.

Individual vs. Group

In addition to making decision about providing group verses individual treatment, clinicians often must assess their patient's functioning as an individual, and within the context of a group. A systemic approach considering familial, peer, cultural, religious, community, and work related influences, is often required to make the most effective interventions (see Chapter 11). Less commonly incorporated into treatment perspectives, however, are some general social psychological principles that often underlie one's experience of trauma. For example, bystanders are more likely to assist someone in distress depending upon various critical cues in the environment (e.g., number of bystanders; time pressure; ambiguity of the situation) than upon their own individual personality traits (Lerner, 1980). The support that survivors of trauma receive is often tied to societal perceptions of the survivor's personal characteristics (e.g., is an individual gay or heterosexual) rather than the nature of the trauma itself (e.g., HIV infection; McBride, 1998), leading many survivors to feel abandoned or inappropriately ashamed of their situation (see Chapter 2).

Female vs. Male

Societal perceptions and expectations also shape the experience of trauma, particularly in regard to gender. For example, many male victims of sexual abuse and domestic abuse fail to report these crimes out of fear that they will receive limited support, be emasculated, and even laughed at, especially by other men (c.f., Whatley & Riggio, 1993). For individual who commit the same crime, their sex can often influence rates of conviction and length of sentence (Zingraff & Randall, 1984). Various aspects of gender, including histories of oppression, sexual expression, job opportunities, and stereotypes can impact upon one's experience of traumatic events. Although an ideal setting would allow practitioners to regard male and female patients in crisis similarly, a careful analysis of gender and sex roles must be performed to provide clients with the most effective treatment.

Youth vs. Advancing Age

The DSM-IV (APA, 1994) now includes information regarding advanced age as a factor in clinical diagnosis and etiology. From the perspective of crisis intervention and trauma counseling, a similar focus upon general developmental issues also is critical. Older adults represent an underserved patient population in the mental health community, and often present with symptoms that differ significantly from other young and middle-aged adults (e.g., Hillman, 2000). In the last decade, older adults also are significantly more likely to die from a suicide attempt than individuals in any other age group (Hendin, 1995; see Chapter 6). Various mental disorders associated with trauma (e.g., PTSD) also have been found to produce increasingly severe and intrusive symptoms with advanced age (Hillman, 2000).

Care also must be taken to acknowledge developmental differences in the processing of trauma among children and adolescents, as well as older adults with cognitive impairments. Dependency issues, ethical issues, legal constraints, and cognitive and emotional processing all can vary significantly between children and adults, and influence various aspects of assessment and treatment (see Chapter 11). Images in the media, including acts of violence and aggression, also appear to affect children quite differently than adults.

Voluntary vs. Involuntary

Questions also can be raised regarding the role of voluntary or involuntary assessment and treatment after the experience of a traumatic event. For example, many emergency service providers who experience a critical incident were required to attend mandatory, small group debriefings. Police officers who experience a traumatic event (e.g., a line of duty shooting; wounding or killing of a perpetrator) currently are required to meet with a police psychologist, and have the resulting report from that meeting become a permanent part of their personnel file. In certain situations, some governmental agencies and private businesses encourage the use of crisis intervention response teams (i.e., CISD) after an adverse event, and will even guarantee the provision of such services to its employees (see Chapter 10). Questions also arise regarding insurance coverage for injured workers, and the mandatory or voluntary nature of primary prevention programs in schools and at work.

Traditional vs. Non-Traditional

Americans' increasing utilization of complementary and alternative medicine (CAM), including herbal remedies, massage therapy, acupuncture, guided prayer (Pelletier, 2000), coupled with recent findings from newly established NIH study centers suggest that clinicians who engage in crisis intervention and trauma counseling may benefit from an examination of these issues and related techniques (e.g., mindful meditation; spirituality; see Chapter 11). Although such approaches may be regarded as non-traditional, empirical investigations will allow practitioners to better evaluate their options. Understanding the pros and cons of alternative medicine can also allow therapists to more effectively counsel patients about their options, as well as the potential side effects of certain CAM approaches.

Flexibility vs. Rigidity

Therapists often encourage their patients to remain open to new experiences, and to flexibility and choice among various life options. The use of "all or nothing thinking" and splitting has been identified as undesirable defense mechanisms. Therapists often encourage patients to avoid seeing things "in black and white," and tolerate ambiguity. However, within the context of crisis intervention and trauma counseling, certain edicts must be followed with virtual disregard for other factors in treatment. For example, if an individual is involved in an abusive relationship, patient safety immediately supercedes all other treatment goals and becomes the number one priority. In contrast to such rigid adherence to formal structure, however, therapists in crisis intervention and trauma counseling constantly must reappraise their patient's mental status, and consider the use of a wide range of therapeutic techniques.

Normal vs. Abnormal

Some debate exists regarding the labeling of certain events and experiences as traumatic, as well as regarding the labeling of certain individuals' responses to traumatic events. Even within a family, significant conflict can erupt concerning members' differential responses to a traumatic event such as a sexual assault, experience of a natural disaster, or death in the family. For example, is it "normal" that one family member becomes withdrawn, whereas another becomes engaged in an appropriate, yet frenetic, activity? Cultural differences often are overlooked as the focal lens through which many individuals view trauma. Some experts even question whether the millions of dollars spent on international (psychological) relief efforts may be misguided, because individuals abroad who are targeted for intervention may typically employ culture-specific rituals in order to cope with traumatic events, with even more success than strictly Western (i.e., mainstream American) approaches.

Action vs. Reaction

Increasing reports of school shootings, domestic violence, workplace violence, and suicide, as well as the terrorist attacks of September 11, 2001, find many communities demanding the development and provision of various violence prevention programs. This focus on prevention is consistent with many aspects of community, health, and positive psychology's focus upon positive behavior and effective coping strategies rather than upon specifically negative behavior and psychopathology. In other words, many mental health providers agree that it is often better to act first, and provide effective prevention, rather than have to react to a crisis later. However, the effectiveness of many primary prevention programs and screening instruments remains unclear, particularly within the context of teenage suicide and work related violence.

TEXT OVERVIEW

An important resource for evaluating empirically based research is that of the Cochrane Collaboration. This non-profit organization has been charged with preparing, maintaining, and disseminating systematic reviews of health related treatments ranging from wound healing to Critical Incident Stress Debriefing (Bero & Rennie, 1995). Independent experts rate all available studies on the quality of their methodology (i.e., does the sample size provide acceptable levels of statistical power; to what extent is the study sample representative of the general population; to what extent is the intervention standardized;

what inclusion criteria were applied; are participants randomly assigned to condition; did independent raters assess clinical outcomes) as well as other factors such as author affiliation (e.g., do the authors have any conflict of interest via their institutional affiliation or other funding source). Most Cochrane reports can be accessed via the internet or through university data sharing agreements.

Chapter 2 presents information germane to the intersection of social and clinical psychology in response to the survivors of trauma. Chapter 3 presents a suggested, step-by-step rubric for working with an individual in crisis. It provides specific information regarding clinical assessment and documentation in work with patients in crisis. Its focus upon the mental status exam as the primary mode of assessment is critical because it engages a common language in interdisciplinary settings, and increased parity among psychologists, social workers, nurses, psychiatrists, clergy, and other professionals. Critical legal and ethical issues for documentation are also presented.

Chapter 4 deals with PTSD, including its origins, assessment, and treatment. Newer and sometimes controversial approaches to treatment, such as EMDR, also are reviewed. Chapter 5 discusses some of the potential, long-term effects of trauma such as dissociative identity disorder and borderline personality disorder. A new paradigm is on the horizon in psychology as more researchers and clinicians posit that repeated exposure to abuse and trauma as a child can lead to devastating mental illness.

Chapter 6 provides detailed information about patient suicide, and Chapter 7 provides detailed information about patient violence. Because patient suicide and threats of physical violence represent one of the more stressful aspects of a clinician's work, Chapter 8 focuses upon the need for therapists to take care of themselves, and how to prevent, recognize, and treat various syndromes such as therapist burn-out and vicarious traumatization. Chapter 9 provides a general overview of some specific subtypes of trauma, including loss, death and dying, domestic abuse, and elder abuse. Although all specific types of trauma cannot be reviewed and discussed appropriately within the scope of this text, effort has been made to report upon the more recent advances in certain areas. (Readers should please note that inclusion or non-inclusion of a specific type of crisis or trauma is not indicative of more or less psychological relevance and importance!)

Chapter 10 discusses the role that clinicians can play in the prevention of violence in social settings such as schools and the workplace, as well as how to best treat those who may be survivors of such violence. The highly controversial role of Critical Incident Stress

Management will be reviewed from both a case study and empirical perspective. Chapter 11 focuses upon crisis intervention and trauma counseling among typically underserved patient populations, including children and adolescents, individuals from various cultural and ethnic groups, and older adults. And, Chapter 12 discusses the future of crisis intervention and counseling, including various topics such as alternative and complementary medicine, wrap-around services, and a renewed focus upon education and primary prevention.

2

The Social Psychology of Trauma
What Clinicians Need to Know

Both laboratory-based and naturalistic research findings suggest that situational factors, rather than personality traits and characteristics, are more likely to influence whether or not we will help someone in distress. An understanding of these powerful situational determinants, typically outside of one's conscious awareness, can greatly aid patients in the midst of crisis or trauma counseling.

OUR FASCINATION WITH CRISIS AND TRAUMA

Even after the vicious terrorist attacks of September 11th, our culture's obsession with death, violence, and fear remains clear. The demand for horror and action movies continues to drive the entertainment industry, and various authors such as Steven King and Anne Rice have made fortunes crafting lines of best selling horror novels. Highly rated, prime time television shows continue to feature many as eight or nine acts of physical violence per episode (Williams, Zabrack, & Joy, 1982). In sum, it appears that many individuals choose to familiarize themselves with the details of grisly stories and frightening events (Goldstein, 1998).

Freud himself discussed man's death drive as a primary motivating force in our existence, and death anxiety has become the subject of various empirical investigations (e.g., Simon, Greenberg, Harmon-Jones, Solomon, & Pyszczynski, 1996). Because death can be considered part

17

of the cycle of life, perhaps it is only natural that humans are obsessed by it. From a more pragmatic perspective, observing traumatic events, including fictitious ones, can provide some relevant information about human suffering, and perhaps allow some people to better prepare for such an event themselves. For example, we may have an opportunity to see what happens when someone drives too fast on a slick roadway or how someone bears up under the pain of a serious injury. Think about the morbid curiosity in effect as drivers slow (i.e., rubber neck) to get a glimpse of the scene of an accident, often resulting in mile long traffic jams. Yet, curiosity about any type of experience is a natural, human trait. And, it is especially important that therapists recognize, process, and accept their own curiosity in response to trauma and crisis.

An element of downward comparison also seems to present itself in consort with our fascination for crisis and trauma. Someone who is "safe" and healthy can develop a conscious or unconscious sense of relief, optimism, or gratitude that they are not currently suffering or in pain. Conscious recognition of this discrepancy between self and other, and accompanying positive, as well as negative, feelings also can elicit feelings of guilt or shame (e.g., How can I possibly feel happy to be alive when my friend was killed in the accident?). It is important to note that clinicians often can help patients in this position of relative safety and security to acknowledge that these types of feelings are natural and often unavoidable in response.

Early Lessons in Trauma

In the glow of flashlights and smoldering camp fires, young children often prod their parents, older siblings, and camp counselors into telling ghost stories that leave them anxious, frightened, jumpy, and huddled against one another. This apparent rite of passage allows children to experience fear and crisis, but only in a brief, time limited context. It also provides them with a socially sanctioned opportunity to call upon an authority figure to protect and care for them at the age when most children are often ambivalent about separation from their parents.

However, the current popularity of ghost stories persists from the earliest of periods of time. Fairy tales have thrilled children and adults alike for centuries. In contrast with relatively benign descriptions of ghosts and spirits in the contemporary children's series, *Goose Bumps* series, tales from earlier centuries were terrifying and graphic. By today's standards, their violent nature would probably prohibit their display in any children's section of any public library or private bookstore. An examination of these original fairy tales, however, as well as their modern counterparts, suggests a number of reasons that may account for their popularity and staying power.

The original tale of Hansel and Gretel recounts the adventures of two young children abandoned by their parents in a dark forest. Tired and hungry, the children find a small house, made themselves at home, and began to gorge themselves on treats. However, the resident of the house, an evil witch, has plans to fatten the children only so that she can eat them for dinner. Thanks to some quick thinking and resourcefulness, Hansel and Gretel push the witch into her own oven, killing her instead. In short, despite being abandoned by the very people who were supposed to protect and care for them, Hansel and Gretel functioned as autonomous individuals and survive a serious death threat (c.f., Ben-Amos, 1994).

Still other popular children's songs and lullabies contain elements of violence. To help children understand that death was a very real possibility for them, their parents, and many other people in their local town or village during the great plague or "Black Death"—songs such as "Ring around the Rosie/A pocket full of posies/Ashes, ashes, we all fall down!" were created to teach children about the disease. The song depicts healers' unsuccessful attempts to protect themselves from the plague by stuffing their pockets with fresh and dried flowers and herbs while tending to plague victims. As noted in the lyric, these posies had no medicinal value and "we all fall down [die]."

Obviously, few child development experts today would dream of composing children's songs about school shootings, terrorist attacks, domestic violence, and AIDS. (Various aspects of popular music, however, do give voice to these very themes.) Despite our culture's current ambivalence about the exposure of children to violence via videogames and other media, we continue to embrace such traditional rhymes and songs without awareness of their true, underlying nature.

Adult Interests in Trauma

Many adults, as well as children, seek out forms of entertainment that include aspects of horror, fantasy, and violence (Goldstein, 1998). Within the context of entertaining horror movies or books, audience members can experience the typically intense feelings associated with crisis and trauma, without having to suffer the literal, physical consequences. For example, some viewers like to experience an adrenaline rush during the anticipatory moments of a horror movie. Experiencing the strong feelings and bodily sensations typically associated with traumatic events, and having the subsequent experience of being able to literally leaving them behind at the theater provides viewers with a sense of hope and optimism that they themselves could indeed survive such a traumatic event.

This practice of becoming familiar with the experience of fear and anxiety, with the benefit of having the opportunity to acknowledge and process those feelings and sensations and feelings rather than being controlled by them, also is replicated outside of the movie theater. Soldiers typically use live ammunition during war games in order to prepare for actual battlefield conditions. Therapists may help patients suffering from panic disorders to self-induce the symptoms of a panic attack by running on a treadmill, for example (also see Chapter 4), to help them experience and manage these sensations in a controlled, "safe" environment.

ESSENTIAL SOCIAL PSYCHOLOGICAL THEORY

Many clinicians receive limited formal education in social psychology. Of course, it is unrealistic to suggest that therapists receive training in every subdiscipline of psychology, particularly when social psychologists do not focus upon abnormal thoughts, feelings, and behavior, but upon the behavior of non-disturbed or "typical" individuals. Fortunately, however, a cursory review of some fundamental social psychological principles will allow clinicians to gain valuable insight into survivors' (and perpetrators') experience of trauma. This differential perspective can be vital in providing more effective assessment and treatment for those in crisis. An examination of various historical and cultural beliefs regarding trauma is similarly informative for clinicians who work with patients in crisis.

The Actor-Observer Bias

According to the actor-observer bias (Jones & Nisbett, 1972; and the related, fundamental attribution error; Ross, 1977), individuals who observe another person's behavior are significantly more likely to think that this person's behavior is representative of his or her personality, and not a function of situational factors. In other words, people manifest a natural tendency to overestimate the role of personality as the driving force behind someone else's actions, while simultaneously underestimating the impact of situational, cultural, and other societal forces upon others' behavior.

To provide an illustration of the actor-observer bias, imagine walking to the train station after a long day of work. Upon entering the station, you see and hear a middle-aged woman dancing on top of a ticket counter, wearing nothing but a bright pink negligee, singing Jingle Bells loudly and off key. Your initial response probably would be that this woman is mentally ill, or under the influence of some unidentified substance. You are significantly less likely to consider that this woman is dancing on top of the counter to win a sizeable bet from a friend or co-worker, or that she is an actress who will appear in a skit for late night television.

Less extreme, but equally effective demonstrations of the actor-observer bias can be commonly observed in many work environments and interpersonal relationships. For example, consider a new employee who shows up late for work two days in a row. In the absence of any additional information, the new employee's boss and co-workers are likely to assume that he is lazy, absent minded, and irresponsible. In contrast, the employee himself is likely to continue to see himself as hard working and responsible because his tardiness occurred in response to a sudden, unexpected disruption in his family's child-care arrangements. He made it into work when many people would have called in sick for the entire day to avoid paying a virtual king's ransom for last minute, quality childcare. (Also consider the hostility and disdain typically directed toward significant others who forget about important events like birthdays and anniversaries.) Of course, most workers are expected to come to work in a timely fashion, and most long-term partners are expected to remember anniversaries and other important events without prodding. Regardless of the underlying personality traits and situational demands for those involved, the actor-observer bias itself results in very different perceptions between parties.

A number of factors appear to drive this pervasive, human tendency to overestimate the role of personality traits and underestimate the impact of situational determinants in our interpretation of others' behavior. First, this cognitive heuristic or "mental short cut" saves a significant amount of time in gathering, reviewing, and processing information. Second, human beings generally seek some measure of predictability and control in their environment to enhance feelings of safety and decrease levels of stress. One way to promote this sense of predictability is to know someone well enough to be able to expect their likes, dislikes, actions, and reactions to various events. And, because situational factors are not easy to predict or identify in advance, and our own internal feelings and beliefs are quite salient, it becomes even easier to presume that other people operate on relatively consistent personality traits, in order to maintain some illusion of control. Once someone has been identified as honest, shy, aggressive,

or any other descriptive personality trait, the natural, and even unconscious, assumption is that an individual will act in accord with her
personality traits *across* different situations and among different
groups of people. Unfortunately, empirical evidence suggests that such
faith in the stability of behavior across time and situations is not
realistic (White & Younger, 1988).

Bias in the Perception of Crisis

The actor-observer bias also can be translated directly into
a crisis paradigm. Consider many individuals' negative attitudes toward
victims of domestic abuse who remain with their abusers. Many laypersons will make comments such as, "How can someone be so stupid?"
and "How am I supposed to feel sorry for someone if they don't even try
to get out of such a bad relationships?" Most of these hostile comments
are fueled by the actor-observer bias, in which people typically fail to
consider related, salient situational and environmental factors.
Consider a young woman with two children who is married to an abusive, older man. This woman may not yet have the current financial
resources or neighborhood contacts established to obtain transportation
to a distant emergency shelter. She also may be worried about threats of
violence against her children if she were to ever leave her abusive
husband. A lack of formal education and marketable job skills also can
make it more challenging for abused partners to start a new life.

Helping patients in crisis recognize the situational factors in their
own experience can help diminish their likelihood of self-blame.
Patients who do not receive appropriate responses from others after
a traumatic event also can be helped to understand the pervasive biases
inherent in most people's interpretation of events. However, just as it
is important to understand the basis for other people's responses to the
survivors of trauma, it remains most important to focus upon our
patients. They must be helped to understand that regardless of the
factors that influenced their experience of crisis or trauma, they are
equally and completely deserving of help, support, and treatment.

Belief in a Just World

Many children grew up hearing the phrase, "good things happen
to good people, and bad things happen to bad people" or some variant
thereof (e.g., Be careful because you will reap what you sow; What goes
around comes around; There's no good luck, only hard work). For
many youngsters, these messages occurred in consort with parental

edicts about being nice to people, performing daily chores, and doing good deeds. In reality, this notion that good things happen to good people performs an important function in society, and encourages our members to act as good citizens. It can also provide a sense of optimism and hope, and increased perceptions of value for sometimes publicly overlooked or unnoticed good works. In addition, this notion that good begets good whereas evil begets evil also may imbue individuals with a rudimentary belief that the performance of good deeds will act as some kind of talisman against wrongdoing, bad karma, and bad luck. At its essence, however, fear about having negative outcomes or punishment is just as much a part of this message as doing good deeds to obtain positive outcomes.

The belief in "good things happen to good people and bad things happen to bad people" is so entrenched in our culture that it has become the focus of extensive study by social psychologists for decades. (Although some theologians debate whether a just and benevolent god could allow events like the holocaust to take place, many religious and social institutions fail to advance this argument.) Lerner was the first psychologists to systematically assess the impact of this supposition upon people's knowledge, attitudes, and behavior. He described his studies of this belief within the context of a belief in a "Just World" (1980). Lerner described this belief, in which people "reap what they sow" as a cognitive heuristic or shortcut that allows individuals to maintain (a sometimes necessary) illusory sense of control over one's often otherwise unstable, unpredictable life.

The impact of one's level of belief in a Just World has been assessed in both laboratory and naturalistic settings. In one striking illustration, participants in one experiment were asked to sit in a small room and observe another person (the experimenter's confederate) behind a one-way mirror receive numerous electrical shocks. Although the participants were told that these shocks would cause no permanent damage, the effect appeared rather painful. Of course, all shocks actually were "faked" by the confederate (Lerner & Simmons, 1966). Participants assigned randomly to one group were asked to watch the person behind the glass receive a shock whenever he made a mistake solving a complicated puzzle. Those in the second group were told that the person behind the glass, attempting to solve a complicated puzzle, would be shocked at random. The findings from this study showed that, even though participants in the second group were told directly that the shocks given to the person solving the puzzle were given at random, they felt that the participant was somehow responsible for receiving the shocks due to their poor performance on the puzzle.

In other words, despite clear explanations to the contrary, the subjects believed that "there just had to be a reason" for the individual solving the puzzle to receive those shocks.

Studies of jury decisions also suggest that the Just World Theory has a robust effect in real life situations. In a classic study, Feldman-Summers and Linder (1976) examined the sentences handed down to criminals convicted of physical assault and rape. Although our justice system suggests that individuals who commit similar crimes should receive similar sentences, the researchers found that criminals who committed rape against a woman identified as a virgin received significantly longer sentences than those who committed rape against a woman identified as a prostitute. Even though the events surrounding the attacks were identical, jury members also regarded the rape victim identified as a prostitute as "more responsible" for the crime than the victim identified as a virgin. Subsequent empirical studies with mock juries have produced similar results (e.g., Foley & Pigott, 2000). In virtually all cases, the assailants of individuals perceived as "bad or unworthy" received significantly shorter sentences and less costly fines than the assailants of those perceived as "good or worthy."

Blaming the Victim

The implications for the Just World Theory for the survivors of trauma are insidious. Strong conscious and unconscious feelings toward survivors, that they are somehow at fault, evil, or contaminated, often leads survivors to experience social isolation, begin to feel obligated toward others (to somehow "make up" for their bad deeds), and even begin to internalize the belief that they are undeserving and weak. In the worst-case scenario, survivors come to believe that they are the only ones to blame for their traumatic experience. The root of the word "victim" itself (note that the term "survivor" is used in this text almost exclusively) comes from Latin, and means a beast carefully selected for sacrifice in a ritualistic dispelling of evil. It does not seem that surprising, then, that a survivor, often identified as a victim, internalizes the belief that they are to blame for the "evil" bestowed upon them, as if they, too, were carefully selected.

Additional responses experienced by survivors, promoted by our society's pervasive belief in a Just World, include, but certainly are not limited to:

- Guilt
- Shame

- Self-Blame
- Humiliation
- Embarrassment
- Fears that they are somehow "bad" or evil
- Idealization of the perpetrator or crisis agent
- Beliefs that "God is giving them punishment"

The survivors of crisis and trauma may benefit from learning that many members of society cling fiercely to a false belief in a Just World because it can provide:

- An illusory sense of control over an otherwise chaotic world
- A sense of personal invulnerability (especially if one thinks they are a "good person")
- A perceived ability to predict possible targets of future trauma and violence
- A belief that justice will somehow prevail
- An opportunity to feel morally superior

Evidence of such feelings of superiority often extends to groups of individuals who are financially disadvantaged, poorly educated, discriminated against, or otherwise marginalized. Such groups include the homeless, the mentally ill, survivors of sexual assault, recipients of welfare (of whom the majority are working mothers), and minority group members among others. Although beyond the scope of this text, much work remains to be done to educate various segments of the population regarding situational factors and "bad luck."

Fears of becoming contaminated by association with a perceived victim of violence (and hence, a "bad person" by definition) also lead many individuals to avoid the survivors of trauma and crisis, as well as individuals from marginalized groups. Such social isolation works to deprive the very people who need help and social support from one of the most effective methods of coping with the aftermath of trauma and crisis. Thus, patients in crisis may learn that other people are indeed avoiding them because of their adherence to irrational beliefs and fears, and *not* because they themselves are somehow damaged, defective, or undeserving.

BYSTANDER INTERVENTION

When someone needs emergency assistance in a public place, a common concern may be whether someone available actually has the proper training or skills to provide help. Of course, this concern is predicated on the belief that people are generally willing and able to respond to accident victims and others in need. However, this notion is seriously flawed. In many instances, people who need help are ignored, abandoned, and even taken advantage of.

One tragedy that prompted the empirical study of bystander intervention occurred in 1964 on Long Island, New York and involved the rape and murder of Kitty Genovese. After arriving home late at night after work, Ms. Genovese was brutally attacked by a man in front of her apartment complex. The man raped her in the middle of the courtyard, and stabbed her once in the chest. Ms. Genovese screamed for help, but no one responded. She managed to drag herself to the front of her apartment door, but her assailant reappeared and stabbed her repeatedly until she died. The entire incident took nearly an hour. After the murder, the police interviewed the residents of the apartment complex. What shocked people around the nation was that more than 50 people said that they heard someone screaming for help, and 38 people said that they actually *saw* Ms. Genovese being attacked as they looked through their windows. However, all of the witnesses made the fatal assumption that someone else had already called the police (Latane & Darley, 1970).

In response to such a heinous story, many people's first reaction is that this event must be highly unusual, and that the apartment dwellers who failed to provide help or assistance of any kind must have been morally bereft or even evil. Certainly, one would assume that most people in the United States would pride themselves on being helpful and supportive, particularly in a time of trouble, and even consider it a moral obligation or civic duty. Unfortunately, findings from naturalistic and laboratory studies suggests the contrary. Bystander apathy (i.e., a lack of helping behavior in response to someone in need of help) is such a pervasive phenomenon that it has been documented among the most upstanding of our country's citizens.

In a classic social psychological experiment (Darley & Batson, 1973), a series of seminary students volunteered to make a speech on campus. The students were assigned randomly to conditions in which they had to rush to make their speech on time, or they had enough time to walk leisurely to make their scheduled appointment. Unbeknownst to the seminary students, a confederate was seated on a bench along the direct route that the students would travel to get across campus. A well-dressed male confederate sat slumped against a bench, eyes closed, and occasionally groaning (presumably in pain.) The experimenters themselves hypothesized that a large number of the students would stop and offer the man assistance, or at least ask him if anything was the matter.

The results of Darley and Batson's study are striking because one would certainly expect that seminary students have a vested interest in serving and helping others. Their findings showed, however, that many of the seminar students failed to help the man in apparent distress, particularly if they were "running late." An even more startling aspect of the study is that when seminary students were asked to make a presentation regarding the parable of the Good Samaritan versus a presentation about recent job prospects, even the relative salience of the moral message to care for others made little difference in the students' helping behaviors. Unfortunately, the majority of rigorous, empirical studies of bystander intervention suggest that people of various ages, from nearly all walks of life, are not always likely to engage in helping (c.f., Latane & Darley, 1970).

Factors that Decrease Helping

Fortunately, a number of studies (e.g., Fritzsche, Finkelstein, & Penner, 2000; Levine, 1999) allow us to identify some factors that influence the likelihood of bystander intervention. Some of the factors identified consistently as a barrier to helping include:

1. A diffusion of responsibility. In most instances, bystanders may truly be alarmed and wish to help or summon help. However, as demonstrated in the tragic case of Kitty Genovese, most bystanders tend to assume that other bystanders have the same thoughts and intentions as they. Many bystanders then conclude falsely, "Surely someone else has called for help by now" or "Someone here must know better how to deal with this than me."

In most cases, the intensity of this phenomenon is directly proportional to the number of bystanders present. In other words, the likelihood of receiving helping behavior in response to a traumatic event decreases as the number of bystanders increases. An individual in crisis is more likely to receive help when in the company of a sole onlooker than among a crowd of potential helpers.

A bike rider. One woman described such an incident in which she was having dinner with friends in a crowded tavern in a large city. When the woman casually glanced out the restaurant window, she saw a man riding across the street on his bike get hit by a van. The rider appeared to smash into a utility pole and slump down onto the sidewalk while the van sped away. It was unclear if the accident victim was conscious or unconscious. The woman pulled at the sleeve of the friend sitting next to her and said, "Oh, my God! Did you see what happened to that guy? Do you think he's OK?"

The woman was shocked that her friends were so nonplussed by the situation. One said, "Oh, yeah, I'm sure he's Ok. He's sitting up now." Another said, "Yeah, if he needed help, someone would have stopped to help him by now. I'm sure it's being taken care of." Frustrated, the woman went up to the maitre d' and demanded, "Could you please call 911 and tell them that someone has been hit by a car out front here?" The maitre d' frowned and said, "Look, lady. We don't have a public phone here!" When the woman again pleaded for the maitre'd to call for help, he responded, "Oh, for God's sake, lady, it's [a big] city! Someone's gonna help the guy!"

2. The perceived potential for discomfort. Bystanders are less likely to offer assistance when they have fears about being embarrassed or looking foolish, or receiving hostile responses in response to their helping. For example, a group of 60 students was sitting in class when a student near the back of the room apparently passed out and slumped to the floor. For a few seconds (the professor had been writing on an overhead and did not notice the girl falling) the students sat in silence. Then one student trained as an EMT moved across the isle to examine the girl's vital signs. Later information revealed that the girl was diabetic, and her blood sugar levels had dropped precipitously during class because she had not eaten properly in the last 48 hours. Ultimately, she was fine.

When discussing the emergency later in the class, a number of students described their initial thoughts when seeing (or first hearing) their classmate slump to the floor. The vast majority made some comment that they did not want to appear foolish or "out there" if they suddenly got up from their seats in the middle of class to see what had happened. Some students stated that they "didn't really know [the girl who fainted], and were afraid that it could be a joke or something. One brave student added, "I guess I didn't want to look stupid."

Still other bystanders may fear some sort of reprisal for helping. One may worry about getting hurt in certain rescue situations (e.g., saving someone from a burning building or cold sea water). One also may worry that others in the general vicinity will express anger if they move to help them (e.g., someone is being attacked by a large number of gang members) or that they themselves will become victim to some kind of scam (e.g., a person feigns an injury in order to lure someone into a dark alley). Still bystanders fear that they will become the subject of an expensive lawsuit if they somehow botch an attempt at help (e.g., giving someone CPR and accidentally breaking a rib; moving an accident victim and accidentally causing some form of spinal injury). At least in response to this concern, many states have enacted so called "Good Samaritan laws" designed to protect well-intentioned bystanders from such litigation.

3. Time required for helping. The perception that helping behavior will require a significant amount of time is associated with a significantly lesser likelihood of bystander intervention (e.g., Fritzsche et al., 2000). For example, one man who witnessed a car accident (neither party appeared hurt, but one driver clearly was at fault) told his therapist that he did not stop to make a report to the police at the scene. When asked why he didn't stop to aid the innocent driver in at least his insurance claim, the man said he was worried about "losing a whole afternoon" and having to serve time as a witness in a possible lawsuit.

4. The "category" or presumed relationship between two or more individuals (e.g., husband and wife, brother and brother, significant other and significant other). An assumption that someone involved in an ambiguous emergency situation is with a significant other or family member significantly decreases the likelihood that a bystander will regard the situation as a true emergency, and contributes to a diffusion of responsibility (i.e., "Oh, their brother will take care of them;" Levine, 1999). In a clear demonstration of this powerful effect, Shotland and Straw (1976) found that after their participants viewed an unfamiliar man strike a unfamiliar woman, more than half of them offered help when they assumed that the man was a stranger, while fewer than one in five of the observers offered when they assumed that the man was the woman's husband. It is as though many individuals still ascribe to the belief that people should "mind their own business," and not try to tell others how to raise their children and treat their partners or spouses. The implications for limited bystander intervention in cases of perceived romantic or domestic relationships are quite insidious (also see Chapter 9).

A review of these aforementioned barriers to bystander intervention suggests that most bystanders who fail to provide help in an emergency situation do not appear to be doing so out of outright lack of concern or maliciousness. For better or worse, overall personality traits, as well as gender, appear to have only limited influence upon the likelihood of helping (Fritzsche et al., 2000; Levine, 1999). Situational determinants often appear to take precedence.

Factors that Foster Intervention

Findings from this area of research can be used to help crisis workers as well as survivors engage in activities designed to promote helping behavior. For example:

- Practice primary prevention. Help yourself and others become educated about bystander apathy and bystander intervention. Individuals who are aware of impediments to helping are more likely to recognize them, and ultimately engage in appropriate, helping behavior. Adults, as well as children, also tend to help others when their previous attempts at helping have met with significant displays of gratitude and thanks (Deutsch & Lamberti, 1986).
- If a situation appears ambiguous, gather information quickly to determine if it represents an actual emergency. Ask direct questions of those immediately involved; do not make assumptions. Also question vague statements from others that "things look OK" or that help is already on the way.
- Decide upon a specific way to help. Identify the necessary skills, personnel, and equipment best suited for intervention. For example, does the person in crisis need CPR, food and water, an ambulance, or suicide assessment?
- Although helping is certainly a priority, be sure to ensure your own safety. You cannot help others if you are in danger, or in need of help yourself. Sometimes a phone call to the proper authorities can be just as helpful.
- Implement your plan for help, and identify people by name when asking them to complete specific tasks. Ask other bystanders for their names if they are not familiar to you.
- If you yourself are in an emergency situation and need help, attempt to draw attention to yourself and indicate that the situation is an emergency. If possible, let others know that you need help immediately. As simplistic as it sounds, bystanders are less likely to intervene when they do not perceive a victim's need for help as urgent (Frizsche et al., 2000).

POSITIVE PSYCHOLOGY

Within the last decade, a new and important field of psychology has emerged, identified as positive psychology (Seligman & Csikszentmihalyi, 2000). This new discipline is intended to celebrate man's potential for adaptation to change, resiliency, and health (e.g., Fredrickson, 2001). Emphasis is placed upon primary assumption that people can significantly affect their own mental health, physical health, and general sense of well being (e.g., Lykken, 1999; Lyubomirsky, 2001). Positive psychology also is aligned closely with social psychology in that both generally operate under the assumption that the vast majority of people are healthy and "normal;" abnormal behavior is relatively uncommon. Various studies suggest that individuals do have some degree of control over their own level of happiness, particularly via the adoption of the belief that love and relatedness are more important than money and material possessions, and a variety of long-term goals that reflect one's personal values (Diener, Suh, Lucas, & Smith, 1999).

Although the information gleaned from positive psychology can be quite beneficial for a variety of reasons, some cautions also must be raised from the perspective of crisis intervention and trauma counseling. Although rigorous empirical studies from positive psychology do suggest that certain life stressors and crises (e.g., getting fired; death of a spouse) can negatively influence survivors' subjective well-being for at least two years, and that these individuals never return to their previous levels of "happiness" (Diener, 2002), little of this information is conveyed accurately to the public due to a lack of specific outreach attempts and the media's propensity to simplify research findings or to report them out of context.

Thus, positive psychology's faith in people's innate ability to remain "happy" and adjusted in the face of adversity is admirable, but also may pose unnecessary burden and guilt upon individuals who trauma and crisis survivors who cannot "return to base-line" without professional intervention. Individuals with serious but treatable mental illness also could be deterred from seeking help, thinking, "Any normal person can make themselves feel better, so why can't I?" Without careful delivery of a wide variety of research findings to the general public, many laypersons may misinterpret positive psychology as glorified support for the often implicitly held Just World Theory.

It thus remains imperative that Psychology as a field retain a sense of balance in its perception and construal of crisis, normality, and mental illness. A multifaceted, dialectical approach, emphasizing the chronicity of certain mental disorders (e.g., major depression; schizophrenia), the seriousness of suicidality, and general lack of social support for survivors of trauma, as well as renewed emphasis upon individuals' innate capacity for resilience, the ability to assume responsibility for one's own happiness, and the utility of positive coping strategies is needed in order to serve people best in the midst of crisis and trauma. Just as the pendulum swings to and fro between medical and psychological theories of mental illness, we must take care that our professional views regarding the innate versus assisted ability of trauma survivors to regain an acceptable level of functioning do not alienate the very people that Psychology intends to help and support.

3

A Step-Wise Plan for Intervention

Psychologists typically must complete four years of coursework, a year of full-time internship, and an additional year of supervised, post-doctoral experience in order to meet minimum licensing requirements. However, virtually no graduate programs or state licensing boards require any specific coursework or training in crisis intervention.

A LACK OF REQUIRED COURSEWORK

Due to a lack of prescribed education in crisis intervention, many mental health practitioners learn about crisis management through formal, structured, expert supervision or, in many cases, through significantly more informal, inconsistent, "on-the-job training." It also is interesting to note that many paraprofessionals, including ombudsmen, grief counselors, and hot line volunteers, obtain more specific education about crisis intervention and trauma counseling than licensed psychologists. The Clinical Psychology division of the American Psychological Association itself did not establish its section on crisis and behavioral emergencies until 2001.

A number of factors may account for this general absence of prescribed crisis coursework in many clinical programs. One critical factor is that many graduate programs in Psychology already require a significant number of prescribed courses in order to address a wide variety of professional issues. For example, psychologists must be trained in a variety of theoretical and pragmatic approaches to clinical assessment and treatment. With additional press from managed care, the need for expert diagnostic skills has become increasingly important. And, psychologists are uniquely trained to engage in psychological testing, including intelligence, personality, projective, neuropsychological, forensic, and achievement testing.

Psychologists also must commonly fulfill course requirements in ethics and cultural diversity. Many state licensing boards now require some minimum amount of formal coursework in those areas. Additional coursework in biopsychology and pharmacology has been added to many graduate programs in order to foster more effective communication and collaborative relations between medical and mental health providers, and to help prepare students for possible, future opportunities to acquire prescription privileges. Thus, just as clinical psychologists cannot be expected to graduate as "experts" in all related subdisciplines of psychology (also see Chapter 2), it can be argued that the time spent in graduate education and training, including the time allotted for crisis intervention and trauma counseling, can be spread only so thinly among diverse areas of study.

Unfortunately, most research findings from industrial and organizational psychology suggest that on the job training is less effective than other, more formal forms of education (Goldstein, 1986). Until graduate programs decide to require additional numbers of course credit or state licensing boards decide to require specific coursework or training in behavioral emergencies, most students should expect to receive more informal, on the job training regarding various life and death issues. Although this statement may appear melodramatic, students, professors, clinical supervisors, and administrators, as well as patients, would benefit from working together to make such critical on the job training more structured and comprehensive.

A STEP-WISE APPROACH

In response, this chapter is designed to offer an integrated, specific, step-wise approach to crisis intervention. The paradigm is intended to offer basic structure for newer practitioners, provide guidelines for clinical supervisors, and provide an analysis of vital issues including overarching legal and ethical considerations for more experienced clinicians. This chapter also is designed to critically examine the use of the mental status exam versus other assessment tools, and offer appropriate guidelines for documentation during treatment.

The following individual steps or stages for crisis intervention will be addressed at length, below.

1. Developing trust and rapport
2. Defining the problem
3. Assessing danger and ensuring safety
4. Assessing coping skills
5. Structuring the therapeutic relationship
6. Providing psychoeducation
7. Collaborating upon goals
8. Mobilizing social supports
9. Supplying a transitional object
10. Maintaining professional boundaries
11. Providing appropriate documentation
12. Acknowledging countertransference
13. Preparing for termination
14. Follow-up (e.g., referrals)

Therapists who provide crisis intervention and trauma counseling have, by definition, a difficult and challenging task. However, the use of such a rubric can imbue therapists with a sense of underlying structure and consistency, even in the mist of helping patients deal with chaotic, overwhelming situations. It also is critical to note that rigid adherence to a preestablished structured plan, without maintaining the ability to make changes and exceptions as needed, can be as detrimental as not having any plan at all.

DEVELOPING TRUST AND RAPPORT

Patients in the midst of crisis are likely to experience initial sessions as emotionally intense. For many patients, these therapeutic encounters may represent the first time they have ever sought help from a mental health professional, who may be identified as a counselor, "shrink," or even "an outsider." Consistent with the release of various hormones and alterations in the functioning of the autonomic nervous system under periods of extreme stress, many patients also will manifest some difficulty with concentration, memory, and affective modulation. Despite these potential barriers to treatment, however, the crisis therapist must work confidently and quickly to establish rapport and develop trust in the therapeutic relationship.

One critically important, typically overlooked aspect of crisis and trauma counseling is that of the physical environment in which patient

and therapist meet. Although the quality of the therapeutic relationship and the quality of clinical interventions are certainly more central
for success in treatment, the "material" aspects of treatment will significantly influence patients' impressions during initial sessions, and
may consciously or unconsciously suggest their therapist is, or is not,
able to provide a safe, secure environment. This supposition is consistent with more general industrial organizational and social psychological findings that various qualities of individuals' home and work
environments can impact significantly upon their productivity, quality
of relationships, and mood (e.g., Hillhouse & Adler, 1997).

Although rather basic, therapists can review the following list to
see if their office or clinic setting provides a formal, symbolic, representation to a patient that they are able to provide them with a momentarily safe and secure setting, even within a period of intense crisis.

- A meeting location away from the crisis location (e.g., if a flood
  has destroyed a patient's home, it would be helpful to meet with
  her in an area of town that was not similarly devastated).
- A temperate temperature and climate. An appropriate room temperature can be essential in order to help patients to focus upon
  their own internal responses associated with their immediate
  stressor, rather than general discomfort associated with sitting in
  a chilly, 55 degree or humid, 95 degree room.
- A waiting area that is quiet and comfortable, furnished with comfortable chairs, some type of artwork or prints, various magazines,
  educational pamphlets, tissues, and even a small pitcher of water.
- Friendly, professional staff, including appropriately trained
  receptionists. Many patient complaints do not involve their
  interaction with their therapist directly, but with staff members
  in the waiting room or on the telephone. One woman stated,
  "I couldn't believe it ... the woman asked me what meds I was
  taking in front of everyone in the waiting room! She didn't even
  call me up to the little window, she just yelled it out like it was
  no big deal for me to tell everyone there that I am taking
  lithium ... this is a small town, and I don't want that kind of shit
  getting around!" Psychologists are responsible for training their
  receptionists, answering service workers, and other employees
  in patient confidentiality; they also can be disciplined for uneth-
  ical behavior if a staff member does not honor patient confidentiality. In general, most staff members (e.g., receptionists; office
  mangers) express a sense of relief when given specific guidelines
  and suggestions for how to handle various clinical situations.

- A sense of privacy. A patient who can hear other conversations taking place in adjacent offices or in different parts of the building cannot be expected to want to reveal anything of a private nature in treatment. Many clinicians in group practice or in make shift, on-site emergency centers have limited options regarding room selection and sound proofing selections. However, a relatively inexpensive, portable white noise machine can mask a multitude of environmental disturbances.

Although it is not always possible to provide patients with this type of idyllic professional setting, it remains vital to strive for such a bucolic setting, to address unexpected disruptions in the environment with patients, and to also allow for a degree of flexibility when required. For example, a small suburban community in Pennsylvania experienced a series of unexpected floods that destroyed many homes and businesses (including a community counseling center) and displaced more than 200 residents. In response to this unexpected increased need for crisis intervention, a local business unaffected by the flooding provided some portable trailers to provide additional office space for counseling. Unfortunately, both therapists and patients at this improvisational clinic quickly realized that they could often hear other patients and therapists in the adjoining rooms quite clearly.

Although many patients acted as though this situation was normal or even expected in such circumstances, all of the therapists acknowledged and apologized for the lack of privacy. Patients were encouraged to discuss the lack of privacy, and if or how they wanted to proceed in treatment. In other words, the therapists did not allow the issue of their physical environment to be ignored or overlooked. Within two days, the clinic director purchased relatively inexpensive white noise machines for each office in the trailer, and the standard of patient privacy was restored.

Another way to help establish rapport in the therapeutic relationship is to immediately support a patient's internal locus of control. Because crises inherently involve some loss of control over something, therapists typically can do a number of things to help their patients experience some sense of control over their immediate environment and treatment. Even a small gesture such as telling a patient, "Please take a seat where you like" or "Would you like me to turn the temperature up or down?" conveys an important message to patients who may feel especially vulnerable or helpless. Giving patients a choice in the first few minutes of the therapeutic interaction also sends the clear message that they are encouraged and even expected to engage in self-selection and decision-making.

The therapeutic relationship is also established with the expectation that both therapists and patients will fulfill certain roles to the best of their abilities. Expectations for these roles must be discussed openly and fully at the beginning of treatment. For example, therapists can be expected to provide professional expertise, empathy, concentration, psychoeducation, attendance at all sessions, referrals to appropriate service agencies, collaboration in treatment planning and intervention, and confidentiality. Expectations for patients may include a willingness to speak openly and honestly, attendance at scheduled meetings, a willingness to collaborate with their therapist upon treatment planning and goals, and a desire to engage in active discussions and problem solving. Articulating such clear expectations increases both patient and therapist motivation, mobilizes patient resistances (which may be unconscious, but are critical for examination), and encourages patients to accept responsibility for, and control over, their own actions.

It also is helpful for therapists to assume a sense of confidence in their abilities, or at least, in the quality of their clinical supervision. Even though a therapist may not feel confident and secure, good modeling is beneficial for patients.

DEFINING THE PROBLEM

Because patients seek crisis counseling for a myriad of reasons, which are not always immediately clear to the therapist or even to some patients themselves, it becomes essential to clearly define the presenting problem. Due to the time-limited nature of crisis intervention, however, therapists must define the problem rapidly, often without the benefit of historical information.

One of the most effective ways to begin to assess the presenting problem is to simply ask a patient, "What brings you here today?" This use of open-ended questions is essential to avoid leading questions or to suggest to patients that there is a typical crisis response. It also is helpful to identify when the precipitating event occurred (e.g., within the past 24 or 48 hours). If a critical incident occurred weeks, months, or even years earlier, it then becomes vital to determine why a patient is seeking help *now*. Many therapists simply ask their patients directly, "So what happened since then that brings you here now?"

Therapist and patient must then work together to generate a concise and accurate statement of the problem. Being specific and clear about the nature of the problem helps keeps the idea of the crisis from spiraling out of control, allows for more objective, balanced perspective of the problem, and helps challenge the presence of any cognitive distortions. For example, a woman who just received divorce papers from her husband may state plaintively, "My whole life is over. Just over! Things will never be the same, and I am left with nothing. I am absolutely, totally, and completely devastated." This statement may certainly capture her feelings at the moment (which must be acknowledged as important and real to her), but they do not necessarily acknowledge the actual, objectively defined, presenting problem.

A more effective way to identify this woman's presenting problem would be to help her articulate the specific changes that have occurred in her life within the last few days. If a patient simply states that they are depressed or "totally devastated," a therapist can respond, "Please tell me what it means to you when you are totally devastated. What happens to you or what kind of things do you find yourself feeling or doing?" After a few minutes of discussion, this patient's presenting problem could be reframed as, "I'm going to lose the most important relationship in my life. I haven't been eating or sleeping well, and I've lost 10 pounds in the last two weeks. I just don't want to lose all of my friends; it seems like all of my friends were 'our' friends, and I don't know who is going to take sides or what. I don't know what I am going to do without him." Working with this patient in treatment would be very different if she responded to the same question by stating, "Wait a minute. I mean, I am so glad that I left; I will never have to worry about him terrorizing me again. I have my self-respect now, and no one will never, ever take that away from me away. I mean that I am financially devastated. I'm going to have to take on a second job and move to some little apartment in a not-so-good neighborhood. It's like I'm getting punished for doing the right thing." Specific articulation of the problem clearly fosters more specific and appropriate treatment planning.

ASSESSING DANGER AND ENSURING SAFETY

When patients reveals that they are in physical danger (e.g., a battering spouse has threatened to kill them if they leave the relationship; a woman engages in unprotected sex for money to maintain a costly heroin addiction; parents do not have enough food to feed themselves or their children after an earthquake destroys their home), the number one priority in treatment must become *patient (as well as therapist) safety*. All other aspects of treatment, including the reflection of feelings, providing psychoeducation, discussing goals for treatment, discussing effective coping strategies, become secondary. Although this may seem initially counterintuitive (i.e., wouldn't it be helpful for a battered spouse to obtain psychoeducation?), therapists must remember that they cannot provide any assistance to a patient who is seriously ill, injured, or dead.

To respond to the potential danger that patients may face, therapists often benefit from having an available list of human resource agencies, including emergency shelters, legal advocacy agencies, police units, along with the name and phone number of individual contact persons for those agencies. Thus, if a patient does indicate that she is in danger of being murdered by a battering, jealous boyfriend, a call can be placed immediately to help obtain protection. A patient who is literally starving for food and a safe place to live must simultaneously receive instrumental assistance; it is almost impossible to imagine doing the often difficult work of psychotherapy when one is preoccupied with a rumbling stomach and thoughts about a next meal is coming from. Just as stated in Maslow's hierarchy of needs (1970), a failure to secure basic physical needs for food, shelter, and safety, preempts an individual's ability to engage in other productive work or relationships.

Similarly, therapists themselves must feel safe from danger in order to properly assist their patients. Just as ambulance crews cannot assist injured victims at a crime scene until the police have secured the area (i.e., the suspect has been apprehended; all gun fire has stopped), therapists who provide crisis intervention are not meant, or expected, to be heroes. They cannot be expected to help a patient if they themselves are so fearful that they cannot think or work properly. A dead therapist also cannot engage in any therapeutic relationships or interventions. Thus, therapists must accept their limitations as a human being and a competent, but not omniscient, professional. Seeking help to avoid potential danger remains essential.

ASSESSING CURRENT COPING

Once the specific problem has been ascertained, and a safe environment is in place, therapists can begin to assess their patients' current and prior coping skills. Simply asking, "So, what, if anything, have you been doing to cope with this problem" or "What kinds of things have you already tried to do about this?" can provide a wealth of information. It also is important to acknowledge that some patients may be reluctant to admit participation in more long-term, negative coping behavior such as substance abuse or violence. The use of a positively structured question, such as "When some people find themselves in the midst of a crisis, they drink, smoke, do drugs, overeat, oversleep, get into arguments or fights, or hit or hurt people or things. Can you tell me about any of these things that you may have done since the crisis occurred?" allows a patient to admit more readily that they engage in such negative coping because the question presupposes that other people engage in those same behaviors.

It also is important to assess the extent to which patients feel that their coping methods are effective. Some patients may have limited insight that the activities they engage in to engender effective coping (e.g., drinking; taking drugs) typically have negative, long-term effects. Similarly, some patients may claim that they are engaging in healthy behavior, such as working or exercising a great deal (i.e., excessively by others' standards) can also be maladaptive in their present situation.

Because many patients become focused on their current situation exclusively, in a type of cognitive "tunnel vision," it also can be vital to elicit information about their ability to cope successfully with previous crises or negative events. Therapists can simply ask their patients, "Have you ever experienced these kinds of feelings before? If so, what happened, and what did you do about those negative feelings? ... How did everything work out?" Sometimes a reminder that a patient has a history of successful coping and adaptation to change provides an increased sense of internal control. For other patients, they may begin to recall effective coping strategies or support persons that they had previously forgotten.

In some instances, however, a patient may have a history of ineffective or maladaptive coping. For a chronic drug user, it would be of no benefit to give that patient the false hope that he could manage his current crisis "just as you have gotten through everything else in your past." To avert an additional, potentially disastrous situation, it becomes essential to help these patients explore the possibility of other specific, generally effective coping strategies. Some patients may not even recognize that listening to music, working out, walking through a park, writing in a journal, praying, or watching a new movie can represent potentially effective coping strategies.

STRUCTURING THE THERAPEUTIC RELATIONSHIP

As noted in the introduction, crisis intervention differs significantly from many traditional forms of therapy. One primary difference between the two is that crisis intervention is time limited, with a maximum of 6 to 8, or sometimes 10, sessions, whereas participation in most other forms of therapy is often open-ended or at least variable in the total number of sessions. The use of time is central in structuring the therapeutic relationship. A time limited approach can be used to increase both patient and therapist motivation (c.f., Mann, 1973). Additional findings suggest that if the number of therapy sessions is made explicit at the beginning of treatment, with treatment goals clearly articulated, patient resistances and maladaptive behaviors often come to the fore (Davanloo, 1980). An examination of patient resistance can be challenging in a short number of sessions, but can be invaluable in helping patients successfully cope. Equally important, however, the use of time limits in treatment should be discussed openly and even determined with patients (within clinical judgment and reason), in order to afford them with an additional sense of control and competence, and to avoid anything that could be as revictimization.

As a critically important caveat, in cases in which patients manifest excessive resistance, high risk for suicidal or homicidal behavior, or recollections of physical, emotional, or sexual abuse, patients should be reminded that after their initial number of prescribed sessions, they can continue to work upon their issues in psychotherapy—with another professional. For practitioners who already engage in psychotherapy, this delineation between crisis intervention and therapy can become blurred. And, therapists certainly have a vested interest in having patients return to them for treatment if it is in their patient's best interest. Some therapists who see patients in therapy for the first time due to a crisis or traumatic event may thus tell them that they will work with them for the next 6 or 8 sessions to reduce their current distress and symptoms associated with their current traumatic event. They also will inform their patients that once those initial 6 or 8 sessions have passed, they can discuss the possibility of continuing in therapy, if they so desire. Thus, patients have the option to continue in therapy to work on other, long-standing personality or relational issues, including those which may arise in exploration during their initial crisis work.

PROVIDING PSYCHOEDUCATION

Therapists, particularly those in training who are immersed in the introspective nature of their training and work, need to remember that many high functioning individuals are not psychologically minded. These individuals may not necessarily associate the recent death of their father with increased GI distress or more fitful sleep. Some individuals may not really understand that there are various physical and emotional responses to trauma, including multiple symptoms (e.g., GI distress, headache, backache, insomnia, increased urination, heightened allergic response, chest pain, muscle weakness, fatigue) impaired concentration, and extreme feelings of fear, anger, helplessness, and sadness.

For patients who are not apt to immediately recognize their mind-body connection, many report a deep sense of relief when they learn that "feeling as if they are going crazy" does not, in fact, mean that they are in danger of becoming psychotic, and that this feeling is well within the normal range of experience among the survivors of trauma. Others who may be unaware of the extreme response that stress can evoke feel relief when they learn that the "feeling of numbness, like I'm not sad or angry or anything" is a normal response to avoid feeling the pain and discomfort associated with loss or change, and not a sign that they are uncaring or even inhuman. (For a sample handout that can be given to patients to augment in-session psychoeducation, please refer to the appendix of Chapter 10.)

For patients who are psychologically minded and insightful, a review of basic stress reactions can still be beneficial. Even patients who appear to understand the mind-body connection may, at that point in time, maintain only a compartmentalized, intellectualized understanding of the concept, and they may be hard pressed to apply these concepts in their own lives. Conversely, some patients may fully understand the nature of the human stress response, but not feel entitled to engage in appropriate help seeking or coping behaviors. Additional psychoeducation often can provide these individuals with a distinct rationale for initiating adapative and helpful responses to their present situation (e.g., take time off from work to visit a seriously ill family member; take the time to exercise; spend the money to purchase healthy food). Other patients who are insightful enough to analyze their own somatic responses to stress may benefit from a review of this information simply because it will reinforce their learning, and because they may benefit from realizing that they already know something that their therapist often must explain to others. In sum, therapists should assume that some degree of psychoeducation is appropriate for all patients in a time of crisis.

FORMULATING APPROPRIATE GOALS

The next step in crisis intervention is to work collaboratively with patients to craft appropriate goals for the immediate future. The formulation of goals is essential for a variety of reasons. Specific goals allow patients to obtain a sense of mastery and control, and also increase patient and therapist motivation. Collaboration between patient and therapist also encourages patients who may temporarily feel helpless and ineffective to assume control and responsibility for their progress, and regain a sense of self-efficacy. The collaborative nature of the work between patient and therapist also certainly fosters increased rapport and trust in the therapeutic relationship.

To help patients identify specific goals for treatment, therapists can ask them, "What do you think you need to have happen in order for you to get through this?" It is critical that the goals are specific rather than global. For example, a patient who just experienced a devastating personal loss may state, "I don't want to be sad anymore." In such an instance, therapists are advised to be honest with patients that it is not possible to be "happy" all of the time, and that unpleasant memories or reminders of a crisis event may remain with them throughout their life, albeit with significantly less intensity. Also telling patients that they are more likely to cope successfully with a tragedy or crisis by couching their goals in positive, or action, terms (e.g., What can I do tomorrow that might help me feel better?) can also be helpful.

When working with patients to formulate treatment goals, the following acronym can be employed as a guide. According to this rubric, the most effective goals for change are "SMART":

- *Specific.* As noted previously, it is helpful for patients to craft specific, action oriented goals such as "I am going to get out of bed by 8 a.m. for the next three mornings in a row" rather than "I am going to work on my sleeping problems."
- *Measurable.* As in cognitive-behavioral therapies, goals must be measurable. In other words, they should be articulated in clear, objective, and preferably numerical terms. For example, instead of "I will make myself eat something for the next few days" a measurable goal would be "To take better care of myself, I will eat at least 400 calories of food for breakfast, 800 for lunch, and 600 for dinner. I also will make sure that I eat at least three pieces of fruit and at least two servings of protein a day."
- *Attainable.* Also as recommended by cognitive-behavioral therapists, specific goals for treatment should be easily attainable, and designed to guarantee patient success, particularly during the early stages of treatment. In other words, therapists do not let patients set themselves up for failure. Positive experiences

must be gathered and collected during times of crisis. Thus, an example of an inappropriate goal would be "I'm not going to just hide in my apartment anymore. I am going to find and make a new, good friend next week," whereas an attainable goal would be "I want to socialize at least 3 times this week with some current friends and acquaintances. If I make a new friend or acquaintance, that's fine. If not, that's fine, too."

- *Realistic.* Treatment goals also need to be realistic. Sometimes patients have unrealistic expectations or fantasies that they will never have bad memories once a crisis has passed, that they will never feel sad or depressed again, or that they can simply will their problems away. For example, one patient who just lost a close sibling stated, "For my goal, I will not cry at all next week." Her therapist was able to help this patient restructure her goal into "I will cry tomorrow if I need to, for has long as I have to or want to. Each time I cry, I will also write down on the same paper when I cried, how long I cried, what triggered my crying, the thoughts I had while crying, and how I felt after crying. I will do the same thing for the next three days." This type of goal, in which patients monitor their own stress reactions and feelings, provides important information gathering, and can help patients cognitively deconstruct an assertion that "I just cry all day, all of the time, for no apparent reason."

- *Time limited.* Goals must also be time limited. Specifically, the most effective goals are time limited for the next 24 hours. Such short periods allow for reassessment of goals, and allow for greater experiences of success. Such an immediate goal also encourages patients to focus on the here-and-now, themselves, and their own recovery.

Patient Resistance

Even after specific, action oriented goals are constructed, therapists must continue to help their patients engage in behavior that helps them to achieve those goals. To preempt resistance to appropriate behavior, therapists should ask patients directly, "What kinds of things can you think of that might make it difficult or at least challenging for you to obtain this goal?" (This process also can be thought of quite simply as trouble shooting; Sells, 1998; 2001.) Posing the question in such a way that it is expected that individuals have obstacles to their goals is important to gather insight into the patient's possible resistance to treatment as well as to help patients acknowledge that making progress is, as they may feel themselves, not always easy. If the impediments to goal directed behavior appear to be pressing or pervasive, the therapist may guide their patients to modify their goal so that is more attainable. It also is critical to examine the nature of the impediment itself (e.g., I don't think my girlfriend would like it if I did that; What would my mom say?; I don't think I can take enough time away from studying to go to that support group; I don't think I can spend that kind of money to join a gym; I am so depressed that I'd rather just kill myself than try to do anything to get better).

In some instances, patients may resist working collaboratively with their therapist to even generate specific goals. Patients may express this resistance via statements such as "Oh, it doesn't matter what I do. I'll probably always feel like this" or "You're the expert here. I think you know much better than me what I should be doing. I'll let you handle this part, OK?" It also is helpful to see patients as *unprepared* for change, rather than consciously or defiantly resisting participation in treatment (Sells, 2001). A number of factors may account for avoidance of goal setting, including:

- Fears about embracing hope (i.e., a positive emotion) for change.
- The impending loss of secondary gains (e.g., sympathy; insurance benefits).
- A conscious or unconscious desire to be taken care of, controlled, or rescued instead of assuming responsibility for themselves.
- Fears that confronting the negative situation will be more difficult than avoiding it.
- Guilt or shame surrounding the crisis event.
- A desire to blame others for the crisis.
- An absence of established, effective coping skills.
- Familial patterns in coping.

Uncovering and processing the bases for patient resistance to treatment represents some of the most important and valuable work in crisis intervention and trauma counseling. An ability to diffuse patient resistance also separates trained mental health providers from paraprofessionals.

MOBILIZING SOCIAL SUPPORT

Another critical component of crisis intervention and trauma counseling is the ability of the patient and therapist to mobilize social supports quickly. Therapists can take an inventory of available resources by asking patients about their friends, family members, neighbors, coaches, health care providers, co-workers, authority figures, and members of their church or other community organizations. Specifically, therapists can ask, "Who in your life do you think might be most helpful to you at this time?" and "If this person were not available for some reason, who else do you think might be helpful?" It also is critical to acknowledge that some individuals from various cultural and ethnic groups (e.g., African-American; Latino) may be more comfortable seeking out community-based, extended family, and spiritual supports than individuals from other groups (e.g., Franklin, Carter, & Grace, 1993). For example, individuals from traditional Eastern cultures may take significant offense at a therapist's request to elicit help and support from members outside of their own immediate family. (Also see Chapter 11 for a discussion of cross-cultural issues.)

Therapists also can inform patients about potential sources of support including social service agencies, formal and informal support groups, legal advocacy groups, foundations that support widows and surviving children of police officers and other civil service workers, appropriate informational web sites, hot lines, emergency shelters, etc. When discussing the role of support personnel, therapists also should be clear to delineate who is responsible for what aspect of the patient's treatment. For example, a patient may learn that a caseworker can be assigned to them to help with finding appropriate school placements for a disabled child. At that time, this patient also would be reminded that they would return to see their therapist for continued work in therapy, to a pediatrician for their child's physical needs and medication prescriptions, and that a therapy support person will come to their home daily will provide care exclusively for the child. It also is critical that patients know who is responsible for making a contact or referral to a specific agency or caseworker. Writing things down can be helpful for many patients, particularly when memory and concentration can be significantly impaired during a time of intense emotional crisis. If at all possible, patients should be encouraged to initiate as many contacts as possible in order to regain a sense of control and mastery.

A wealth of rigorous, empirical studies provides valuable evidence that both the actual and perceived quality of an individual's social support can bear significantly upon a patient's response to a crisis or transitional life event (e.g., Brissette, Scheier, & Carver, 2002). Thus, although therapists certainly would want to encourage their patients to garner actual, instrumental support from others in their midst, "just knowing" that people care seems to be enough to help many people regain a sense of community and self-worth. Even among non-clinical

samples, the presence of quality social relationships appears requisite
for general perceptions of happiness (Diener & Seligman, 2002).

SUPPLYING A TRANSITIONAL OBJECT

Another tenant of crisis intervention is that patients should literally come away with something after their initial session with something. This "something" could represent an actual item such as an
appointment card, a list of available support agencies and their
addresses and phone numbers, or more intangible items such as a plan
for recovery or, preferably, a specific instructions for performing relaxation exercises, self-hypnosis, or other forms of meditation. Giving
patients something concrete, such as an appointment card or learnable
skill helps patients feel that they are worthy of instrumental health and
support, elicits the norm of reciprocity (in which patients may be
encouraged to engage openly and actively in therapy), and can serve as
a transitional object (c.f., Winnicott, 1971) for patients during times of
stress. Some therapists will even tell their patients, "If you want to call
my machine to just to hear my voice, without having to leave a message, that's OK, too."

MAINTAINING PROFESSIONAL BOUNDARIES

Another important consideration in crisis intervention, as well as
in work with all patients in psychotherapy, is the effort that must be
expended to monitor and maintain professional boundaries in the
patient-therapist relationship. Therapists also must consider disruption in both psychological (e.g., a patient calls his therapist six times a
day in hopes of having extended conversations over the telephone) and
physical boundaries (e.g., holding a patient in an embrace). To illustrate the problematic nature of therapeutic interactions that violate
various patient-therapist boundaries, please consider the following
passage drawn from a textbook in abnormal psychology and crisis
intervention.

Betty's Therapist: An Unfortunate Example

"Betty, a 19 year-old university student, came to see me unexpectedly. I had met her once, when she accompanied her roommate to my
office; but I had no direct contact with her. She was in obvious distress

and incoherently blurted out that she had some pills and was seriously thinking about taking them because she 'didn't want to live anymore.' I immediately notified my secretary to hold all calls and appointments and *spent the next couple of hours* [emphasis added] talking with her. She told me that her fiancé and brother had been killed in an automobile accident six weeks before that and that she just couldn't get over it. She didn't feel that she had anything to live for. She cried. *I held her* [emphasis added]. We went over her loss and her anger at being left alone over and over again. Finally, when she was completely exhausted, I asked her if she thought we could work together to find some meaning in her life. When she tearfully agreed, I pushed for some commitment: would she give me the pills and promise not to do anything to herself until I could see her the next day at 3:30? I asked her to look me in the eye and promise that much. It took some time for her to be able to do that."

General Prohibitions against Physical Contact

This purported example of exemplary therapeutic technique is quite disconcerting. For example, the presence of the simple statement, "I held her" is quite problematic. In general, therapists should not touch their patients, especially through hugs or "holding." Although there is some controversy regarding the decision to touch or not touch patients, particularly when the patient is a child, is medically ill, or dying, therapists must have a clear, specific reason *for* touching a patient (Hillman, 2000), particularly in crisis intervention. When under duress, patients can be even more vulnerable to therapeutic suggestion, or to make inappropriate assumptions about their therapist's underlying motivation. In the excerpt above, Betty could have easily interpreted her therapist's embrace as a sign of romantic affection.

Of course, every rule has its exception. In the aforementioned passage, it remains unclear whether Betty attempted to embrace her therapist first. In that case, the therapist could have hesitated for a fleeting second, so that she would not feel completely rejected, and then draw back, placing her hands gently by her side. Once can also consider a patient in hospice, dying of terminal lung cancer. If the patient and therapist have worked together for an extended period of time, holding hands in greeting may be extremely comforting and appropriate.

Therapists must consider various issues, including the sex of the therapist and patient, the length of the relationship, the type of touch requested, and the patient's ability to process the interaction. In sum, therapists must have a specific reason, and clear rationale, for touching a patient at any time in treatment. It also is better to be more conservative than liberal when making any such determination.

Time Constraints

Another problematic aspect of Betty's case is her therapist's immediate call to his secretary to hold his calls and cancel all other appointments for the afternoon. At that point in time, has had not even met with Betty to interview her and assess her mental status. It is as though he has already decided that Betty is actively and acutely suicidal, and that extreme measures must be taken. Although therapists can expect to spend up to two hours with a suicidal patient during an initial intake, most clinicians are able to focus upon critical issues regarding danger to self or other; sitting with a suicidal patient for five hours could actually prove detrimental, and even encourage the expression of preexisting character pathology. For example, Betty could be led to feel "special" and worthy of this special treatment, and expect such extended sessions in the future. Conversely, Betty could be left thinking, "Wow. I must be majorly messed up if he thinks I need to be here all afternoon...I guess I'm even worse than I thought I was." Such a patient may begin to doubt her ability to gauge her own level of internal distress (i.e., observing ego).

Encouraging an Internal Locus of Control

Although Betty's therapist received her permission to telephone her roommate, he also usurped any belief that Betty may have in being able to control her own actions for the next 24 hours. (Also see Chapter 6 for an in-depth exploration of many of the popular myths surrounding suicide, including this inappropriate plea for friends and family members to provide around-the-clock supervision.) If Betty herself wanted to have some company for the evenings, which represents a positive step in her desire to activate a support system rather than be the passive recipient of a monitoring system, the therapist could encourage Betty to call her roommate in the moment, from his own office. Her therapist would be there to provide emotional support, and to help Betty process her feelings and brainstorm about other ways to engage social supports if her roommate were unavailable. In sum, whenever possible, encouraging patients to have control over their own treatment (i.e., their lives) represents a desirable and highly effective therapeutic intervention.

PROVIDING APPROPRIATE DOCUMENTATION

A number of documentation issues exist in any clinical context, but they have become increasingly salient in crisis situations, due in part to the presence of managed care and the increasing use of litigation in our society (see Soisson, VandeCreek, & Knapp, 1987). Most experts in ethics and legal issues (e.g., the American Psychological Association's Guidelines for Record Keeping; 1993) suggest that well documented sessions, which including specific, detailed information regarding clinical assessment, provide significantly better protection from litigation than poorly documented, or even absent, reports. Another critical reason to provide appropriate record keeping is to satisfy the criteria for various agencies, typically including the Joint Commission on Accreditation of Hospitals (JCAH), Medicaid, and Medicare. Satisfying JCAH audits can make the difference between the continued federal and state funding for large hospital clinics and units, as well as continued community-wide trust and support. As well as keeping records for more "defensive" reasons, good record keeping also allows therapists to orient themselves for future sessions, remember important details from prior sessions, and help identify core issues in treatment.

Additional considerations in the construction of chart notes, progress reports, and other material (e.g., testing results; requests for consultation) are that patients have a legal right to look at their medical charts at any time. One way to protect therapists and patients from misinterpretation of these legal documents is for therapists to simply remember that everything that they write in their patients' chart may be read by their patient, at any time, either with or without their presence. In support of this somewhat simplistic guideline, in virtually all cases, the notes contained in patients' charts would not share any clinically significant differences. The knowledge that patients may view their chart notes also may aid therapists in maintaining a greater sense of empathy and respect for their patient's difficulties, as well as to provide additional incentives to document sessions clearly and accurately.

Another reason that therapists should assume that their chart notes and entries may not remain confidential, is that therapists may be required to turn over or testify upon their chart notes in certain court cases and ruling. Some HMOs also require a release of specific information about patients and their progress in therapy, which is not consistent with general APA guidelines. It also is important to note that these mandates for disclosure can be enforced legally in certain cases, even if both the patient and therapist contest the ruling. However, although the APA requires psychologists to uphold the ethical standards of their profession, includes attempts to block the revelation of confidential patient records, this professional organization also instructs psychologists to obey any legal mandates when presented with an conflict between ethical and legal standards. Additional legal and ethical considerations are involved in work with suicidal and homicidal patients. Specific information and ethical guidelines in work with such patients are presented in Chapters 6 and 7, respectively.

SOAP Notes

Although sometimes criticized for their close approximation to medical notes (Baird, 1999) and rigid format, SOAP notes (see Weed, 1971) satisfy all JCAH standards, meet ethical guidelines for the APA (1992), and can be adapted easily for use in a myriad of clinical settings and can be completed in a reasonable amount of time. The acronym SOAP stands for:

- *S*ubjective: a narrative overview of the session's content, including the date, time, participants, and type of professional service (e.g., martial therapy; individual therapy; crisis intervention; group therapy).
- *O*bjective: mental status indicators
- *A*ssessment: diagnosis; clear notation if patient is at risk to self or other
- *P*lan: treatment plan, including specific goals and objectives, and strategies for patient safety and risk management, when necessary

This type of semi-structured progress note also can foster increased communication and parity among a variety of professionals.

The Mental Status Exam

The mental status exam (MSE) represents one of the most fundamental tools in a crisis therapists' arsenal for both assessment and documentation. It provides a thumbnail sketch of a person at a specific moment in time, and helps organize indicators of suicide and homicide. It also provides, as well as can be expected in any interpersonal context, a relatively objective, structured assessment of a patient's current psychological status. No clinical judgments or explanations or offered for a patient's mood, behavior, or symptoms. Thus, other professionals could be asked to evaluate the patient without being influenced by another practitioner's theoretical orientation or clinical interpretations.

Although the mental status exam is really not a formal exam, the terminology arose from its origins in psychiatry. Its terminology is recognized consistently across a number of disciplines, including general medicine, psychiatry, psychology, social work, occupational therapy, physical therapy, criminal justice, law, and forensics. Although a number of other systems of assessment exist, including the Triage Assessment Form (Myer, Williams, Ottens, & Schmidt, 1992), these have not achieved the popularity or level of professional acceptance as the mental status exam. See this chapter's Appendix for a brief overview of the MSE.

ACKNOWLEDGING COUNTERTRANSFERENCE

Because the risk for burnout and vicarious traumatization is so pronounced for therapists who engage in crisis intervention on a regular basis (also see Chapter 8 for a review), therapists must be sure to process their own internal responses to recollections of patient trauma and potentially stressful or dangerous interactions with patients. Acknowledging both positive and negative countertransference (in relation to the therapist, and generally *not* to the patient) is essential in order to help therapists engage more effectively and objectively in their work with patients. In other words, management of countertransference is a central feature of competent crisis intervention and trauma counseling.

The identification and processing of countertransferential reactions also can serve as a valuable therapeutic aid. Lakovics (1983) purports that the countertransference that therapists experiences can be placed in one of six categories, including concordant and complementary identification. In concordant identification, the therapist experiences thoughts and feelings that are consistent with those that their patient may experience. Acknowledging such concordant identification can help foster empathy in the therapeutic relationship, and can sometimes help therapists allow patients to express emotions that they had been reluctant to share or identify.

In complementary identification, the therapist experiences countertransferential responses that are quite different from the thoughts and feelings expressed by their patient. Therapists may feel surprised, startled, or initially disappointed by their reactions to certain patients (e.g., feelings of boredom, anger, or amusement; fantasies about abandoning the patient; sympathy for individuals whom the patient expresses anger or irritation). When such complementary identification occurs, it typically reflects the experience of others who are closely associated with their patient. This parallel process in the therapeutic relationship can provide practitioners (as well as clinical supervisors; Lakovics, 1983) with a significantly better understanding of the interpersonal dynamics in their patients' relationships.

In addition, an intense countertransferential response also can signal a need for additional support and resources—for the patient and therapist. Specifically, therapists may consider seeking additional support through consultation with legal experts, peer consultation, psychiatric referrals, results from personality, intelligence, and neuropsychological testing, as well as social workers, caseworkers, therapeutic support staff, clergy, and other professionals and para-professionals. Therapists who seek such consultation and support, when indicated, enable themselves to provide competent professional care.

PREPARING FOR TERMINATION

A commonly overlooked aspect of crisis intervention is the formal discussion of termination with patients. Some practitioners are led to believe that termination is only something to be worked through when the patient and therapist have worked together extensively, and have forged a relationship that has lasted for many months or even years. However paradoxical, the importance of discussing termination may be just as, or even more critical within the context of short-term (e.g., crisis intervention) versus long-term therapy.

Many practitioners even choose to broach the subject the topic of termination during the initial crisis session. This emphasis upon a definitive time-line is consistent with general beliefs that the time needed for productive "work" in therapy will expand or contract in order to fit the time allotted (Appelbaum, 1975; Baldwin, 1979). Even though the therapist may be reminding patients that their relationship may end almost as soon as it appears to get started, reminders of a specific time line also provides patients in the midst of chaotic life or personal circumstances with some clear, established structure and limits.

Common statements to address termination may include, "I know that we are meeting here for the first time today and we have a lot of things to work on, but I also want to remind you that we will have approximately eight more [weekly] meetings after this one...I will help us keep track of how many sessions we have left together as we continue working in the next few weeks." Although concerns may arise that the discussion of termination so early in treatment may cripple the development of a therapeutic alliance (e.g., "How can I talk to someone about the innermost secrets of my life when she's already reminding me that we are going to be 'done' in two months?"), many patients describe this explicit discussion of the beginning and end of the therapeutic relationship somewhat liberating. One woman stated, "I think it actually made it easier for me to 'spill my guts' to someone when I knew I wouldn't be seeing them [in long term therapy] for the rest of my life... it was like [the crisis therapist] was giving me the message that I would make it, and that I could move on without his help."

Many rounds of crisis counseling end in referrals to different therapists, agencies, or groups for supportive or insight oriented psychotherapy (sometimes short term or long term in duration). However, many therapists will see patients in order to address critical incidents via crisis counseling, and then expect to continue with those patients in some form of psychotherapy after the initial crisis is over. Consistent with general principles of eclectic therapy, therapists certainly may, and often do, continue on with their patients after an initial round of crisis intervention or counseling. However, from the perspective of integrative therapy, in which choices about moving between techniques or orientations have a theoretical basis or demonstrated necessity (c.f., Hillman & Stricker, in press; Gold & Stricker, 2001), therapists would be advised to formally address the issue of "switching gears" with their patients, for example, from an initially supportive, consultative crisis stance to a more insight oriented, client-focused process.

REFERRALS AND FOLLOW-UP

For many patients in crisis counseling, their time in therapy often is limited by time, number of available sessions (via managed care or organizational constraints), or other extenuating circumstances. For such patients, appropriate referrals and follow-up is essential, both in order to maintain any therapeutic gains and to avoid abandoning or "dumping" a patient. APA ethical principles (1992) make it clear that patients must not be abandoned in the midst of a crisis. One way to help a patient transition to a community agency or other provider is to have that patient call from the crisis counselor's office to set up an initial appointment. The crisis counselor then can make a follow-up phone call to the provider to see if they attended their first session. Of course, obtaining the patient's permission to contact the new therapist for this expressed purpose, and that purpose only, is required.

CONCLUSION

Because the APA's section of Behavioral Emergencies suggests that practitioners have limited education and formal guidelines regarding crisis intervention, this general rubric is offered as a starting point for future discussion and empirical research, as well as an overall review for both novice and experienced clinicians.

APPENDIX

An Overview of The Mental Status Exam

1. General Description. The purpose of an appropriate description is to allow for the identification of someone in a public place. In some crisis situations, the police or other authorities may be asked to identify a patient who poses imminent homicidal risk, or a patient with severe dementia who has wandered from their nursing home.

- Appearance
- Behavior
- Speech
- Attitude

2. Mood and Affect. (M/A)

- Range and appropriateness of affect
- Subjective and objective mood

3. Thought Content. (T/C)
- Suicidality. The presence or absence of any of these factors is indicated typically with the use of a + or − sign. All positive indicators must receive additional explanation, typically with patient quotes.

   (1) Suicidal ideation. Thoughts about suicide or death (e.g., I wish I were dead; I wish I would get hit by a car; I think everyone else would be better off without me around, if you know what I mean.) Suicidal ideation can also be characterized in its frequency and level of preoccupation (e.g., intermittent, recurrent, constant preoccupation).

   (2) Suicidal intent. The extent to which a patient actually intends to carry out a suicidal wish or plan. For example, a patient may state overtly, "I am going to kill myself tomorrow if it's the last thing I do" or "With my husband and children dead,

I have nothing else to live for. I'm going to do it." In the majority of cases, patients are not so direct about their level of intent, for a variety of reasons. Some may wish to hide their intent in order to carry out their plans, whereas other patients may be more ambivalent about their intent to commit suicide. Thus, other patient statements regarding intent may include" I really want to die, but I don't know if I can do it while my son is still alive" or "The feeling comes and goes. I mean, sometimes I feel like I could go one way or another, especially when I've been drinking" or "I want to kill myself so badly, but I don't know if I can go through with it because of my religious beliefs." Anything cited by a patient as a concrete or abstract barrier against suicide also should be documented via patient quotes.

(3) Suicidal plan. Specific information as possible about a patient's plans for suicide, if any such plan is present. Critical information to assess is the intended mode of suicide (e.g., hanging, shooting, jumping from a high building or bridge, taking an overdose—including the number and type of pills expected, having a car accident, suffocation), the specific date and time they plan to commit suicide (e.g., the anniversary date of a specific event such as a loved one's death, murder, or suicide; a time when a roommate is away on business; a Monday morning), the targeted location (e.g., in their bedroom; at a wooded campsite, in an office), and how close or distant other people would be during their attempt (e.g., they want to commit suicide in front of a girlfriend; in school while students and teachers are in class). For specific guidelines on suicide assessment, see Chapter 6.

- Preoccupation with fears, excessive guilt, or feelings of worthlessness.
- A/V (i.e., auditory or visual) hallucinations or delusions. Obtaining and documenting accurate and detailed information about this type of thought content is essential. Note the content, type, and frequency.
- Paranoia. "Do you believe that anyone in particular wants to hurt you or your loved ones, or that you may be in significant danger?" It also is important to determine if a patient's reported paranoia has any foundation in reality. For example, a police officer may have legitimate fears that a previously incarcerated criminal may wish to harm her family members, and a person living in an impoverished neighborhood may have legitimate fears of being subject to random acts of gang violence.

- Dissociation (depersonalization or derealization)

   (1) Depersonalization. Unusual feelings of detachment. Patients may have an unusual perceptual experience, but they readily identify themselves and the reality of the situation. Therapists may ask, "Do you ever feel like you are watching yourself doing something from a distance, like you are on a movie or a train?" and "Do you ever feel disconnected from your body and sensations like cold or pain?"

   (2) Derealization represents the more extreme form of dissociation. Patients not only experience a degree of detachment and distancing from the perception of their own bodies and experiences, but they typically fail to maintain ego boundaries, or, more aptly, their own sense of identity. Most examples sound bizarre and extreme. Patients may describe waking up someplace and not knowing how they got there or looking in the mirror and not recognizing themselves. Typically associated with serious psychopathology.

- Somatic preoccupations. Usually associated with some form of hypochondriasis.

4. Thought Process (T/P)

- Goal directed. Is a patient able to engage in purposeful, everyday activities. For example, can a patient cook a meal for himself, get dressed, apply for a job, and follow through on basic tasks?
- Alertness. Is a patient alert enough to acknowledge changes in their immediate environment, do they appear able to respond quickly to a crisis situation?
- Orientation. The assessment of patient orientation is requisite. Therapists must determine if patients are aware (i.e., oriented) of person, place, and time.
- Concentration. Can ask a patient to count backwards from 100 by 7's, and ask them to spell "world" backwards.
- Abstract thought. The ability to engage in symbolic thought. Many therapists ask patients to identify the meaning of various culturally relevant sayings such as, "Don't count your chickens before they're hatched" or "What comes around goes around."
- Memory. The general qualities of patients' long and short term memory can be described as good, fair, or poor.
- Coping strategies. What do patients do when under a lot of stress? They may represent confabulation, denial, avoidance,

sublimation, intellectualization, and rationalization. If a patient identifies adaptive coping strategies, these too should be noted.

* Insight. The extent to which patients are aware of, and have insight into the nature of their problems and the role that they may play in them; poor, limited, fair, or good.
* Judgment. The extent to which an individual can understand and ascribe to social convention and rules, and to understand what is dangerous to self and other. One question that can be posed to patients is "Imagine that you find yourself stranded in the [Denver] airport. The only thing you have is five dollars in your pocket. What would you do?" Patients who appear to be higher functioning individuals also can have impaired or circumscribed judgment. May be described as WAL; within acceptable limits.
* Perseveration. If present, note the repetitive actions or behavior.
* Impulse control. Patients must be evaluated in terms of their purported ability to control aggressive and sexual impulses. If a patient has only fair or poor impulse control, the specific type of problem (i.e., control of sexual or violent impulses) also should be noted.
* Reliability as a reporter.

5. Vegetative Symptoms. This section of the mental status exam is most closely aligned with traditional medical assessment. These potential symptoms are identified typically as present or absent within the last two weeks.

* Change in appetite.
* Quality of sleep/insomnia.
* Diurnal variation. Symptoms may worsen in the morning or evening.
* Energy diminished/increased.
* Psychomotor agitation/slowing.
* Weight change. A gain or loss of more than 5 pounds within the last two weeks can be considered clinically significant.
* Loss of libido. Even patients who do not have a sex partner (including those who may be older adults) should be asked to consider if they have been *thinking* more or less about sex than usual in the last two weeks.
* Somatic symptoms: headaches; GI distress; increased urination; excessive sighing; muscle aches, back pain; hives; high blood pressure; dizziness; and increasingly intense asthma attacks among others.

4

Post Traumatic Stress
The Need for a Multidimensional Approach

More than three out of four Americans can expect to be exposed to a traumatic event at least once in their lives. Conservative estimates, made before the tragic events of September 11th, also suggest that one in four Americans exposed to a traumatic event will develop chronic or at least transient symptoms of PTSD

A BRIEF HISTORY

Post Traumatic Stress Disorder (PTSD) represents a considerable presence in American life. Conservative estimates suggest that between 5 and 10% of our population will suffer from PTSD at some point in their lives (e.g., Foa, Keane, & Friedman, 2000). Even within the last century, however, PTSD was often misdiagnosed or treated as a hysterical disorder. Early investigations of PTSD typically revolved around the experience of soldiers in combat. During the civil war, soldiers who could not seem to recover after a bloody conflict were labeled with "soldier's heart," in which their tremors, difficulties with sleeping, and fears of returning to the battlefield were seen as a function of personal weakness and a lack of military discipline (Herman, 1997). During World War I, individuals with PTSD were called shell shocked, because military officers believed that the blasts from high power guns and explosives literally disrupted normal brain function, leaving their men dazed and confused.

During World War II, soldiers who displayed depression, tremors, and exaggerated startle responses after traumatic battle events were called "psychos" by their commanding officers. However, in response to information that soldiers were more likely to return to the battlefield if some level of compassion were shown to them, their ailments were then referred to as war neurosis or combat exhaustion. Some military advisors also posited that these unusual symptoms resulted from a conflict between a soldier's id (e.g., drive to survive) versus their superego (e.g., sense of patriotic obligation). Thus, some degree of blame was taken from the men who experienced these disruptive symptoms.

During the Korean War, the DSM-I formally identified "gross stress reactions" as a psychological disorder in 1952. The disorder was said to arise from "situations in which the individual ... had been exposed to severe physical demands or extreme emotional stress, including combat." Interestingly, all references to combat stress were removed from the DSM-II without any official statement or comment during the Vietnam War. And, it was not until *1980* when the DSM-III categorized PTSD a specific psychological disorder that could be characterized as acute or chronic, and caused by any traumatic event (Herman, 1997).

More importantly, the diagnostic criteria in the DSM-III made it clear that both women and men can suffer from PTSD. It also emphasized that extreme psychological responses to stress were no longer limited to wartime events. Although many therapists may feel comfortable with the diagnosis of PTSD, it also remains important to note that this diagnosis was introduced little more than two decades, or one generation, ago.

INSTIGATING EVENTS

When asked to identify the type of traumatic event responsible for the majority of cases of PTSD in our country, many students in psychology classes (as well as laypersons) posit that combat, natural disasters, and rape account for the majority of cases. Thus, many of these students are surprised to learn that automobile accidents represent the primary critical incident for most cases of PTSD (e.g., Blanchard & Hickling, 1997). Of course, this statistic is not meant in any way to minimize the immense toll that war, natural disasters, and rape can take upon its survivors. What is important to note from this finding is that a wide variety of personal experiences, which may or may not be viewed typically as traumatic by all people all times, can engender significant and long-term psychological distress. Although factors such as the extent of one's injuries and the intensity of fear experienced during an event are related to the emergence of psychiatric symptoms (Blanchard & Hickling, 1997), it is the individual, unique perception of the event that is most important in determining the impact of PTSD, and *not* the perception of friends, relatives, co-workers, therapists, physicians, or others.

Similarly, PTSD can result from secondary exposure to a traumatic event. For example, some individuals who witness a traumatic event from a "safe" distance may develop PTSD. Other patients with PTSD describe the start of their symptoms in conjunction with learning that a close friend or family members was injured, assaulted, or killed. Patients often need to be helped to understand that the interpretation of trauma is unique to the individual, and that each traumatic event is relative to one another.

Therapists should help patients understand that any reaction to a stressful event is normal, and no one else can or should force their opinion upon them. Some common statements made by other, sometimes well intentioned individuals in survivors' lives include variations of, "Oh, come on … It wasn't that bad," "What's your problem? You were just mugged, I got shot," "If you hadn't gone out alone by yourself at night, I bet that wouldn't have happened," "The same thing happened to me and I'm not having any problem with it," and "You should be ashamed of yourself. Other people died after that accident, and you were one of the lucky ones who lived." (Also see Chapter 2 for a social psychological analysis of such responses to trauma.) Whether or not a patient suffers from PTSD, therapists should discourage individual in treatment who experienced or witnessed a traumatic event from being drawn into any type of emotional comparison (i.e., a pissing contest) or "justification" of their experience with others.

PRIMARY SYMPTOMS AND DIAGNOSTIC CRITERIA

Although the DSM-IV (APA, 1994) has its limitations, including its calculated focus upon meeting specific diagnostic criteria (e.g., symptoms must be present for at least one month before a diagnosis can be made) a general review of the DSM-IV criteria remains essential. To receive a formal diagnosis of PTSD, an individual must be exposed to a traumatic event by experiencing, witnessing, or being confronted with a threat to health or safety of self or other. Second, the individual must display three or more dissociative symptoms. These include a subjective sense of numbing or a lack of emotional responsiveness, a reduction in awareness of one's surroundings (e.g., being in a daze), derealization, depersonalization, and dissociative amnesia in which specific aspects of the trauma cannot be recalled. Third, the traumatic event must be reexperienced in at least one of the following ways: recurrent images, thoughts, dreams, flashbacks, and distress on exposure to reminders of the traumatic event.

As noted in the DSM-IV, individuals with PTSD also must avoid stimuli that remind them of the trauma. For example, individuals with PTSD may avoid certain thoughts, feelings, conversations, people, places, and activities. To illustrate, one survivor of sexual assault described driving more than 40 miles out of her way to get to work in order to avoid the highway where her assault took place. A Vietnam veteran in treatment described the increasing severity of his avoidance behavior. He reported that after suffering from terrifying symptoms for more than 10 years without significant relief, he spent most of his day in his basement "bunker," and only went out of the house if he had to (i.e., to buy food; got to the doctor). His wife finally demanded that he seek counseling upon threat of divorce.

Other identified symptoms of PTSD include those that are associated with anxiety or increased arousal: sleep problems; irritability; poor concentration; hypervigilance; an exaggerated startle response; and psychomotor agitation. One girlfriend of a man who had been beaten and robbed noted that she learned not to come up and hug him from behind because his tendency was to turn and blindly punch before being able to identify his "possible assailant." In sum, these symptoms tend to be quite disruptive to patients' lives.

PTSD also tends to appear in consort with other mental disorders. Although the nature of the relationship sometimes appears in question (e.g., does one disorder really increase the propensity to develop another?), epidemiological studies suggest that 80% of individuals diagnosed with PTSD have concomitant diagnoses of depression, anxiety, and substance abuse (Foa et al., 2000). Accordingly, therapists must make differential diagnoses with care, and rule out symptom presentations due to underlying medical conditions or substance abuse. Therapists also should use extreme care when reviewing diagnostic criteria in general; the very brief overview provided here is certainly not sufficient to use as a basis for diagnosis. It is unfortunate that many patients' diagnoses of PTSD, an extremely serious mental illness, tend to be made somewhat indiscriminately.

THE PSYCHOBIOLOGY OF TRAUMA

Patients diagnosed with PTSD often describe intense fears that they are "going crazy" or describe intense self-hate and loathing because they attribute their symptoms to "mental weakness" and a general lack of character. In response to these negative beliefs, patients often begin to identify themselves through their diagnostic label, engage in negative, self-punishing behavior, and possess only a limited sense of self-efficacy and faith in treatment. However, recent findings suggest that personality characteristics, with the possible exception of IQ (Buckley, Blanchard, & Neill, 2000), have no virtually ability to predict whether an individual will, or will not, develop PTSD.

In contrast, recent findings from neuropsychology suggest that PTSD arises from generally unavoidable physiological responses to stress—especially if those responses occur at heightened levels over prolonged periods of time (Sapolsky, 1996). Thus, psychoeducation for patients about the underlying psychobiology associated with PTSD, including actual, physical changes in brain structure and function, becomes extremely important and valuable. In essence, patients can be assured that they are not "a weak person" who is "just imagining things" or "making things up." Allowing men and women with PTSD to make appropriate attributions for their symptoms often empowers them to alter previous patterns of ruminative self-blame into more active participation in therapy, and subsequent reduction in their more disruptive symptoms.

Adaptive Responses to Stress

During stressful events, the body releases a number of hormones or glucocorticoids, including epinephrine (i.e., adrenaline), norepinephrine (i.e., noradrenaline), and cortisol. As a result, individuals experience a classic "adrenaline rush," including a rapid heart beat, pupil dilation (which increases visual acuity), and reductions in digestion (c.f., Herman, 1997). Many individuals also experience increased alertness and a reduction in their sensitivity to pain. (Physicians often use the drug hydrocortisone, which is virtually identical to humans' own, naturally produced cortisol, to reduce acute pain and inflammation in joints.) When called upon to use physical strength and speed in a moment of crisis, this naturally occurring "fight or flight" response can provide individuals with a competitive advantage.

During times of crisis, many individuals experience minor (and major) injuries, but only realize later that they have been hurt. Stories abound in which young mothers lift cars from atop their babies after an accident, and emergency service workers rescue people from burning buildings, despite sustaining serious injuries themselves. In reality, most people actually have the strength required to lift a car for a brief period of time. What prevents people from doing this under normal circumstances is that the deep pressure receptors associated with our joints and ligaments generate extreme sensations of pain in order to dissuade us from lifting or moving objects heavy enough to cause permanent physical damage. Under periods of extreme stress, however, the body may produce enough cortisol and adrenaline to override this natural warning system.

Maladaptive Responses to Stress

In large doses, or under extended periods of stress, this normally adaptive stress response, with its flood of glucocorticoids, prevents the body from returning to normal homeostasis. In response, individuals may experience somatic distress such as constipation, diarrhea, stomach cramps, headaches, and insomnia. (Epinephrine and norepinephrine tend to diminish blood flow to the extremities and the digestive system.) Individuals also may experience confusion, a narrowing of attention, impairments in learning, and a catatonic like state, similar to that often exhibited by individuals in shock after a serious injury or accident.

In chronic doses, these stress induced hormonal changes can cause significant impairment in mental and physical health. Lesser amounts of epinephrine can provoke a full-blown stress reaction. And, individuals with PTSD typically show higher levels of these stress-related hormones in their bloodstream when compared to controls, even in a state of rest (Sapolsky, 1996). This heightened state of physiological alertness is consistent with the exaggerated startle response often observed among individuals suffering from PTSD. The amount of cortisol produced during periods of stress becomes so great that it also provides extensive pain relief, which may be adaptive in specific moments of crisis or trauma, but not on a prolonged basis. A landmark study by Van der Kolk and colleagues (Pitman, Van der Kolk, Orr, & Greenberg, 1990) revealed that Vietnam vets diagnosed with PTSD, compared to a matched sample of veterans without the diagnosis, experienced a 30% reduction in their sensitivity to pain after watching just 15 minutes of the film, "Platoon." This change in sensitivity to painful stimulation was equivalent to an 8 mg dose of morphine.

Changes in Brain Function

Sophisticated neuroimaging technology has introduced startling evidence that chronic exposure to stress related hormones also causes significant changes in brain activity or metabolism. For example,

Vietnam veterans with PTSD who were injected with yohimbine hydrochloride, a chemical designed to interfere with normal sympathetic nervous system functioning, experienced flashbacks and panic attacks, whereas Vietnam veterans without a diagnosis of PTSD experienced virtually no flashbacks after injection (Southwick, Krystal, Morgan, & Johnson, 1993). In addition, PET scans of veterans with PTSD revealed that during flashbacks, the Broca's area of their brains (i.e., responsible primarily for language production) did not actively metabolize traditional sources of energy. Thus, Broca's area remained essentially inactive. In contrast, during periods of rest or while contemplating "boring," every day events, the veterans' Brocas areas displayed metabolic activity within a clinically normal range range.

Flashbacks also appear to be associated with changes in blood flow to the brain's visual association and motor cortex (Bremner, Narayan, Staib, Southwick, McGlashan, & Charney, 1999). Because these areas of the brain are inactive during flashbacks, as well as Broca's area, individuals with PTSD appear to re-experience their traumatic memories sensorimotorically (i.e., through sensory perceptions such as vision, hearing, smell, taste, and even unpleasant bodily sensations such as anxiety, fear, and pressure), without access to language. In other words, individuals with PTSD appear to experience flashbacks in the midst of indescribable, abject terror. During some of their most vulnerable moments, these trauma survivors are literally unable to put their feelings into words.

Changes in Brain Structure

The physical changes to actual brain structures in response to chronic stress appear most pronounced in the hippocampus. A number of empirical studies report that sexually abused women and Vietnam veterans suffering from PTSD display hippocampal atrophy, in which this critical brain structure actually shrinks in size (Bremner, 1999; e.g., Sapolsky, 1996). Vietnam veterans have been shown to lose an average of 8% of hippocampal mass. Other studies suggest that survivors of long-term sexual abuse experience a reduction in the size of their hippocampus of more than 10% (e.g., Bremner, 1999).

The hippocampus itself is such a vital structure in the brain because it is associated with learning, memory (including the conversion of short-term into long-term memory), and even the modulation of depressive affect (c.f., Buckley et al., 2000). Individuals with reductions in the size of their hippocampus have been found to manifest significantly more, and more intense, symptoms of PTSD including dissociative symptoms (e.g., feeling numb, detached, or wooden), impairments in verbal memory (Bremner, 1999), and vivid flashbacks (Bremner et al., 1999). It is as though PTSD prevents individuals from logically and systematically processing their experience, and disrupts the appropriate transfer of that experience into long-term memory (Van der Kolk, Burbridge, & Suzuki, 1997). What remains available in memory appears to be a conglomeration of vague, frightening sensations and perceptions, coupled with heightened levels of anxiety, depression, and dissociation.

Comorbid Medical Problems

It has become widely recognized that the survivors of trauma, when compared to nontraumatized individuals, are significantly more likely to seek out medical services and receive a significantly higher number of diagnosed medical problems during a routine checkup (Foa et al., 2000). The presence of additional, potentially life threatening medical conditions have been linked to PTSD, particularly among women. A number of researchers have identified specific forms of hormonal dysregulation among female survivors of trauma. In addition to increased levels of cortisol production, PTSD also appears related to the dysregulation of the hormones oxytocin (Liberzon & Young, 1997) and vasopressin. These two hormones are linked intimately with menstruation, fertility, and fetal growth. Changes in their production and metabolism are typically associated with serious medical problems during pregnancy and delivery, including ectopic pregnancy and miscarriage (c.f., Seng, Oakley, Sampselle, Killion, Graham-Bermann, & Liberzon, 2001).

Findings from a carefully controlled study of more than 2,200 pregnant women (Seng et al., 2001) offer evidence that the hormonal changes associated with PTSD can significantly threaten a woman's reproductive health. When Seng et al. compared Medicaid records of pregnant women diagnosed with PTSD with a randomly selected subsample of pregnant women without a diagnosis of PTSD, the women with PTSD were significantly more likely to require hospitalization for spontaneous abortion, ectopic pregnancy, preterm contractions, and excessive vomiting (i.e., morning sickness). What makes these findings even more dramatic is that these relationships remained significant even after controlling for a variety of demographic and psychosocial factors including age, ethnicity, and reason for Medicaid eligibility. Although Seng et al.'s (2001) findings are subject to limitations regarding the generalizability of these findings to women who are not in their child-bearing years or with different insurance options, they highlight a critical need for early detection and treatment of PTSD.

EVIDENCE-BASED APPROACHES TO TREATMENT

Clinicians and researchers cite a variety of treatment approaches that have been employed in the treatment of PTSD. These include a myriad of treatment modalities and techniques, such as group therapy, inpatient treatment, behavioral therapy, cognitive-behavioral therapy, hypnosis, art therapy, psychosocial rehabilitation, and skills training. Although a number of these approaches hold promise in the amelioration of PTSD symptoms and can be supported by anecdotal evidence and case studies (e.g., art therapy; group therapy; psychosocial rehabilitation; Shalev, Friedman, Foa, & Keane, 2000), significantly fewer have consistent, empirical evidence to back their claims of treatment benefit. These evidence-based therapies, supported by various professional groups including the International Society for Traumatic Stress (Shalev et al., 2000) and Cochrane reviews (Wessley, Rose, & Bisson, 1988) include

- behavioral therapy (e.g., flooding)
- cognitive-behavioral therapy (e.g., systematic desensitization)
- pharmacotherapy (e.g., SSRIs)
- Eye Movement Desensitization and Reprocessing (EMDR)

In general, therapists often employ a variety of treatment approaches in order to best help their patients. Although these aforementioned, evidence-based therapies will be reviewed here, mental health professionals certainly should not abandon the use of additional, adjunctive techniques if they reduce patient distress, do not interfere with potential forensic issues (e.g., hypnosis generally should not be employed if a patient expects to become engaged in litigation regarding the traumatic event; Feldman-Summers, 1996), are culturally appropriate, and met with patient consent (Shalev et al., 2000). Clinicians also must note that these evidence-based treatments are not be appropriate for all patients at all times, and that clinical judgment must supercede any written, organizational guidelines. In addition, the rapidly changing body of work regarding empirically validated treatments makes it vital to engage in continued review.

Behavioral and Cognitive-Behavioral Treatment

Various professional groups recommend exposure theory as an effective treatment for PTSD, with an average time requirement of six months, with opportunities for continued, long-term follow-up (Ballenger, Davidson, Lecrubier, Nutt, Foa, Kessler, & McFarlane, 2000). Although behavioral treatment such as flooding and in vivo exposure has empirical evidence to support its use, its use may not always be appropriate for every patient with posttraumatic symptoms. Because flooding literally involves exposure to overwhelming, traumatic affect, many patients either decline to participate in treatment or terminate before any positive effects are obtained. Also due to the intense affect typically associated with flooding is considered so intense, many VA hospitals provide PTSD treatment primarily on an inpatient basis in order to provide additional patient support. Still other therapists encourage their patients to participate in group therapy as an adjunct to behavioral treatments such as flooding (c.f., Saigh, 1998) in order to elicit peer support and decrease feelings of isolation. In contrast with flooding, many patients are more amenable to some type of graded exposure (i.e., a variant of cognitive-behavioral treatment), in which therapists guide patients through recollections of a traumatic event at a slower pace, with significant reliance upon relaxation techniques to quell disturbing affect.

Coupled with graded exposure to traumatic memories or stimuli, many cognitive-behavioral approaches include the construction of a personal narrative regarding the traumatic event. In addition to demonstrating the ability to recall aspects of the trauma at will, without succumbing to extreme levels of stress (i.e., become desensitized), patients are able to critically examine any related cognitions or beliefs they have regarding the experience of the traumatic event. For example, a patient who thinks that "only weak people, like me" become overwhelmed after surviving a mugging or other traumatic event can be made aware of his cognitive distortions and helped to challenge them. Working through survivor guilt is often a central feature in work with individuals suffering from PTSD (Khouzam & Kissmeyer, 1997).

An Example of Survivor Guilt.   Every summer, Jonathan looked forward to attending a month long, residential summer camp for swimmers. During the summer when he was 14 years-old, Jonathan developed a high fever and chest cold, and knocked on the door of his camp counselor for help. When the counselor opened the door, he welcomed Jonathan into his room, had him lie down on the bed (presumably while he would go to the infirmary and get him medicine), and then attempted to molest Jonathan. With a start, Jonathan fought off the counselor, struggled with the door, and fled from the counselor's room in a panic. For the next two weeks of camp he told no one about what happened, but slept on the floor of his room against the door jam so that he would not be surprised by the counselor's entry. He also would only take a shower and use the toilet if at least two other boys were in the bathroom. (The staff members had keys to all of the rooms in case a resident lost their key.) Jonathan also developed stomach problems and lost weight.

A few weeks after Jonathan returned home after camp, he casually mentioned to his mother that "something weird happened" with one of the counselors, and that "he tried to hug me and kiss me and stuff." His mother's response was to deny what had happened, "Oh, maybe you were imagining things, Honey. I mean, you said you had a high fever and didn't feel good. I can't imagine that really happened... it's such a good camp and I know you look forward to going there every year." Jonathan told no one else about the attack.

At age 18, Jonathan sought counseling for "having trouble with school" at the university-based treatment center where he attended college. As he grew up and matured physically, Jonathan became very interested in girls, and became a real "womanizer" as he called it. After a brief scare regarding an STD in his first semester at college, he became concerned about his promiscuous behavior, and that he seemed more interested, and even crazed, about dating girls than studying.

A few sessions later, Jonathan told his therapist about the attack he experienced during summer camp as a teenager. Tears rolled down his cheeks as he said, "I just couldn't do it, could I? I can't believe it." When his therapist responded, "What do you mean, Jonathan; "I couldn't do it?", he stated, "If I had only done something about it... I mean, if I told the people running the camp about what he did, then maybe he couldn't have done that to someone else. What if he molested other boys... and it's all my fault because I was too much of a wimp to stop him?!"

Jonathan had inadvertently taken full responsibility upon himself to control the actions of his adult attacker. To him, the logic was clear; "I should have done something. It was up to me to stop him, and I didn't. I never told anyone else about it. So now maybe a whole bunch of other kids suffered because I was too weak to do anything about it." Jonathan's cognitions of himself as a failure were so rigid that he was unable to acknowledge his mother's inability (as an adult no less) to help *him* most when *he* needed it, that he himself deserved help as much as "some other kid who might have been attacked by the same counselor," and that he, in fact, had limited control over the actions of a grown man, especially when he was a physically ill teenager who was turning to an identified authority figure for help.

In later sessions, Jonathan was helped to recognize and appreciate his own intense will for survival. As a young teen, he fought off an adult attacker and was able to remain safe for the duration of his stay at camp. Jonathan also was able to recognize that some of his survivor guilt (e.g., "I am a terrible person. Why didn't I stop him and keep this from happening to someone else?") masked his own anger and fury that the attack happened to him, and that he had no one to come to his aid in a time of need. He also was able to express the anger, fear, and confusion regarding his subsequent concerns about his own sexual orientation (i.e., "So am I gay but I don't know it since this guy attacked me?), and his attempt to "overcompensate" by actively pursuing women.

Additional Empirical Approaches. Foa and colleagues (Foa, Hearst-Ikeda, & Perry, 1995) conducted a model program in which female survivors of recent assault (sexual and non-sexual) received a brief (four session) course of cognitive-behavioral treatment, including psychoeducation about normal stress reactions, instruction on deep breathing and relaxation, imaginal exposure to the critical incident, in vivo exposure, and cognitive restructuring in response to self-blame and any perceived loss of control (Foa, Rothbaum, Riggs, & Murdock, 1991). These survivors who received cognitive-behavioral treatment were matched and statistically compared with other women who experienced a recent assault, but received only repeated assessment of their PTSD related symptoms.

More than five months after the delivery of cognitive-behavioral treatment, the women in Foa et al.'s (1995) study reported significantly less intense reexperiencing of the event (e.g., flashbacks; nightmares) and were significantly less depressed than the women who received only assessment of their symptoms. In addition, only 10% of the women who received cognitive-behavioral treatment met full diagnostic criteria for PTSD whereas more than 70% of the women in the control condition met diagnostic criteria for PTSD. However, due to the multifaceted nature of the treatment intervention, the extent to which psychoeducation, in vivo exposure, imaginal exposure, and cognitive restructuring each contributed uniquely to symptom reduction remains unclear.

Psychopharmacology

A number of studies and anecdotal reports (e.g., Khouzam & Kissmeyer, 1997) also suggest that psychotropic medication can serve as a useful adjunct in treatment of PTSD. The most recently updated Cohrane review available (Stein, Zungu-Kirwayi, van der Linden, & Seedat, 2001) recommends the use of psychotropic medication such as selective serotonin reuptake inhibitors (SSRIs) such as Prozac, Zoloft, and Paxil in treatment. These antidepressant medications appear useful in reducing some primary symptoms of PTSD such as anxiety and hyperarousal, as well as comorbid disorders such as anxiety and clinical depression (Friedman, Davidson, Mellman, & Southwick, 2000).

All of these aforementioned experts also make it clear that while psychopharmacology can be an effective tool in the treatment of PTSD, addressing underlying issues (such as survivor guilt and spirituality; Khouzam & Kissmeyer, 1997) by engaging in traditional therapy (e.g., cognitive-behavioral therapy) with long-term follow-up (Ballenger et al., 2000) remains essential. Specifically, while various professional groups concur that while psychopharmacology may represent an effective treatment, they also support the use of SSRIs for at least a two (Friedman et al., 2000) to 12 month period (Ballenger et al., 2000). The danger of employing psychotropic medication as a sole treatment modality is that a patient will come to locate their locus of control externally, within their medication, instead of internally, within themselves.

EYE MOVEMENT DESENSITIZATION REPROCESSING

The first empirical findings to support the use of EMDR were published by the procedure's founder, Francine Shapiro, in 1989. Within a decade, practice guidelines from the International Society for Traumatic Stress Studies (Chemtob, Tolin, Van der Kolk, & Pitman, 2000) and rigorous Cochrane reviews (e.g., Wessely, Rose, & Bisson, 1998) suggested that EMDR does represent an effective, evidence based form of treatment for PTSD. However, many members of the scientific community (e.g., Herbert, Lilienfeld, Lohr, Montgomery, O'Donohue, Rosen, & Tolin, 2000) maintain serious reservations about the use of this nontraditional treatment and its highly commercial nature. Before deciding to use EMDR as a treatment modality with their own patients, therapists are encouraged to examine some of the myths regarding this nontraditional treatment, and to review available empirical evidence that both promotes and cautions against its use in clinical practice. Thus, this portion of the text is designed to describe the overall treatment protocol, examine public perceptions of the protocol, and examine scientific evidence regarding its efficacy for the treatment of PTSD as well as other psychological disorders.

General Misconceptions

Televised documentaries often promote EMDR as a mystical or even magical "quick fix." Patients typically are shown in the middle of a session, with their therapist sitting directly across from them, waving a finger rapidly, back and forth, in front of the patients' eyes. The therapist may stop occasionally to ask the patient to "stop...blow it out...and tell me what you are getting now." Additional, narrative statements regarding the "previous, retractable symptoms of this patient...alleviated in only one treatment session" often add to the mystique. (EMDR typically requires "typical" therapy or "talk sessions" before, during, and after the eye movement protocols.) Out of context, the procedure appears bizarre, irrational, and even nonsensical. Such overly dramatic and simplistic presentations of EMDR are probably related to the rigorous editing often required to meet network time demands as well as the investigative reporters' general interest in creating some degree of sensationalism. Although numerous clinical trials have shown that EMDR is more effective than placebo (Chemtob et al., 2000), one can probably assume that the fantastic nature of the procedure, as portrayed to the general public, only adds to its effectiveness.

Although EMDR is touted as a short-term therapy, most proponents of EMDR indicate that single sessions may be helpful, but that the use of a single session should be limited primarily to an emergency situation (e.g., Solomon, 1994). The effects of EMDR appear optimal when practiced within the context of a formal therapeutic relationship over a number of weeks, and even months (e.g., Shapiro, 1995). Furthermore, EMDR is designed to serve as an *adjunct* to more traditional psychotherapy. It is not meant to replace the therapeutic relationship or the primacy of a therapist's clinical skills, experience, and judgment (Shapiro, 1995; 1996). Client safety is paramount. In many cases, EMDR is not even initiated until a number of sessions have passed, and patient and therapist begin to share a working relationship based upon open lines of communication and trust. Still other therapists introduce the use of EMDR only when more traditional cognitive-behavioral approaches fail to produce significant symptom relief. The practice of EMDR itself often involves the use of a variety of therapeutic techniques, including an analysis of dynamic issues (including possible secondary gains for symptom maintenance), journal writing, and hypothesis testing.

An additional misconception about EMDR is that it enables patients to recall specific, factual details about early traumatic events or repressed memories. In contrast, EMDR is not designed to reclaim repressed memories or employ the use of hypnotic regression. In direct opposition to the typical goal of hypnotic regression, in which patients are instructed to recall specific, accurate details of previously repressed events, the aim of EMDR is to *transform* previously unpleasant memories and related, negative cognitions surrounding traumatic events into more realistic perceptions of oneself and a related experience of a trauma. However, as with hypnosis, patients must be cautioned *before* engaging in EMDR that the use of this procedure is likely to render anything that they recall in relation to a previous trauma inadmissible as evidence in any American court of law.

Treatment Protocol

The overall treatment protocol for EMDR has eight primary components or stages.

1. History of trauma
2. Preparation
3. Assessment of negative cognition
4. Desensitization
5. Installation of positive cognitions
6. Body Scan
7. Closure
8. Reevaluation

In respect to general cautions about self-instruction in EMDR (e.g., Shapiro, 1995; 1996), only a general overview of the procedure is provided here.

The first component of treatment represents the early stages of therapy and the initiation of a working relationship. Possible impediments to success, including secondary gains, entrenched negative beliefs, and environmental stressors are investigated and addressed. In essence, the history of the patient and the presenting problem are thoroughly explored. The second stage educates the patient about EMDR and allows them to assent to the procedure. To prepare for intense emotional reactions, therapists increase patients' ego strength by teaching specific relaxation exercises, reviewing realistic expectations, and creating a "safe place" through mental imagery. Therapy sessions that incorporate EMDR generally require 90 minutes (Shapiro, 1996), representing a significantly greater amount of time than in the traditional 45 or 50 minute "therapy hour."

In the third stage, therapist and patient work together to determine the specific negative cognitions, emotions, and bodily sensations associated with a specific traumatic memory (e.g., I can still see those eyes, peering out at me behind the ski mask; I can still hear the screams of the people trapped in the car) and related, negative cognition (e.g., I am a horrible person because I was too scared to even try to fight back; I should have been the one who was hurt instead) to target for change. Patients are asked to rate how stressful they find that unpleasant memory, and how believable they find a more constructive, objective cognition (e.g., I am a good person, regardless of how I responded to my attacker; I did the best I could) and to rate the extent to which they believe a more appropriate cognition.

In the fourth stage, various "sets" of eye movements are begun. Patients are asked to recall their disturbing image or memory while engaging in saccadic, or rapid eye movements. At various intervals, patients are asked to stop and report upon their experience. Most patients experience a decrease in subjective distress, and report significant changes in their perceptions (versus recall) of events. This fourth stage is the one typically featured in television documentaries, often at the expense of more comprehensive coverage. In the next, or fifth, stage another series of eye movements are used to "install" positive cognitions (i.e., make them feel more valid) in place of negative ones. Therapists also ask patients to engage in a body scan (i.e., an internal assessment of bodily tension or strain) during the sixth phase of EMDR, to address through additional sets of saccades. It is important to note that EMDR actively works to explore patients' visual, auditory, olfactory, tactile, and kinesthetic associations to a trauma.

The seventh stage of the procedure, in which some degree of closure is generated in session, typically receives little attention in the media. Therapists assess their patients carefully to ensure that they do not leave the session in the midst of an intense abreaction. Part of this process includes debriefing, including reiterating the fact that important material is likely to emerge in between sessions. Patients are asked to keep a journal or log regarding these emergent issues for processing and discussion in further sessions. In the eighth, or final, stage of the protocol, patients continue to be reevaluated for maintenance of symptom relief in a structured series of follow-up sessions.

Critical Considerations

Some critiques of EMDR include its aggressive commercial promotion (e.g., Herbert et al., 2000) and the relative ownership of the procedure by a small number of organizations. In order to practice EMDR, therapists are directed to complete one or more formal training courses, typically through the EMDR Institute, Incorporated. As noted by Shaprio, "trying to teach EMDR yourself [to friends or colleagues] renders a disservice to both them and the procedure ... please send them to be officially trained [so that] we can assure that they can best receive and contribute to the knowledge base of this new area of psychology" (inside front cover; 1996). Concerns have been raised that the use of EMDR by untrained clinicians can result in significant patient distress.

To quality for training, therapists must be registered as a licensed mental health professional, travel to a specific location for training (usually a large city), and pay a few hundred dollars for each level of training. Groups of professionals also can arrange for on-site training. Training sessions are typically offered in two-day blocks for initial, or Level I training, Level II training, and Advanced Topics in EMDR. Individuals who complete Level I and Level II training become eligible to join the EMDR Network and receive patient referrals via a provided listing in their national register.

Proponents of EMDR argue that training is mandatory for appropriate treatment delivery, as well as ethically necessary (e.g., Shapiro, 1995; 1996). For example, most clinicians who integrate biofeedback or hypnosis into their practice often take extensive training courses. Still others can argue that although psychologists are encouraged to engage in pro bono work by the APA, mental health practitioners are entitled to operate successful businesses, earn a decent living, and profit from the development of specific treatment protocols and tests. However, detractors speculate that the process of creating a specialized in-group of practitioners that use EMDR actually minimizes the ability of those practitioners to be skeptical or objective about the process (Herbert et al., 2000).

Another potential concern is that EMDR is overused, and promoted as a virtual panacea for a multitude of disorders. Although EMDR has demonstrated efficacy in the treatment of many disorders including PTSD, panic disorder (Goldstein & Feske, 1994), complicated bereavement (Solomon & Shapiro, 1997), and dissociative disorders (Young, 1994), some clinicians appear to use EMDR indiscriminately. One such practitioner described her experience with EMDR stating, "Oh, yes. EMDR is great. I use it for practically everything—depression, sexual dysfunction, you name it. My clients love it." Although only limited information is available regarding the decision-making used by therapists to determine whether or not they will use EMDR in their practice (e.g., Herbert et al., 2000), Shapiro also states that EMDR is not a "cookie cutter" procedure, and that it is not designed for use with all patients at all times (Shapiro, 1995; 1996).

In sum, a number of professional organizations endorse the use of EMDR as a preferred mode of treatment for most patients who suffer from PTSD. Because PTSD represents a chronic, pervasive, and

destructive mental illness, many therapists have been willing to experiment with the technique because it represents a clearly evidenced-
based treatment. Many therapists also are willing to explore the use of
EMDR in order to help patients who often experience unmitigated suffering in the aftermath of a traumatic event. Even though the specific
method of action in EMDR responsible for symptom relief remains
unknown (Zabukovec, Lazrove, & Shapiro, 2000) and may actually
produce such positive outcomes due to its similarity with other
evidence-based treatments (e.g., cognitive-behavioral therapy; Herbert
et al., 2000), many proponents argue that identifying the corrective
mechanism in EMDR becomes moot if patients with previously
intractable symptoms are able to experience some measure of symptom
relief and treatment success.

NON-TRADITIONAL APPROACHES

A number of additional treatments for PTSD have been explored
throughout the last decade. Some of these include culturally modified
rituals and various forms of alternative medicine such as therapeutic
massage, Yoga, Ti Chi, and mindful meditation. (Please see Chapter 11
for a critical review of complementary and alternative medicine in
relation to the experience of trauma.) Others incorporate unique
aspects of the patient's culture into a comprehensive treatment "pack-
age." Unfortunately, few empirical findings are available to affirm the
effectiveness of many of these alternative approaches in the treatment
of PTSD.

Culture-Based Rituals

One non-traditional approach that has garnered empirical support
in the treatment of PTSD is that of culturally derived rituals. Native
American Indians have long established practices in which their survivors of war and combat are recognized in a series of elaborate tribal
ceremonies. As noted by Johnson and colleagues (Johnson, Feldman,
Lubin, & Southwick, 1995), these ceremonies often include distinctive
songs, dancing, and role-plays of the battle itself. A hallmark feature of
these ceremonies is the indoctrination of the survivors into a special
group of warriors, who receive venerated titles and distinctive head-
dress. In other tribes, warriors wounded in battle also received membership into a small, selective group that must accept tribal prohibitions

against drinking alcohol and using other psychoactive substances. This mandated avoidance of substance use by Native Americans certainly is consistent with current recommendations for trauma survivors (e.g., Mitchell, 1988).

Based upon the apparent success of these rituals among Native Americans, coupled with mainstream American culture's relative dearth of traditions and rituals, a number of researchers (e.g., Johnson et al., 1995; Silver & Wilson, 1988) have successfully modified these Native rituals for use among Vietnam veterans, a current cohort of American warriors. Veterans engaged in various ceremonies that included family members, therapists and other staff members, and veterans from World War II and Korea. To encourage a sense of acceptance, the veterans from other wars formally welcomed the Vietnam veterans into a brotherhood of survivors. The veterans also made written records of their experiences on the inpatient PTSD unit, and burnt them in a ceremonial fire to indicate their symbolic release from the past and return to the future, and their waiting families.

Community-Based Interventions

In some close-knit communities, including those that may be physically isolated from other groups of people, traditional approaches to the treatment of trauma may be limited due to a lack of formally trained professionals. Thus, more radical, specifically crafted approaches may be required to meet the needs of such isolated communities. Terry (1999) skillfully describes one such approach with a small community in the Alaskan outback or "Bush," in which 45,000 Native Alaskans live in … 171 small, remote villages … located on more than 600,000 square miles of land and water … without [access to] roads, hospitals, or physicians" (p. 150; Terry, 1999). Access to health care was obviously limited.

In response, the Indian Health Service and the state of Alaska provided funding for the training of "Community Health Aides," mostly middle-aged, female residents, who provided emergency and adjunctive medical care within their own, local village. The program was initially well received, but one the attrition rate for these Health Aids was nearly 33%. Terry (1999) hypothesized that secondary stress reactions predicated most of these resignations. Because these Alaskan villages had such small populations, the Health Aides's patients typically were their own friends, neighbors, and family members rather than strangers. The Aides also had to engage in multiple roles such as therapist, physician, EMT, and even undertaker. Many of these women earned significantly more money than their husbands, which also tended to cause considerable distress within the context of a traditionally defined marriage. In addition, villagers tended to blame the Health Aides for failed treatments and rescue attempt, rather than acknowledge the Aides' limited training and supplies.

To address the impact of such secondary trauma upon the Health Aides, a series of traditional approaches to trauma survivors were employed. For example, a formal Critical Incident Stress Debriefing (CIDS; also see Chapter 10) program was instituted. The Health Service sponsored various in depth training seminars on topics such as stress management, grief, traumatic stress, depression, and substance abuse. An employee assistance program also was instituted for Health Aides, as well as other state employees. However, Terry (1999) also noted that the program still did not work.

Cultural and community issues appeared to doom the initial attempts at mediating Health Aide stress. The Native Alaskan worldview is at odds with the psychobiological reasoning for stress reactions typically offered during traditional crisis debriefings (Terry, 1999; Mander, 1992). The traditional Western approach to treatment, which relies heavily upon an individual approach to self-care and healing, is in direct opposition to many Native beliefs and emphases upon collective rather than individual undertakings. In addition, long-standing support groups for stress management or sobriety were nonexistent.

Change only came when members from the Traditional (Native) and City Councils agreed to work together on a potential solution. After discussing their deviation from traditional values, the group rallied around the concept of Kelengakutelleghpat, a term employed on group whaling trips that translated loosely into "watching out for each other" (Terry, 1999). The Native community also responded positively to public service initiatives that explained the specialized training and experience of the village Health Aides, and identified them as a limited but valuable community resource.

Health Aides also utilized electronic communication (e-mail) to communicate frequently with physicians, physician assistants, mental health counselors, and other Health Aides. Medical decision-making also was made via an interdisciplinary treatment team, which helped the community view "failures" as a system, rather than individual, problem. This return to a traditional focus on collective rather than individual functioning helped alleviate a significant amount of Health Aide attrition and stress (Terry, 1999). Similar, community based programs have been instituted in various locations including Canada and other locations (see Ramsey, 1993).

Final Cautions

The aforementioned information regarding the Alaskan Health Aide program, as well as any other community-based program, illustrates the critical need to tend to cross-cultural issues in the treatment of PTSD. As a nation, we also spend millions of dollars on international relief efforts for PTSD, in a myriad of countries for a myriad of very important reasons. However, we, as a profession, may not ask ourselves often enough whether we really are promoting the most effective treatment for those traumatized individuals, within the context of their own geography and culture.

5

Long-Term Sequela of Trauma

A number of theorists have initiated a powerful paradigm shift in which chronic exposure to trauma is believed to underlie the development of serious psychological disorders including Borderline Personality Disorder and Dissociative Identity Disorder.

BORDERLINE PERSONALITY DISORDER

Patients suffering from borderline personality disorder (BPD) often present health care providers with some of their most challenging clinical work. Patients with PBD have been described as manipulative, suicidal, reckless, impulsive, and coercive. Therapists have described their work with patients suffering from BPD as intense, draining, and even frightening. Common accounts of clinical scenarios include repeated, late night phone calls, threats of suicide, episodes of self-injurious behavior (i.e., cutting), erratic attendance in therapy sessions, requests for special favors or preferential treatment, and visits to the ER. Anecdotes also emerge in work with patients with BPD regarding "splitting" among treatment team members, patients who overturn desks upon hearing that their therapist is going on vacation, and clinicians who openly state, "I will only work with one borderline [patient] at a time" or "You can't pay me enough to work with a borderline [patient]." The use of the term "borderline," to describe a patient in their entirety, further illustrates the tendency of many therapists to narrow their focus (Zweig & Hillman, 1999), perhaps unintentionally, upon the problematic symptoms of the disorder rather than upon patients themselves.

Clinical Presentation

Estimates of the prevalence of BPD among the general population vary. Many experts estimate that 2% of the general population, and up to 20% of psychiatric patients, suffer from BPD. Patients diagnosed with BPD also appear to account for a significant proportion of all patients (between 30–60%) diagnosed with any type of personality disorder. Significantly more women are diagnosed with BPD than men (Zweig & Hillman, 1999). According to the DSM-IV, individuals must display symptoms consistent with at least five out of the nine following criteria to receive a diagnosis of BPD:

1. Frantic efforts to avoid real or imagined abandonment (e.g., many accounts exist in which a patient threatens suicide the day before their therapist is scheduled to leave on vacation).
2. Patterns of unstable and intense personal relationships characterized by extremes of idealization and devaluation (e.g., one patient could not understand why her boyfriends "always went from being the best boyfriend in the world to a bunch of total assholes—virtually overnight").
3. Identity disturbance; markedly and persistently unstable self-image or sense of self (e.g., one patient stated, "It's like there's just nothing in here...It's like I don't even exist unless other people are around").
4. Impulsivity in at least two areas that are potentially self-damaging (e.g., spending, sex, substance abuse, reckless driving, binge eating; one impoverished elderly patient in a state supported nursing home ran up a credit card bill of more than $7,000 dollars ordering merchandise from the Home Shopping Channel).
5. Recurrent suicidal behavior, gestures, threats, or self-mutilating behavior.
6. Affective instability due to a marked reactivity of mood (e.g., intense episodic dysphoria, irritability, or anxiety with transient states; one patient stated, "It's like my skin is crawling...everything just seems to bug the living shit out of me").
7. chronic feelings of emptiness (e.g., "I'm just so bored. I don't know what I'm supposed to be doing anywhere).
8. inappropriate, intense anger or difficulty controlling anger (e.g., frequent displays of temper, constant anger, recurrent physical fights; one patient with BPD was fired from her job as a customer service representative because she threw a telephone at a customer and told him to "get the fuck out of the building").
9. transient, stress-related paranoid ideation or severe dissociative symptoms (e.g., one patient described sitting in front of the TV

watching a police drama, and suddenly watching herself in the television program, taking a loaded gun and putting it to her own head).

Classic Theories

A number of theories exist regarding the origins of this interpersonally devastating disorder. The three theorists cited most often are Kernberg, Adler, and Masterson. Their views on the etiology of BPD will be reviewed here briefly.

- Kernberg believed that BPD results from "excessive early aggression" coupled with poor mothering or frustration. He believes that the experience of trauma has nothing to do with the development of the disorder—it comes "from within." Kernberg used this internally based rationale to explain why some individuals who suffer under extremely abusive conditions fail to develop BPD, whereas others who suffer similar traumatic events develop severe BPD.
- Adler (1993) believed that inconsistent, insensitive, and nonempathic mothering fostered the development of BPD. Specifically, he posited that children of these mothers developed without the benefit of stable, internalized objects (e.g., internally maintained conceptions of a significant personal relationship), and thus engage in impulsive behavior in a desperate attempt to replace their lack of emotional connectedness with instant gratification
- Masterson believed that problems with separation and individuation (c.f., Mahler, 1971) underlie the development of BPD. He reasoned that when mothering interfered with a child's natural strivings (i.e., a mother could only tolerate a child who provided a reflection of her own needs, wants, and interests), a natural response is to become emotionally withdrawn. These children were believed to experience profound feelings of emptiness and loneliness, in part because they were not afforded the opportunity to explore and develop their own identity.

All three of these traditional theories minimize the impact of trauma upon personality development.

Revised Theories: The Centrality of Trauma

Within the last decade, a small of theorists (e.g., Davies & Frawley, 1994; Kroll, 1993) began to note considerable similarities between patients suffering from BPD and PTSD, including persistent experiences

of irritability, suicidality, dissociation, and contradictory self-percep-
tions. An examination of the social histories for patients diagnosed with
BPD suggests up to 80% of these individuals report a history of physical
or sexual abuse, and 75% report a history of childhood verbal abuse (e.g.,
Morey & Zanarini, 2000). The majority of patients with BPD also appear
to have been raised in a household with at least one parent suffering from
a serious psychological disorder (e.g., depression, substance abuse, character disorder; Zweig & Hillman, 1999). Thus, trauma appears to represent a common thread among most individuals diagnosed with BPD.

Within the last decade, a significant paradigm shift has occurred
in the conceptualization of borderline PD and its treatment options.
For example, Davies and Frawley (1994) postulated that childhood
trauma represents the causal factor in virtually all cases of borderline
personality disorder. These experts describe individuals who "protect"
their parents or abusers, and avoid acknowledging the presence of
abuse themselves, via denial and dissociation. When exposure to
trauma remains chronic, severe, or unacknowledged, patients may
remember details about abusive events in "bits and pieces," without
the benefit of a personal narrative. Consistent with the symptom presentation in PTSD, various distortions in perception also are noted commonly among patients with BPD:

- problems focusing attention (i.e., patients may defensively learn
  not to pay attention to their environment because certain stimuli may trigger memories or intrusive thoughts)
- global, impressionistic perceptions (Learning or remembering
  vague details about a traumatic event may seem less threatening
  than specific details)
- imprecision or exaggeration of events (e.g., heightened startle
  responses; a tendency to respond to even minor, negative events,
  such as a run in a pair of stockings, in an extreme fashion
  because psychic energy is focused upon daily issues versus
  repressed, severe trauma.
- disturbing somatic symptoms and sensations, similar to those
  experienced during flashbacks. In response to these overwhelming feelings and perceptions, patients often engage in self-
  mutilation or cutting. Paradoxically, patients often describe this
  self-harm as a release from tension; a release of naturally occurring opiates and a sense of control over one's own body may
  account for this perception.

Davies and Frawley thus assert that BPD actually represents a severe,
chronic form of PTSD. Professionals involved in this paradigm shift,

unlike their predecessors, also assert that patients' experiences of trauma must be addressed in order to offer effective treatment.

Evidence Based Treatment Approaches

Unfortunately, treatment outcomes with traditional, individual psychotherapy for BPD appear quite variable. Patients often enter and exit treatment with multiple therapists, and continue to manifest symptomatic behavior. As noted, many clinicians describe feeling overwhelmed and even powerless in response to some of the disorder's most severe symptoms. However, a growing body of research provides empirical support for the use of a recently developed integrative therapy with chronically suicidal, substance-dependent and severely disordered individuals with BPD (McMain, Korman, & Kimeff, 2001). Preliminary evidence also supports its use among individuals with binge eating disorders (Telch, Agras, & Linehan, 2000). This evidence-based treatment for BPD is referred to as Dialectical Behavioral Therapy (DBT; Linehan, Armstrong, Suarez, & Allmon, 1991).

The History of Dialectical Behavior Theory. Linehan, the therapist and researcher who developed DBT, generated her approach to treatment using a combination of trial-and-error and outside observation. Because Linehan appeared significantly more successful in her work with chronically suicidal patients than many of her colleagues, a group of investigators observed her to identify some of her specific techniques and to articulate her approach to the disorder. This qualitative research approach revealed that Linehan's conceptualization of psychopathology is BPD is significantly different from that of more traditional theorists (e.g., Kernberg, Masterson) and more similar to that of Davies, Frawley, and Kroll. Specifically, Linehan postulated that pathological symptoms originated from problems with

- emotional dysregulation (e.g., patients typically have a low threshold for emotional reactions, and often employ blunting or escalating in typically failed attempts to cope)
- invalidating environments (e.g., systemic problems in which a child does not learn to trust in her own assessment of affective experience; a child learns that the only way to get attention is to escalate behaviorally or emotionally)
- deficiencies in adaptive behavior—not deficiencies in character or psychophysiology (i.e., patients never learned effective coping skills; treatment must be adapted to individual patients)

The team also discovered that Linehan's atypical approach to treatment incorporated aspects of behavioral, cognitive-behavioral, interpersonal, family (i.e., systems), and group therapies, and social psychological and Buddhist principles. The crux of DBT is its focus upon dialectics. Linehan asserts that traditional therapy primarily emphasizes *change*, which can make a patient feel ridiculed or blamed for her current situation. In contrast, she noted that Zen philosophy emphasizes *acceptance*, which can alleviate concerns about constantly correcting oneself, but also foster feelings of hopelessness and stagnation in treatment. Rather than aligning herself with either of these approaches, Linehan regarded them as dialectic in which nothing is viewed in absolutes (e.g., splitting; all-or-nothing thinking; perceiving in "black and white") and opposites often co-exist. Thus, Linehan developed DBT in order to address both sides of any conflict simultaneously, and to emphasize the importance, and simultaneous function, of both internal (i.e., biochemical, affective, cognitive processing) and interpersonal (i.e., family, cultural, environmental) systems.

Treatment Overview. DBT has four requisite or mandatory components, which share some similarity, but more dissimilarity, with traditional individual treatment approaches. These essential components include:

1. Individual therapy for one hour per week
2. Skills training in a small group for two and a half hours per week
3. Between session phone contact, to encourage the generalization of skills training to real world, rather than classroom, settings
4. Group supervision for all therapists, for one and a half hours each week

Treatment begins with a series of paper-and-pencil measures designed to determine the presence of BPD. The primary therapist then informs her patient directly, "You have borderline personality disorder" (Koerner & Linehan, 1992). The diagnosis is written upon a chalkboard, and the patient and therapist review each of the DSM-IV inclusion criteria to discuss the extent to which the patient feels she experiences or engages in those behaviors. Linehan reports that clients typically express relief that their problem can be identified, and that it even has a *name*. This approach, in which patients are presented with their diagnosis in order to instill a sense of hope and mastery, is similar to that employed by Ryle and Low (1993) in their Cognitive Analytic Therapy.

Before the DBT can be initiated, however, both the "client" and therapist are required to make a formal one year commitment to therapy—in writing. The client makes a commitment to decrease their parasuicidal behaviors and any behaviors that could interfere with the course of treatment. Therapists make a commitment to function as coach, educator, cheerleader, and consultant. Patient and therapist then work to discuss the clearly delineated goals of DBT. Identified sequentially, in order of their importance, specific targets for behavioral change include:

1. a reduction in suicidal and self-injurious behaviors
2. a reduction in therapy-interfering behaviors (e.g., missing sessions, excessive between session contact)
3. a reduction in quality of life problems (e.g., homelessness, unemployment, substance use)
4. an increase in successful coping
5. a reduction in PTSD symptoms (e.g., dissociation, panic attacks)
6. an enhancement of self-respect
7. any other goals as determined by the client

It also is important to note that treatment goals in DBT are based entirely upon changes in overt behavior in comparison to changes in underlying affect, mood, and cognition.

Goals for each individual therapy session are based upon the client's behaviors exhibited during the prior week; weekly diary cards provide important information about parasuicidal behavior and thoughts, the daily use of prescribed and elicit substances, and the use of adaptive behavioral techniques. If a patient fails to complete her weekly diary card, this would be viewed as therapy-interferring behavior. If this patient reported an absence of parasuicidal behavior during the past week, this therapy interfering behavior would take precedence in the session, and be addressed immediately.

As with any other approach to therapy, suicidal behavior of course takes precedence in any therapy session. DBT differs from other, traditional approaches in its approach to suicidal behavior. Self-injurious behavior is viewed as a maladaptive attempt at problem solving and communication, often in response to emotional dysregulation. In other words, suicidal gestures are not viewed as manipulative or attention seeking. Therapists who have attempted suicide are visited in the ER in order to help provide them with alternative cognitions and behaviors, as well as to examine their individual reinforcement contingencies. In other words, therapists may make patients review again and again, in specific detail, everything that led up to their suicide attempt and all of their actions during the attempt in order to generate insight into maladaptive behavioral responses and to provide negative reinforcement for future behavioral analyses. Therapists also may use the therapeutic relationship as reinforcer itself, with the use of statements such as, "Well, I'm not helping you, so I have to see you less, unless you can prove to me that this therapy is working!"

Overall techniques in therapy revolve around the primary dialectic of validation (i.e., acceptance) versus problem solving (i.e., change). Some of these related techniques include "extending," based upon principles of Japanese Aikido (e.g., meet force with resistance) and social psychology (i.e., paradoxical persuasion; Swann, Pelham, & Chidester 1988). In "extending," therapists do not engage patients who make extreme statements or threats (e.g., Oh! I'm so mad at you that I am going to quit [therapy] right now!) in any serious debate. Rather than usurping a patient's superego or decision making process, therapists literally "step aside" and let patients consider the consequences of their own actions without evoking feelings of shame or blame. For example, in response to a patient who threatens to terminate treatment in response to unprocessed anger, a therapist may reply, without any hint of anger or insult, "Wow. I guess you are really serious about this. Let me get you a referral."

According to many therapists who practice DBT, patients often are able to summon their own resources to realistically approach their problem, rather than engage in an emotionally driven, escalating decision. Similarly, DBT endorses the use of "irreverent communication," similar to that employed in Ellis's Rational Emotive Therapy (e.g., "Oh, so if you go ahead and kill yourself, how are you going to continue to honor your commitment to remain in therapy?" Other dialectical approaches include playing devil's advocate, focusing on current events, decisions, sensations, and perceptions rather than past or future perceptions, praise (i.e., positive reinforcement), operant shaping of desired responses, and "reciprocal communication," which involves a significant amount of therapist self-disclosure (e.g., "When you [my patient] call me five times a day, I feel like I don't want to work with you. So, what are we going to do about it.)

The second primary component, which deviates significantly from most traditional approaches, is that of a small group skills training class for two and a half hours each week. The course itself is highly structured and workbook driven. The four primary "modules" identified as

- Mindfulness (i.e., a focusing of attention and labeling of current experiences and feelings)

- Distress Tolerance (i.e., striving for "radical acceptance" of current events, in which a patient does not give up or give into anything or anyone, but works to engage in coping in the moment, without discrimination or judging of oneself)
- Emotion Regulation (i.e., using behavioral techniques such as guided imagery and deep breathing to prevent both negative and positive emotions from escalating)
- Interpersonal Effectiveness (i.e., assertiveness training that includes role playing and communication strategies)

The use of a group setting also can provide patients with a sense of hope, and prevent feelings of social isolation.

The third component of DBT, which deviates significantly from most traditional approaches to treatment, is that of encouraging patient-therapist contact between individual sessions during regularly scheduled and unscheduled phone calls. DBT encourages this outside contact to the extent that therapists are encouraged to provide their patients with phone numbers when they are traveling, and to send them postcards even during brief vacations. Although this interaction outside of the context of a typically recommended, highly structured therapeutic environment appears paradoxical, DBT views distortions in the frame and an absence of therapeutic neutrality as excellent opportunities for clients to generalize their skills, and to adapt to "the real world" (Linehan & Kehrer, 1993).

The fourth, and final component of DBT is group supervision for all individual therapists and group leaders. These sessions are held for one and a half hours per week. Attendance in this group is required, even for experienced therapists; no exceptions are made under any circumstances. Supervision is designed to:

- help monitor therapists' actions
- buoy therapist morale
- process countertransference
- engage in problem solving
- reduce splitting among team members.

Even though licensed practitioners can freely take training sessions in the use of DBT, individual practitioners cannot effectively engage in DBT unless they are working within the context of a larger therapeutic system.

Although DBT originated via the context of discovery, Linehan and her colleagues employed the context of justification (Spence, 1956) in order to assess the outcomes of their therapeutic work. Randomized clinical trials of more than fifty patients assigned to DBT or treatment-as-usual revealed that patients who received DBT exhibited less suicidal behavior, had fewer inpatient treatment days, (Linehan, Tutek, Heard, & Armstrong, 1994a) reported less displays of anger, and reported better social adjustment after one year of treatment (Linehan, Tutek, Heard, & Armstrong, 1994b? check on "a and b" stuff—see previous ref). DBT also appeared to provide decreases in suicidality among adolescents, an increasingly challenging patient population (Miller, 1999). However, most patients who received DBT reported similar levels of depression, feelings of hopelessness, and suicidal ideation, with no increase in reasons for living (Linehan, Armstrong, Suarez, & Allmon, 1991). Thus, DBT appears to accomplish what it sets out to do, and decreases the frequency parasuicidal behaviors among clients. However, it appears that their emotional suffering lingers, despite their best interpersonal efforts (and successes). At least among individuals suffering from borderline pathology, it appears that improvement in behavior alone via DBT is not sufficient to promote insight or emotional change. Despite these limitations in DBT outcomes, patients who remain healthy and alive at least have the opportunity for future, internal change. It also remains unclear to what extent Linehan's charismatic personality, rather than these specific behavioral interventions, enacts change in her clients. Regardless, Wolf (1988) suggests that charismatic therapists may heal patients by introducing idealized, easily internalized, self-object experiences.

DISSOCIATIVE IDENTITY DISORDER

The term multiple personality disorder (MPD) became a mainstay in popular culture during 1970–1980. Best selling books and feature films like *The Three Faces of Eve* and *Sybil* presented dramatically the lives of heinously abused young women who later developed a number of individual personalities or "alters" to help them cope with their abuse. Most media portrayals of MPD, especially during the late 1970's, featured peculiar situations in which some alter ego states (i.e., alters) engaged in behavior that remained virtually unknown to others, fostering an increasing sense of chaos in the featured women's lives. At that time, MPD also was considered extremely rare in the scientific community, and therapists who chose to work with patients with dissociative disorders, or who professed some belief in the existence of dissociative disorders were regarded as weirdoes or quacks.

It was not until the mid 1980's that empirically based, systematic inquires were conducted into the validity, etiology, and epidemiology regarding dissociative disorders such as MPD. Systematic investigation into the characteristic features of dissociative disorders, including dissociative amnesia and dissociative fugue led one expert, Kluft, to conclude that MPD currently represents a "hidden," but not rare, disorder (1995). Kluft noted that MPD did not appear to be a modern manifestation; examinations of various case studies by Freud and Charcot suggest that these analysts probably engaged in therapy with patients suffering from dissociative disorders (Herman, 1997). (Historical accounts of demonic and spiritual possession among peoples throughout the world also may represent dissociative episodes.) In 1994, the DSM-IV sanctioned a change in diagnostic nomenclature. Specifically, the term MPD was replaced by the more explanatory and inclusive diagnostic label, Dissociative Identity Disorder or DID.

Proposed Etiology

Kluft was one of the first analysts to articulate the belief that multiple or independent personality states develop as a maladaptive extension of a previously adaptive psychological response, dissociation (1995). As humans, we all engage in dissociation to one degree or another. Dissociation is often helpful and adaptive in our everyday lives. It can help us to ignore competing external stimuli (e.g., being able to study for an exam in the middle of a crowded room) and to better tolerate mildly unpleasant situations (e.g., being able to daydream vividly about weekend plans while stuck in traffic during Monday morning rush hour). Anytime someone has to be tapped on the shoulder to get their attention during an engaging movie or television program, or anytime someone drives by their designated highway exit because they were engrossed in thought (also referred to as highway hypnotism), that person is engaging in dissociation, albeit at a low level of intensity. Kluft reasoned that individuals with DID use dissociation in its most extreme forms (e.g., depersonalization; also see Chapter 3 for a review) as a defense against the pain, humiliation, and shame typically associated with severe abuse.

Assuming that the presence of alternative ego states is possible, at the time of the tragedy or abuse, a dissociative strategy appears to make sense. In many instances, children may not have any immediate options to remove themselves from an abusive situation. Children typically are vulnerable because of their size, unfamiliarity with healthy interpersonal relationships, and limited resources. An eight-year-old boy is not able to tell his parents, "OK, folks, I've had enough. I'm going to move out to the west coast and get me a good lawyer to prosecute you to the fullest extent of the law. By the way, I'm taking the car."

On a psychological level, the development of cognitive sophistication takes time and exposure to a variety of life events.

Children who suffer from abuse often fall victim to primitive thinking, as a result of their age-appropriate cognitive ability. For example, an abused child may reason, "Mommy is good. She feeds me most of the time, gives me toys and clothes, and a place to sleep. Moms are supposed to be good, so she must beat me because I am doing something wrong... Good mommies don't beat up their kids unless they do something really, really wrong. I must have done a lot of bad things. I don't understand everything that I did, but I must deserve it. Mommies and daddies always know better than kids. That's because they are the ones who take care of us. Maybe I can try harder to please her next time." This type of dichotomous thinking (i.e., all or none thinking; splitting) represents a primitive defense among adults. However, it often represents the only available, age appropriate defense for a child who has no other means to cognitively evaluate their situation, and recognize that some things that "mom" does are "good," but that some things she does are "bad," and even unacceptable. In other words, because children often cannot physically escape from their abusers physically, their only resort is to do so mentally.

Picca (1999) posits that during times of severe stress or abuse, children employ alternative ego states (i.e., imaginary friends, the presence of which is generally considered normal or even desirable in child development; Somers & Yawkey, 1984) to shoulder the abuse, allowing their primary identity or ego state to dissociate enough to avoid the experience of physical and emotional pain (Pica, 1999). Over time, this experience of abuse, or lack thereof, becomes fragmented so that each "alter" often serves a different function or purpose.

Regarding the etiology of DID, most researchers (e.g., Kluft, 1995; 1999; Putnam, 2000) suggest that four specific factors or conditions are typically present in the development of the disorder. These factors will be presented here briefly.

1. The individual has a high dissociative potential, including a high level of intelligence, creativity, capacity to enter a trance state, hypnotizability, and suggestibility (Putnam, 2000).
2. The individual has suffered severe trauma, typically in childhood (Putnam, 2000), including neglect, emotional abuse, physical abuse, and sexual abuse (e.g., Sar, Tutkun, Alyanak, Bakim, & Baral, 2000).
3. The individual presents with ongoing dissociative phenomena including fantasy-proneness (Putnam, 2000) or beliefs in some type of imaginary world.

4. The individual does not have access to corrective emotional experiences or relationships. The individual feels isolated and alone, and often literally is isolated and alone within the context of their physical environment.

Symptom Presentations and Diagnostic Features

Epidemiological information regarding the symptom presentation of individuals diagnosed with DID shows a relative degree of variation and uncertainty regarding its validity. However, a number of symptom patterns or clusters have emerged from studies of independent reports. A common theme is that most individuals who suffer from DID do not receive a formal diagnosis until they are in their third of fourth decade of life; it remains unclear whether this statistic will change according to practitioners' level of acceptance, and education of, DID as a true disorder. The following information represents some of the common symptoms, themes, and diagnostic features observed among individuals diagnosed with DID (see Putnam, 2000, for a review):

- a high level of education and high IQ, coupled with a sporadic or poor job history
- participation in a current, or prior, abusive romantic or familial relationship
- initial diagnosis of DID typically made when the patient is 30 or 40 years of age
- the patient often spends six to eight years in the mental health system before a diagnosis is made. Early diagnoses often include Cluster B personality disorders, bipolar disorder, schizophrenia, and factitious disorder
- suicidal ideation, intent, and plan. Estimates suggest that 75% of all patients with DID are actively suicidal. Twenty-five percent of patients with DID appear to display self-inflicted abuse such as cutting or burning.
- night terrors and hypnogogic (e.g., unpleasant sensations falling when entering sleep) and hypnopompic experienced (e.g., being alarmed and startled upon wakening for no apparent reason)
- panic attacks
- somatic pains, which may represent somatic memories of abuse. For example a patient may report severe pain in the throat, chest, or vagina in the absence of any identifiable medical cause.
- A high percentage of men diagnosed with DID are incarcerated, whereas a high proportion of women diagnosed with DID are in some type of mental health system or institution. These

differential features may be a result of socialization and gender roles and expectations.

- Feelings of unreality, including numbness and tingling
- One third of patients with DID appear to have some form of substance abuse, possibly in an attempt to self-medicate
- Evidence of a thought disorder, including word salad and pressured speech. Some therapists believe that the individual presents as psychotic when rapid switching occurs among alternative personalities or ego states.
- Auditory hallucinations, with their origin clearly identified within the individual (e.g., "I hear voices sometimes, but I know they are inside my head," versus "I hear a space alien talking.")
- Persistent or constantly occurring headaches
- Psychosomatic disorders including irritable bowel syndrome and asthma.

Dissociation as a Defense

As noted, dissociation can provide moments of reprieve during horrific experiences when no other means of coping is available. However, the long term use of dissociation as a defense can appear to result in the formation of alternative ego states, which continue to function independently from one another even after the abuse has stopped. (These ego states may allow a survivor of abuse to "forget" that it ever happened, and avoid dealing with the intense abreactions often association with any form of traumatic event, as well as the implications for current and prior relationships.) A number of features appear to be association with the presentation of these alters. Until recently, due to more accurate portrayals in the media, forensic psychologists often used this information to help determine whether a defendant was malingering or "creating" their own alters. Some general information about alternative ego states includes:

- Most individuals with DID appear to have both male and female alters. Some experts posit that patients' opposite sex alters often possess disavowed aspects of the self (e.g., being too aggressive or too weak) or internalized characteristics of an abuser.
- Alternative ego states can be perceived along a continuum from "a vague sense of someone else being here" to individuals with distinct names, histories, personalities, needs, wants, fears, and desires.
- Individuals' alters have been shown to range widely in age, from infancy through adulthood.

- A wide range in reported number of alters.
- Alters may engage in supportive or self-destructive behavior.
- The patient (i.e., primary personality) may or may not be aware of some or all of her alternative ego states.

In addition, many patients may not recognize that they are actively dissociating, whether or not they appear to have separate, independently functioning ego states. For example, one patient commented, "Well, I always thought that kind of stuff [an absence of memory for both important and every day events] just happened to everyone. You know, like when someone says, 'Oh, I don't remember a thing about my wedding,' so you think that it's not such a big deal then that you can't remember your wedding, or your high school graduation, or the first time you had sex, where you had lunch yesterday, or whatever." In the majority of cases, any perception of time loss (e.g., I have no idea what I did yesterday) indicates the need for additional investigation.

Other potential signals for dissociative episodes include finding unusual personal possessions, and not knowing where they came from. For example, one patient noted, "I knew something weird was going on when I kept pulling Marlboros out of my coat pocket...I only smoke Slims, and I don't remember who would have given me those things." Other patients describe being greeted by people who they do not know, or being called repeatedly by the wrong name by someone who claims to know them. Still other patients indicate that they were often blamed for things as a child when they had no recollection of doing something wrong. Many describe being frustrated by bad grades in school, even though they feel they are reasonably intelligent. (Most individuals diagnosed with DID do appear to have above average intelligence as measured by IQ.)

Assessment

Before bestowing the relatively uncommon diagnosis of DID, which carries significant social, clinical, legal, ethical, and insurance implications, clinicians are advised to perform extensive assessment protocols and work closely with other medical and mental health providers. In other words, *significant care* must be taken to avoid the unwarranted diagnosis of such acute disorders (i.e., DID, as well as BPD and PTSD), which seem to have become quite popular and even faddish in recent years. Practitioners must first rule out organic brain injury (e.g., Cantagallo, Grassi, & Della Sala, 1999), poisoning with toxic chemicals, rare metabolic disorders (Putnam, 2000), epilepsy, and other seizure disorders (Bowman & Coons, 2000). The use of video-EEG monitoring can be beneficial in ruling out numerous underlying medical problems (Bowman & Coons, 2000).

Thus, before making a diagnosis of DID, practitioners are advised to use the following assessment instruments (Steinberg et al., 1991):

- clinical interviews
- behavioral observation
- personality testing (both projective and objective measures)
- intelligence testing
- neuropsychological testing
- the DES
- the SCID

With any clinical interview, it remains vital to acknowledge the critical impact of culture (including culturally acceptable role enactments; Lilienfeld, Kirsch, Sarbin, Lynn, Chaves, Ganaway, & Powell, 1999), ethnicity, SES, and religiosity, as well as a history of childhood abuse, upon the possible assessment of DID. In a handful of cases, interviews with other friends and family members may provide collaborating evidence of abuse or dissociative symptoms, as well a better sense of the patient's interpersonal relationships. The critical danger, however, is that an interviewee may be someone who subjected the patient to abuse, or who continues to subject the patient to abuse. Many assailants are unlikely to admit their role in any abusive activity, and confrontations can result in significant, negative abreactions among patients. Another realistic concern is that an interviewee may be someone significant in the patient's life who "covered up," minimized, or denied the presence of abusive behaviors in the past, and potentially in the present. Thus, such interviews of family members and friends should be conducted with extreme care, and only under very specific circumstances. The use of these interviews must take place only with full patient permission and support.

Although limited empirical evidence is reported in the literature, a number of behavioral indicators may help clinicians identify individuals with DID. For example, Silberg (1998) trained blind raters to evaluate the testing protocols of 60 patients, of whom 30 received a psychiatric diagnosis of DID or Dissociative Disorder NOS, for the presence or absence of specific responses to testing. The blind raters were able to identify 93% of the individuals with a dissociative disorder, based upon the presence of memory impairment, staring, dramatic fluctuations in mood and behavior, fearful and angry responses to testing materials, and somatic complaints during testing. Patients with a dissociative disorder, compared to those without such a diagnosis, also were more likely to provide testing responses consistent with dissociation, including depersonalized imagery, dichotomous thinking (i.e., splitting), images of mutilation and torture, magical transformation, malevolent religiosity, and emotional confusion (Silber, 1998).

The Dissociative Experiences Scale (DES; Carlson & Putnam, 1993) is a brief self-report measure designed to assess the presence of dissociative phenomenon, ranging on a continuum from minor, adaptive processes and defenses (i.e., highway hypnotism; pleasant day-dreaming) to severe, pathological processes and defenses (i.e., persistent depersonalization or derealization.) Please see Table 1 for sample items.

Patients also are instructed to exclude experiences encountered while under the influence of drugs or alcohol. Regarding its use as a diagnostic instrument, researchers have shown that psychiatric patients' scores on the DES could be used to differentiate between those patients who had been diagnosed with dissociative disorders versus those who had not (Steinberg, Rounsaville, & Cicchetti, 1991). Please see this chapter's Appendix for excerpts of a testing report for a patient later diagnosed with DID.

Continued Controversy

The diagnosis of DID remains highly controversial. Investigations of most mental health practitioners' attitudes toward DID, including those of board certified psychiatrists (e.g., Pope, Oliva, Hudson, Bodkin, Alexander, & Gruber, 1999), suggest that little professional

TABLE 1. Sample Items from the Dissociative Experiences Scale

1. Some people have the experience of driving a car and suddenly realizing that they don't remember what has happened during all or part of the trip. Mark the line to show what percentage of the time this happens to you.
5. Some people have the experience of finding new things among their belongings that they do not remember buying. Mark the line...
6. Some people sometimes find that they are approached by people that they do not know who call them by another name or insist that they have met them before.
9. Some people find that they have no memory for some important events in their lives (for example, a wedding or graduation).
15. Some people have the experience of not being sure whether things that they remember happening really did happen or whether they just dreamed them.
19. Some people find that they sometimes are able to ignore pain.

Note. From Carlson and Putnam (1993) and reprinted with permission. Individuals are asked to respond to each item by drawing a vertical slash on a provided, 100 mm horizontal line to indicate what percent of the time (0–100%) they have that specific experience in their daily life. Higher mean scores indicate the presence of more dissociative experiences. The DES has a total of 28 items.

consensus exists regarding the diagnosis of DID and other dissociative disorders (e.g., dissociative amnesia). For example, less than one half of surveyed psychiatrists believed that DID and dissociative amnesia should be included in the DSM-IV without reservation, and only one quarter believed that enough empirical evidence exists to support the diagnosis. Other experts suggest that some of the most widely publicized cases of DID, including that of Sybil, represent the "fraudulent construction" of false memories and alters that arose from therapists' leading questions (Rieber, 1999). Differential rates of diagnosis of DID in other cultures and countries (e.g., Britian, Ireland, the United States, Germany, Turkey) also raise questions about the validity of the disorder (Lilienfeld, Kirsch, Sarbin, Lynn, Chaves, Ganaway, & Powell, 1999). Questions also have been raised regarding a negative bias in the literature toward DID (Van Velduizen, 2000), when researchers (e.g., two of the authors from Pope et al., 1999) experience a conflict of interest by receiving payment for expert testimony in opposition to the diagnosis.

In contrast, an extensive survey of psychologists, regarding the presence corroborative evidence about their patients' dissociative symptoms (via family reports and medical record), revealed that nearly three out of four patients diagnosed with DID had evidence of dissociative symptoms before their diagnosis, and more than two out of three patients had evidence of dissociative symptoms before their entry in psychotherapy (Gleaves, Hernandez, & Warner, 1999). Although some interesting anecdotal evidence suggests that individuals with DID show differential physiological responses when in different alters' states (Putnam, 1984), recent functional MRI findings provide more objective, corroborative evidence for the validity of DID in certain individual cases, and further support the hypothesis that severe trauma may foster the disorder. Tsai, Condie, Wu, and Chang (1999) reported in the Harvard Medical Review that the apparent switch of alter ego states for a patient under fMRI was associated with differential metabolic activity in the hippocampus and portions of the temporal lobe, consistent with overall changes in brain function typically observed among patients with PTSD. Clinicians also should note that it is not uncommon to see any combination of DID, factitious disorder, and underlying medical problems among any one patient (Kluft, 1995); a diagnosis of DID does not preclude the presence of other disorders.

Treatment

Assuming that DID does exist as a true clinical phenomenon, one promising aspect of this tragic disorder is that individuals with DID are believed to have a good prognosis if they receive appropriate treatment. Patients with DID or other dissociative disorders are not psychotic (or "crazy" in the words of one patient), and their typically high level of intelligence can often aid them in treatment success. A number of approaches to treatment have been offered, and some appear more controversial than others. For example, one of the most potentially dangerous and destructive approaches to treatment for patients with DID is that of sedation and injection with sodium pentathol or other "truth agent" in order to retrieve previous memories of abuse. Such invasive procedures, which strip patients of any sense of control and often appear to repeat various aspects of their victimization, are rarely discussed in the literature, but have been shown on televised documentaries as an appropriate mode of treatment. The use of hypnosis and group therapy in treatment of DID remains controversial (Kluft, 1999); unfortunately, little empirical evidence is available to evaluate its effectiveness. Other specialized treatment modalities, including EMDR (Young, 1994) and art therapy (Kluft, 1999) have been employed with some degree of reported, empirically validated success.

Currently, a number of experts identify psychodynamic psychotherapy as the optimal approach to treatment (e.g., Kluft, 1999). The goal of psychodynamic treatment is to help patients suffering from dissociative disorders to metabolize their both their early and current life experiences, and become better equipped to feel and function like an effective adult, primarily because internal and external information now appear consistent with one another. It is important to note that a primary goal of therapy is not to recover previous memories of abuse or to engage in intense, overwhelming abreaction. Early work involves the discussion of informed consent, pragmatic issues (e.g., when to meet; how to reach a therapist outside of regularly scheduled sessions), informed consent, interaction with alters (e.g., who will be addressed; when will control be passed from one alter to another; secrets among alters) and the use of techniques such as deep breathing exercises and EMDR. In the initial stages of treatment, supportive psychotherapy is essential. Patients are helped to muster various internal and external resources, practice more adaptive coping skills, and engage in basic problem solving. (This process is similar to that employed with individuals in a current state of crisis; Kluft, 1999).

Later stages in psychodynamic treatment involve exploring the function of various ego states (some therapists help patients construct a genogram-type mapping of their alters), acknowledging the impact of previous trauma upon their lives, and ultimately causing a cease to amnestic barriers. It also is interesting to note that while many experts

strive for the integration of all ego states (Fine, 1999) into one comprehensive whole (i.e., the individual!), others note that this is not always
possible. Some therapists report that treatment success also can be
achieved if a patient maintains some alternative ego states, but that one
alter remains in control, and is always aware of the others. In this
instance, dissociation still remains available as a defense against horrific memories of abuse or current as well as stressful, current life
event. This treatment outcome has been referred to as unification.

Final Cautions and Recommendations

Some potential pitfalls in such psychodynamic treatment include
intense countertransference, increased risk of patient suicide, and potential legal problems. Regarding countertransference, processing and bearing witness to profound stories of patient abuse can be extremely
challenging for even the most experienced therapists. Some recommendations for practitioners managing such intense countertransference
include peer supervision or consultation, and scrupulous self-care.
Therapists also are cautioned against becoming enamored with the diagnosis, and the interesting differences often reported or observed among
various ego states. Also critically, therapists must remain alert to possible symptoms of PTSD themselves, as a function of vicarious traumatization, in order to seek professional help immediately.

Estimates rates of patient suicide and self-harm are quite high
among individuals diagnosed with DID. To help manage patient suicidality, therapists are encouraged to be direct and straightforward in
treatment. Some experts recommend working with patients in therapy
three times a week in order to assess patient suicidality more often, and
provide increased patient support. Working with patients to identify
and discuss firm patient-therapist boundaries, which is a necessity in
treatment of DID as well as a general standard for practice, also can foster beneficial, increased patient perceptions of order, predictability,
and security. Therapists also are encouraged to spend a significant
amount of time during the end of each session to alert patients that the
session will be ending, and assist them in identifying and decreasing
the intensity of any emotional abreactions. The use of metaphors can
be helpful in this regard, including the closing or storing of distressing
memories or overwhelming affect in a mental "box."

A number of legal issues also are central to any discussion of DID.
This surge in legal concerns is associated primarily with costly
increases in lawsuits regarding the treatment of patients with DID.
When working with this patient population, the consideration of

various risk management strategies (e.g., meticulous documentation; securing legal counsel; Scheflin, 2000) becomes essential. Many legal problems also arise in response to current controversies regarding the validity of recovered patient memories (i.e., are they false memories). For example, some patients who elect to press charges against their abuser often learn that hypnotic inductions, EMDR, and even partici-pation in psychotherapy itself, may render their testimony about the abuse inadmissible or questionable. Thus, one highly advocated approach is to ask patients to sign some kind of consent form in which they acknowledge that participation in therapy may negatively affect the credibility of their testimony, and that therapists may be forced to reveal all treatment information, rather than selective information, in certain court proceedings. Other general recommendations include focusing upon a patient's experience of the traumatic event, rather than upon the factual accuracy of that event. However, as an important, additional consideration, other researchers suggest that rigid mainte-nance of therapeutic neutrality may actually impair patients' reality testing, and prevent them from the correction of cognitive disortions and the completion of an integrated, personal narrative (van der Hart & Nijenhuis, 1999).

APPENDIX

Clinical Illustration of Assessment Issues in the Differential Diagnosis of DID: Excerpts from a Psychological Evaluation.

Date of Report: 07/94

Reason for Referral

Ms. B was referred for testing to clarify her diagnosis and assess her suicidality. She previously has been diagnosed with major depres-sive disorder, dysthymic disorder, fictitious disorder, dissociative identity disorder, bipolar disorder, adjustment disorder, and substance abuse. She also has received numerous character diagnoses including borderline, narcissistic, and mixed personality disorders.

History of Present Illness

Ms. B graduated from high school, and attended one year of community college to take courses in nursing. She was employed as a nursing assistant in a local nursing home before her first inpatient hospitalization in November of 1992. She has not worked in that capacity, or in any other, since that time. Ms. B currently is divorced, and lives in her home with her son ... She reports that on most days she "stares at the walls," has severe headaches, and eats little more than coffee and cake.

Ms. B has a lengthy and complicated case history, which may be summarized here only briefly. Ms. B began outpatient treatment at X Hospital on 7/29/92 ... At the psychiatric outpatient clinic, Ms. B presented with feelings of depression and anxiety, weight loss, insomnia, poor concentration, and suicidal ideation. She described that emotional outbursts and poor concentration were interfering with her performance at work ... On 11/8/92, Ms. B was admitted to a hospital medical unit to treat a severely infected bite wound inflicted by one of her patients. According to the medical staff, Ms. B showed impaired judgment and had not tended to this wound herself. Although Ms. B denied substance use, marijuana was detected in her blood upon admission. While in the hospital, Ms. B exacerbated her condition by forcing lipstick into her wound and using a cigarette lighter to inflate thermometer readings. When confronted, she denied these behaviors. While hospitalized, Ms. B also had two episodes of "non-responsiveness" which were evaluated medically as psychogenic.

On 1/5/93, because Ms. B's arm had become infected again and she expressed significant suicidal intent, she was involuntarily admitted to the inpatient psychiatric unit. Upon this admission, Ms. B displayed a 20 pound weight loss, poor ADL's, and reported that her "mind hurt all over." Her impulse control and judgment were limited, and she showed an impaired ability to understand the meaning of simple proverbs. On 1/22/93 she was sent to the E.R. for seizures and unresponsiveness. These episodes also were deemed psychogenic in nature. She was prescribed numerous medications including Trazodone, Zoloft, Klonopin, and Thorazine ... Upon her release from the unit, Ms. B damaged hospital property and was escorted back to the clinic where she was readmitted to the inpatient unit for marked suicidal ideation. After this discharge, Ms. B continued with individual psychotherapy in the outpatient clinic ... she revealed that at ages six through seven, she was raped and abused repeatedly by a family friend.

Test Behavior

Ms. B is a 44 year old ... Caucasian female. She is above average in height and significantly below average in weight. (She has lost more than 20 pounds since her initial hospitalization ... She wore no make-up, and her hair appeared stringy and only lightly brushed. During the first testing session, dirt was clearly visible under her fingernails ... Ms. B accosted her examiner angrily and described how furious she was that she had to attend the session, and how she found it nearly impossible to locate the examining room. After this outburst, Ms. B engaged the examiner in little, if any, spontaneous conversation. Throughout the remainder of the sessions Ms. B's mood remained fairly consistent; she typically sat slumped against the back of her chair, and either gazed downward or appeared to look off into space with a distant expression. Sometimes she would hold her head very still, and her eyelids would flicker strangely back and forth. At this time she would not respond immediately to questions or prompts from the examiner.... Ms. B occasionally spoke in a soft, low voice that was difficult for the examiner to understand ... Ms. B typically took a very long time to respond to questions from the examiner, and to complete most test items. Additionally, after she appeared to recognize repeated failures on a series of structured tasks, Ms. B sat quietly while a tear ran down her cheek. It thus was unclear whether Ms. B was being oppositional, or was genuinely unable to engage in tasks in a timely, meaningful way.

Test Results

Cognitive Functioning.   As measured on the WAIS-R intelligence test, a Full-Scale IQ of 65, a Verbal IQ of 70, and a Performance IQ of 68 suggest that Ms. B may be functioning in the mentally retarded range of overall, verbal, and performance intellectual functioning .... However, it is crucial to note that when asked to perform other structured and non-structured tasks, Ms. B displayed at least average abilities to comprehend and to use language, to identify objects and the relationships between them, and to attend to and follow moderately complicated directions ... What is most notable about Ms. B's cognitive abilities is their extreme fluctuation. It remains unclear whether this variability in performance may be due to oppositionality, organicity, dissociation, or some combination of these three.

Personality Functioning.   The poor interpersonal relationships that Ms. B does have may be heavily distorted, and grounded more in fantasy than in reality. Her views of others are distorted by her typically negative views of herself, and her underlying feelings of anger and frustration. Individuals are seen as either victims or victimizers, as good or evil; little thought is given to others as unique individuals.

Women are viewed as either defenseless, hapless victims of male abuse, or as naive, confused creatures craving male attention. Even when women try to confront a situation, their attempts are not taken seriously by those around them, and result in no lasting changes. Men are seen alternatively as hardworking simpletons, or as unnamed, repeat abusers. Relationships between men and women are epitomized by miscommunication, abuse, separation, secrecy, and betrayal. There is no perception of a functional family unit; mothers are portrayed as ineffective, unwilling protectors, and fathers are nowhere to be seen.

Differential Diagnosis

Because Ms. B's case is so complex, further, extensive evaluation will be necessary to determine Ms. B's diagnosis or diagnoses. The following differentials should be considered; it is unclear to what extent her psychotic features are driven by major depression, schizoaffective disorder, organic impairments, dissociation, or any combination of these. It also is recommended that Ms. B receive further medical attention to rule out the possibility of underlying organic problems, including those that may have resulted from substance abuse, seizures, and/or poor nutrition ... From her test performance and behavior, it is unclear to what extent Ms. B is actively dissociating (e.g., brief episodes of derealization versus distinct ego organizations) ... However, it is clear that Ms. B is in a severe major depressive episode. Consonant with this diagnosis and her articulated hopelessness and despair, the test data suggest that Ms. B is actively suicidal. Thus, despite the aforementioned difficulties in arriving at a specific, clear-cut diagnosis for Ms. B, it is clear that her suicidality should be a focal point in current treatment planning.

Recommendations

... Regardless of her ability to arouse powerful feelings in others, Ms. B's health care providers must guard against being lulled into complacency, or being led into denial about her problem; her suicide potential is great ... Despite these barriers to treatment, Ms. B's ability to tolerate significant amounts of situational stress, and her potential to be involved in personal relationships will be assets in therapy. Because many of Ms. B's conflicts revolve around issues of unrecognized personal boundaries and space, it also appears vital to provide her with a "safe" therapeutic environment, with clearly delineated and enforced limits, structure, and boundaries. Because some of her impairments in reality testing appear to result from raw, intensely overwhelming negative affects, her therapist also could provide Ms. B with auxiliary reality testing, while helping her to identify and process her own underlying, negative affects. This affective labeling function should be especially helpful in allowing Ms. B to identify the functions that her primitive defenses provide.

Diagnosis

Axis I:	296.33 Major Depressive Disorder
	296.43 R/O Major Depressive Disorder with Psychotic Features
	195.70 R/O Schizoaffective Disorder
	300.15 R/O Dissociative Disorder, NOS
	300.19 R/O Fictitious Disorder
Axis II:	301.83 R/O Borderline Personality Disorder
Axis III:	R/O Organic Impairment
	R/O Nutritional Deficiencies
Axis IV:	Severe: Living with physically abusive son; Unemployed
Axis V:	GAF = 25 (current)
	GAF = 45 (past year)

6

Patient Suicide
Clinical Assessment and Management

A seriously depressed patient stated that she had taken to driving past police cars at more than 90 miles an hour on the highway in hopes of being stopped and asked, "So, what seems to be the problem?" She did not think anyone would be willing to talk with her about suicide if she brought it up on her own.

A number of pervasive societal myths exist regarding important issues related to suicide. These persistent misunderstandings influence the portrayal of suicide in the media, the perceptions of individuals who seek treatment, and the beliefs of family members and friends of those who attempt and complete suicide. Increased awareness of the factual information regarding suicide allows therapists to better understand the world-view of our patients, to provide appropriate psychoeducation to those who need it, and to aid others in the development and evaluation of more effective suicide prevention programs (e.g., Richards & Range, 2001). Laypersons such as teachers also appear to benefit from suicide education (Davidson & Range, 1999). A number of clinical case studies and findings from various research programs will be used as the basis to explore these persistent myths, as well as to illustrate overall principles for suicide assessment and management.

THE PREVALENCE OF PSYCHOPATHOLOGY

Myth: People who commit suicide are basically "normal," everyday people who were pushed over the edge by some terrible event. A common misconception among the general public is that individuals who commit suicide typically do so in response to one specific, devastating loss (e.g., the sudden break-up of a romantic relationship; being fired from a job) or humiliation (e.g., accidentally learning that one's spouse is having an affair; being taunted or rejected by classmates at school). However, this notion that people who commit suicide were only temporarily over-whelmed, but are otherwise "just like you and me" (i.e., "normal;" generally well-adjusted) is *unequivocally false*. Virtually all rigorous, epidemiological studies from countries around the world including the United States, United Kingdom, Korea, China, Japan, Germany, France, and Australia suggest that at least 90 percent of people who commit suicide suffer from some form of often untreated mental illness.

In addition, certain types of mental illness are associated with increased suicide risk (see Jamison, 1999, for a review, 1999). In comparison to the expected risk of suicide for the average American, individuals who suffer from major depression are 20 times more likely to commit suicide. Individuals with bipolar disorder (i.e., manic depression) are at least 15 times more likely to commit suicide. Substance abuse carries a 6–14 time increased risk of suicide; although the underlying reasons remain unclear, individuals who abuse heroin and other opiates appear to exhibit greater risk than those who abuse alcohol or other drugs. For individuals with a dual diagnosis (i.e., the presence of an Axis I mental illness in conjunction with some form of substance abuse), their risk of suicide is nearly doubled from the suicide risk associated with substance abuse alone.

Other types of psychopathology are associated with increased suicide rates, but at somewhat lower risk than that observed for substance abuse and mood disorders. For example, schizophrenia is associated with a 10 times greater risk of for suicide than that expected among the general population. Both borderline and antisocial personality disorders (i.e., Cluster B disorders, characterized by impulsivity and high emotion; Zweig & Hillman, 1999) also carry a risk for suicide that is appropriately 5 times greater than the national average. The presence of an anxiety disorder (e.g., PTSD; generalized panic attacks; obsessive compulsive disorder) is linked to a three times greater risk of suicide than that observed among members of the general population (Jamison, 1999).

In contrast, individuals suffering from extremely serious, debilitating, and typically painful physical illness such as Huntington's chorea, multiple sclerosis, and cancer, appear to have a comparatively lower risk for suicide—only 3 to 4 times that of the expected population rate (Jamison, 1999). Certainly, this comparison of statistically determined risk is no way construed to suggest that individuals with physical illness suffer any less psychological distress than individuals with any of the other aforementioned mental illnesses, or that they should be evaluated any less judiciously for suicidal risk. For example, many experts encourage the education of primary health care providers in suicide risk to help prevent intended deaths among medically ill patients (Kleespies, 2001). However, such epidemiological findings do make one thing clear: when compared to some of mankind's most debilitating and devastating physical illnesses, certain types of mental illness (i.e., mood disorders, substance abuse, and schizophrenia) appear to place individuals at more than 20 times the expected risk for suicide among the general population.

EVIDENCE BASED PREDICTORS

Various epidemiological studies, psychological autopsies, and prospective studies (e.g., Brown, Beck, Steer, & Grisham, 2000) have identified a number of patient characteristics as empirically based predictors of both attempted and completed suicide. Fortunately, many of these related factors, including increased feelings of hopelessness, clinical depression, and unemployment, can be addressed in treatment (Brown et al., 2000). Although invaluable, however, the correlational, quasi-experimental, and retrospective designs of the studies that provide information about these predictors cannot provide specific information about the extent to which those predictors actually *cause* suicidal behavior.

We can only consider the relationship or association between those predictors and suicide risk. (Obvious ethical constraints do not allow for randomized protocols in which participants are assigned randomly to conditions in which they are asked to shoot heroin, keep a loaded gun in their home, or experience a psychotic episode.) Thus, due to the limitations inherent in our available research methodology, *it remains impossible to predict with 100% accuracy* which patients will or will not commit suicide.

Demographic Characteristics

A number of demographic characteristics, including age, gender, marital status, employment status, and ethnicity, are associated with suicide risk. As noted previously, however, care must be taken to acknowledge that these predictors represent statistical values, and not real people. Any patient can present a significant suicide risk even if they are not part of a statistically identified, high-risk group.

Myth: Of all age groups, teenagers are most likely to commit suicide. Epidemiological studies reveal consistently that adults over the age of 65 are more likely to use highly lethal methods of suicide such as firearms and falls from high buildings, and are thus more likely to complete a suicide attempt (i.e., die from it) when compared to individuals in any other age group (Richman, 1999). The presence of a chronic medical illness also is linked to increased suicide risk in old age (Jamison, 1999). On average, teenagers are more likely to attempt less lethal means of suicide, such as taking pills or cutting themselves. Overall, findings from epidemiological studies suggest that White, elderly, medically ill, males who live alone are at greatest statistical risk.

Myth: Many adolescents say that they are going to kill themselves as a way to get attention. Although studies do suggest that teenagers are more likely to be rescued or resuscitated after a suicide attempt than older adults, any statements about suicidal intent by any individual must be taken seriously. Many parents and laypersons do not realize that many suicide-related deaths among teenagers are related to untreated mental illness or to the impact of drug or alcohol abuse. The numbers of multiple psychiatric diagnoses among suicidal teenagers also is increasing, and requires very careful attention and monitoring (Miller, 1999).

A young person who plans on attempting suicide via a relatively non-lethal method (i.e., slashing one's wrist; taking a few pills) with plans of being "rescued" could easily underestimate the dangerousness of their attempt, or act impulsively after drinking or taking recreational drugs. This could mean cutting one's wrist deeper, taking more pills than originally intended, or not recalling correctly when a friend or family member is returning home. Other adolescents (or individuals from any age group, for that matter) may plan on taking a certain number of pills that will only "put them in the hospital," but underestimate the toxic nature of those drugs and end up seriously injured or killed. Any mention of suicide in any context, particularly by a child or adolescent, must be taken seriously. Parents, teachers, and coaches could all benefit from acquiring this knowledge. (Please see Chapter 11 for additional information about developmental issues in relation to crisis and trauma.)

Because we cannot predict suicidality with 100% certainty, however, therapists are ethically bound to take any patient's suicidal intent seriously. Thus, if a young, educated, financially secure married woman mentions thoughts of suicide, her status should be assessed just as assiduously as a widowed elderly man with major depression in a statistically identified "high risk group." Although knowledge of these predictors of suicidal risk is responsible and helpful, it cannot nor should not replace clinical interviewing, assessment, judgment, and skill.

Mental Status Indicators

Careful assessment of a patient's mental status also can provide invaluable clues regarding their suicidal risk (e.g., Brown et al., 2000; Yufit, 1991). Many of these characteristics are related to the presence of specific forms of psychopathology (e.g., major depression, substance abuse, anxiety disorders), but others appear to be more situation specific. Some of these vital characteristics for assessment include, but are not limited to:

- Feelings of unrelenting hopelessness (e.g., I can't take one more day of this. I just can't do it. Things are never going to change, no matter what I do.)
- Intense feelings of guilt (e.g., I can feel guilty about something I said to someone ten years ago. I mean … that's just nuts, but I really do.)
- Anhedonia (e.g., lack of pleasure; I knew I was in bad shape when I didn't even want to see my grandchildren.)
- Suicidal ideation (e.g., "Yeah, I sure wish I could be dead.")
- Feelings of worthlessness (e.g., I'm just taking up space here. Who am I kidding?)
- An increase in violent dreams
- Idyllic thoughts of death as a release (e.g., I'll be up in heaven with my wings just looking down at everyone; No one will be able to hurt me anymore.)
- Excessive anger or irritability
- Loss of libido (e.g., My husband is beginning to get pretty upset with me, but I just can't bear it. I can't even stand him touching me anymore; [sex] just feels like such an annoying, tedious thing.)
- Attempts to give away previously prized possessions
- Enrollment in or renewal of insurance policies
- A sudden decrease or increase in energy (e.g., I had a ball the day I decided to kill myself. I made dinner for my kids and cleaned the house. It's like a weight was lifted from my shoulders … I knew I would be free from this shit at the end of the day.)

- Impulsive or reckless behavior such as engaging in illegal activities like high-stakes gambling, drug and alcohol binges, needle sharing, and unprotected sex. It is also important to include speeding and reckless driving as potentially dangerous behaviors.

The Presence of Firearms

Regardless of patient age, occupation, or mental status, the presence of firearms is associated with significant suicide risk. Most individuals who attempt to kill themselves with a gun often succeed, and those who fail often survive in a vegetative state or with horrific facial deformities and cognitive impairment. There is limited time for "changing one's mind" or for getting help.

Various questions also arise regarding differential suicide rates among professionals who train with and use firearms. Some studies suggest that police officers and security guards have a significantly higher rate of suicide than member of other professions. Yet, other studies suggest that high rates of job stress or alcoholism are associated with increased levels of suicide among emergency support personnel, not the simple presence of firearms. Still other studies suggest that police officers are no more likely to commit suicide than members of any other profession. Due to the methodological flaws and small sample sizes associated with many studies (Hem, Berg, & Ekeberg, 2001), the question essentially remains unanswered. What is clear, however, is that many emergency service providers are not given ample opportunity or access to a mental health professional. Any police officer who speaks to a police psychologist risks having all information disclosed during any session become a permanent part of their service record.

Although the connection between the practice of psychology and participation in public policy remains tenuous and controversial at best, some experts in the field, such as Jamison (1999), implore other mental health professionals to take a firm political stance, call for rigorous gun control laws, and eliminate sales of high caliber, automatic weapons. At least psychologists could explain clearly to their patients the clear link between the presence of firearms and the risk of suicide. Clinicians also can direct their patients to have someone they know and trust remove their own guns for a period of safekeeping during any suicidal (or homicidal) crisis.

Previous Suicide Attempts

The number one predictor of future suicide is the presence of previous suicide attempts (Brown et al., 2000). This finding, supported by numerous empirical studies of psychological autopsies, is consistent with the general social psychological principle that the best predictor of future behavior is past behavior (c.f., Nisbett & Ross, 1991.) Because the presence of a previous suicide attempt is such a statistically significant predictor of future attempts, it becomes critical to gather as much information as possible about that attempt. Beck, Morris, and Beck developed the Suicide Intent Scale (SIS; 1974) for the specific purpose of gathering such important data.

The SIS is a 20-item questionnaire that can be completed within a matter of minutes, and can be self-administered or administered verbally by a therapist. Even a cursory review of items from the SIS suggests the importance of assessing both the clear, objective facts surrounding an attempt (e.g., whether the patient slashed his wrists in an unlocked, upstairs bathroom while his parents and sister were eating dinner in the kitchen, or in a small pup tent pitched at a secluded camp site more than three miles away from a main road) and the underlying behavioral intentions (e.g., subjective perceptions) of the attempter.

Of course, the use of a questionnaire cannot, and should not, attempt to replace clinical interviewing. The following information should be obtained from any patient who has made a suicide attempt. Although it can sometimes seem difficult to speak so directly and candidly about such a life threatening event, the process of working together to gather these details can significantly strengthen the therapeutic relationship, and give patients an opportunity to more objectively review the issues surrounding their attempt. Vital information to gather about any and *all* previous suicide attempts include:

1. The month, date, and year of the attempt (anniversary dates often trigger extreme stress for patients, and may coincide with future attempts)
2. Exactly where the suicide attempt took place.
3. How old the patient was at the time of the attempt.
4. What they hoped to accomplish (e.g., revenge, a release from pain, resolution of self-object confusion)
5. What precipitated the attempt (e.g., separation, clinical depression, anger, fear, time of year, mania, anniversary events).
6. Specific details about the method used to attempt suicide. For example, if a patient attempted a drug overdose, one should ascertain: the kind of pills they took, how many they took, how they obtained the drugs, the number (mg) of drugs taken, whether they hoarded the drugs, their thoughts about what exactly the drugs would do to them, whether they took the

drugs with alcohol or other drugs, and whether they took the drugs all at once or over a period of time, among others.)

7. The patient's perception of how lethal their attempt would be.
8. The patient's social support system at the time of attempt, including friends, family members, co-workers, mental health care providers, and community or social groups (e.g., church; support groups).
9. How they were rescued
10. How others close to them responded to their attempt
11. Whether the patient considered or attempted to abort the attempt at any point in time, including what they did and when.
12. Whether the patient left a suicide note, and its specific contents.
13. How the patient views their attempt now, in comparison to how they felt about it then (e.g., are they ashamed; relieved that they lived; upset that they didn't die).

It also is essential determine if the patient knows a close or distant relative, friend, neighbor, classmate, co-worker, or acquaintance who has attempted or committed suicide. If a patient reports positively to such a query, the same kind of exacting, detailed information should be gathered for that attempt as for an attempt that the patient made herself, including information about the public response to that individual's death, and any funeral arrangements or ceremonies.

Carol. Carol was a 19 year-old woman who was self-referred to her university counseling center for feelings of depression, and worries about "fitting in" on campus. During her initial intake, Carol reluctantly described harboring suicidal ideation in which she "wanted to die and show everyone else how miserable she was." However, she flatly denied any suicidal intent or plan, citing her strong Catholic prohibitions against suicide. She also denied the presence of any prior suicide attempts.

Despite Carol's strong admonitions against suicide, and her lack of a specific plan, her therapist was somehow unconvinced that Carol was not a significant suicidal risk. She was unsure if these feelings arose in response to Carol's cool, detached manner or her limited amount of eye contact during conversation. At any rate, Carol's therapist continued to ask her pointed questions about suicide, even though she seemed clearly bored by the topic.

Carol's therapist asked her if anyone in her immediate family attempted or committed suicide. Carol replied, "nope." Carol's therapist asked if she had friends or distant family members who tried to kill themselves. Carol again replied, "nope." However, Carol's therapist still felt uneasy. She took a deep breath and asked Carol knew *anyone* who tried to kill themselves. Carol looked up and her therapist and stated plainly, "Well, my neighbor, Timmy, down the street killed himself a few months ago, when I was finishing high school."

When pressed for details, Carol told how she heard about Timmy's death during a lunch period at school. From her description, Timmy appeared to be a shy, unassuming 9th grader who was having difficulty making friends at school. He often sat alone at lunch, and was bullied by older students. Carol said that she heard that Timmy hung himself in his room at home. She said that most of the kids at school were "really freaked out," and that "some of the mean ones, the ones that were mean to him, felt really bad about it." Carol continued and described how her parents made her attend the viewing and the funeral "because he was our neighbor, and all" even though I didn't really know him. She described the viewing as "really creepy, with "Timmy just lying there, and everyone else just standing around."

Carol continued in her description of the funeral ceremony without pausing for even a second. She simply continued, "it was awful, but I guess he really found out how many people he affected, and who really noticed him and cared about him ... After the funeral, when everyone went back to Timmy's house for food and stuff—my parents didn't make me go to that, though—the line of people to get in his house all the way around the block. There were so many people, and he really got to see who cared about him or not. I hope that many people show up at my funeral." This critical piece of information, that Carol had a school-aged peer who broke the social taboo about suicide, coupled with her idealistic view that one can "look down from above" to acknowledge the sorrow and concern of those left behind, added greatly to an understanding of Carol's suicidal ideation. However, this vital information was obtained only after repeated, in-depth questioning about her knowledge of other individual's suicide attempts.

CLINICAL ASSESSMENT

One of the most challenging tasks for both novice and even experienced therapists is the assessment of patients' suicide risk. Because this topic is so affectively charged, it sometimes can seem difficult to ask critical questions in a straightforward manner, without fears of offending the patient or goading them into action. As in Chapter 2, a pervasive myth in our culture suggests that talking about a private problem only serves to exacerbate it. Therapists must model their willingness to discuss difficult, emotionally charged topics with candor and sensitivity. It also is essential to speak to patients in terms that they understand (without being patronizing in any way), rather than using a clinical or highly intellectualized vocabulary.

Myth: Talking with someone about suicide who is really upset will probably just make things worse, and can even "put ideas in their heads." Many patients describe an incredible sense of relief when given the opportunity to talk about their wish to die, or their developing plans to die. It is as though talking about suicide breaks this social taboo, and allows for the processing of intense emotions and beliefs without the fear that their therapist views them as a "weak character." Talking openly about suicide, an experience that most people describe only having within the context of psychotherapy, also allows someone with suicidal thoughts to openly express those thoughts without fears of a "hysterical" or inappropriate affective response. Patients also describe being comforted by the fact that their therapist "can handle it...even if it is something this bad." Thus, although somewhat paradoxical (i.e., to convince someone not to commit suicide, someone should talk to them about all aspects of their thoughts and plans in depth), case studies, anecdotal reports, and empirical research studies all describe the benefits of talking openly about suicide in psychotherapy, thus dispelling this pervasive, and often destructive, societal myth.

In essence, a therapist must always ask a patient directly, "Have you been thinking about committing suicide?; What exactly do you think about doing? How frequently—and when—do you think about killing yourself?" Some therapists preface these pointed question with, "I ask everyone I see this next series of questions" in order to help normalize the experience. This type of direct questioning also is helpful if a therapist suspects that her patient is reluctant to engage in self-disclosure, or even the process of talking to a mental health practitioner. Asking patients more ambiguous questions, such as, "Have you been thinking about hurting yourself or causing damage to yourself?" can be interpreted in various ways, and does not help to convey the seriousness and danger involved in any suicide attempt.

Suicidal Ideation, Intent, and Plan

Three essential, primary constructs in the clinical assessment (and documentation) of suicide risk include a thorough review of a patient's suicidal ideation, intent, and plan. Each of these constructs, a requisite feature in any mental status exam (see Chapter 3), must be identified clearly, and in as much detail as possible. If a patient does present with some form of suicidal ideation, intent, or plan, the use of direct patient quotes must be included in any progress note and reports to justify and illustrate the clinical risk associated with that factor.

Suicidal ideation indicates the extent to which a patient wishes to die or "be dead." Note that suicidal ideation can be active or passive, and appear with or without out a specific plan or intent to engage a plan. For example, a patient may say, "I wish I were dead" or "I want to die," which indicates the presence of suicidal ideation, but may expand upon their response differently in accord with differing levels of suicide risk. For example, in response to a therapist's question to "tell me more about that," the patient may state, "I just wish God would take me," or "I wish I could just be minding my own business and get hit by a bus." Such statements represent *passive suicidal ideation*, in which the patient expresses a desire to die, but no wish to engage in an active attempt. In contrast, the same patient might state, "I can't wait to get this [my life] over with" or "I've got to figure out some way to do it" which represents *active suicidal ideation*, which generally is associated with significantly greater risk.

Suicidal intent is somewhat similar to suicidal ideation in that suicidal ideation must generally be present in order to possess suicidal intent, but suicidal intent specifically reflects the level of motivation and ability of a patient to follow through with a specified (or non specific) suicide plan. For example, a patient might say, "I want to die so much," representing the presence of suicidal ideation, but respond to additional questions with statements like "I don't think I can get up the nerve to go through with it," "I don't think I will be ready to really do it until my daughter is a little older; I would feel so guilty," or "I wish I had enough sleeping pills to do it but I can't get another prescription from my doctor and I don't know an easy way to get them" indicating a relative lack of intent. In contrast, the same patient may expand upon his previous statement with comments such as "I want to die so badly that I will do whatever it takes to get it done. I don't care what it is, but no one is going to stop me," or "I have all of the pills I need counted out in a bottle in my top dresser drawer, just waiting for me" which represent significant suicidal intent. The presence of the intent to commit suicide is associated with significant clinical risk, and must be explored carefully and thoroughly with all patients.

Suicidal plan represents the extent to which a patient has constructed and prepared a specific plan for suicide. Suicide plans are typically regarded as present or absent, and any plan mentioned is typically rated as vague, general, or very specific. For example, a patient may state that they want to kill themselves, but when asked specifically (and repeatedly, if necessarily) how they intended to kill themselves, they make vague references to "getting in some kind of accident" or "doing something stupid, like maybe staying out too late and drinking a lot." This type of plan would be regarded as vague. (Some patients may report, "I want to die, yeah, but I don't have any idea of what I would really do to kill myself." This statement qualifies for an absence of a suicide plan.) In contrast, some patients may report that they have "some pills in the medicine cabinet and some JD in the liquor cabinet, just great for mixing," or that they "will drive off of an embankment near the top of a mountain," which qualify as general suicide plans. In other words, the individual identifies a specific mode of death, but does not provide specific details about how, when, and where they plan to kill themselves.

Specific suicide plans, on the other hand, do provide detailed information regarding how, when, and where the patient intends to kill herself. One example of a detailed suicide plan (constructed by the owner of an older model car) is: "I've got about a twelve length foot of heavy duty hose, and I was thinking of stuffing that into the muffler and running the tube around to the front seat of the car, tucking it into the window. I know I have a few holes in the back wall of the garage, where the squirrels burrowed through to get at some nuts or birdseed or something, but I've got some spackle and concrete patch to take care of that. I know the car itself will hold up pretty tight, except for where the hose will come in the window. I figure if I sit in there with the radio on, around nine or ten at night, noone will come to bother me, and I will just drift off into that sweet night, and meet up with Nancy [his deceased wife.]" As noted previously, it is absolutely essential that all noted details and direct patient quotes are used included in any form of documentation, and to aid in additional risk evaluation and management.

Yvonne The consequences of being vague during clinical assessment can be catastrophic. Consider the comments of Yvonne, a new patient in psychotherapy who remarked, "Yeah, [my prior therapist] asked me if I thought about hurting myself...I sure was planning on cutting myself later that day. I did it almost every day since it always made me feel better...I didn't cut deep or anything, just enough to feel it...It kind of surprised me she never asked if I wanted to kill myself...And, since she never asked, I never told her about it, even though I started thinking about it a lot more...I'm not totally sure if I would have told her if she asked me, but I might have, because I think her asking me straight up would have shocked the hell out of me."

These statements come from a 27 year-old divorced woman with a college degree who had locked herself in her bathroom, taken 31 aspirin, 25 Tylenol, and 39 prescription sleeping pills, "topping it all off" with eight shots of whiskey. (Yvonne knew exactly how many pills she took because she had been hoarding them.) This young woman was resuscitated at a local hospital after being discovered semi-comatose by her roommate, who returned home early from a three-day business trip. Yvonne sought help in psychotherapy, trying to ease her depression and "make some sense of [her] life." Her current therapist asks Yvonne clearly and directly about the presence of any suicidal thoughts or plans.

The Presence of Warning Signs

Myth: People who commit suicide always give off some kind of clear warning sign or call for help. Adherence to this belief grants the desirable, and certainly less anxiety provoking, perception that family members, friends, and co-workers, as well as mental health practitioners have some degree of control in both predicting and averting suicide attempts. It also posits that people who commit suicide always want someone to intercede on their behalf, and prevent them from carrying out their plan. Unfortunately, a number of research findings suggest that the overwhelming majority of people who do commit suicide do not broadcast such clear, direct signals (i.e., "cries for help") before their attempt. Some patients who appear to be recovering well after a serious depressive episode actually may appear so upbeat and goal directed because they have resigned themselves to a serious, future suicide attempt, and now have the energy to commit it. Such individuals, in particular, may present a happy, content persona in order to deflect suspicion from their underlying suicidal intent.

Rudestam (1977) found in his seminal review of psychological autopsies that only 62% of people who completed suicide communicated their intent to someone before carrying out the act. Warning signs that were identified included changes in language such as specific references to suicide (e.g., You don't have to worry about me much longer...When I die, you can have a nice party for me; Ebert, 1987), requests to have others "take care of my kids if something happens to me," making gifts of family heirlooms and jewelry unrelated to any recipients' birthday or holiday celebrations, and detailed discussions of newly acquired or updated life insurance policies and wills.

In discussions with patients who made serious, failed suicide attempts, some describe with anguish and disbelief their attempts to make obvious "calls for help" that appeared to fall on proverbial, deaf ears. For many of these patients, this lack of acknowledgement served as further evidence that no one cared about or even noticed them, and that they might as well kill themselves anyway. However, although based a relatively small number of case studies, when these survivors of failed suicide attempts are asked to describe exactly what they said or did to give friends and family members "warning signs," their messages could be interpreted as indirect, equivocal, or cryptic at best.

Cathy. Discussions with Cathy, a patient currently seen in psychotherapy after being cut down by paramedics after a serious suicide attempt by hanging, illustrates the ambivalence often surrounding patient's purportedly expected "warning signs." Cathy suffered with untreated clinical depression for three years, prior to her suicide attempt. She explained that in her profession (fire fighting), seeking psychological help or counseling was viewed as a shameful weakness of character. Thus, Cathy described to endure her depression alone, without any social support for more than two years. She provided details about her attempts to self-treat (i.e., "I tried to exercise more for a while, and then try to eat right") and self-medicate (i.e., "I thought that maybe drinking more, especially with everyone else after work might help me deal with things better"), which appeared unable to break the cycle of her "nearly constant" unbearable emotional suffering.

Cathy said that after this initial two-year period, she began to consider and then plan her own death. She fantasized about her death, and primarily being freed from her feelings of worthlessness and emptiness, and her increasing physical discomfort from constant tension headaches and insomnia. Cathy described her decision to die as "completely rational, like it made total sense...I had, like, tunnel vision... It was the only option that made any sense...but in the back of my mind I wished there was something else..." Cathy also described trying to reach out to her friends and family members for help in the week before her attempt, but to no avail.

After her suicide attempt, Cathy felt betrayed and dismissed by those closest to her. She said, "I gave [my friends and co-workers] clear signs and calls for help...There is no way they could have missed them...Jesus Christ, it was so god damn obvious!" When asked to describe the clues she gave them, however, it was difficult for Cathy's therapist to understand how Cathy could be so adamant about the clarity of her calls for help. When asked to describe exactly what she said or did, Cathy remarked, "Instead of saying 'see ya' like I always do, you know, I'm always laughing and friendly with everyone at work, so nobody probably thought I was depressed, either, 'cause I could hide everything so well, but when leaving work that day, I said 'good-bye' to everybody. I even said, 'good-bye' and their name ... I mean, I always say 'see ya;' that's my thing I do every time I leave work. I never, I've never said good-bye to anyone at work. I just don't do that ... I just can't believe they didn't get it."

Cathy truly was stunned that her co-workers failed to acknowledge what she perceived to be blatant calls for help. When her therapist attempted to discuss the indirect nature of Cathy's call for help, which took the form of a two word change to her typical social greeting, conveyed once to her co-workers during a hectic time of day (i.e., a shift change), she had great difficulty understanding how her remarks could not be obvious. It is as though being steeped in her own pain for so long depleted Cathy's normal ability to perceive and evaluate social situations and events, providing only a remaining, incredibly narrow self-focus. This type of "rational ... tunnel vision," to quote Cathy's own words, would certainly allow a suicidal individual to believe that her calls for help are as obvious and salient to others *as they are to herself.*

Cathy met with a psychiatrist for an evaluation and agreed to begin a trial of anti-depressant medication. She also began participation in psychotherapy at an outpatient clinic, located outside the catchment area of her own emergency department. In therapy, Cathy began to acknowledge her rescue fantasies (e.g., You know, I'll just wake up one day and meet Mr. Right, and just work for fun, and have enough money for my kids) and take more responsibility for her own actions. More importantly, Cathy began to internalize the belief that she had enough intrinsic value as a human being to ask for, and even demand, help when she needed it.

Thus, acceptance that not all suicidal individuals provide clear, easily recognizable "warning signs" is essential for the friends, family members, and co-workers, and therapists of people who attempt or commit suicide. This knowledge can sometimes help survivors avoid feelings of additional, ruminative guilt. It can also help allow them to place some responsibility for the suicide attempt upon a victims' probable, narrow cognitive focus upon their own suffering.

Psychological Testing

Even though a number of factors have been identified as evidence-based predictors of heightened suicide risk, clinicians and researchers continue to look for additional forms of assessment that can provide additional clues or information. Current research suggests that scores on the Beck Depression Inventory (BDI) are predictive of suicidal intension (Cochrane, Kate, Lofchy, & Sakinofsky, 2000; Gilbar & Eden, 2001; Kingsbury, Hawton, Steinhardt, & James, 1999). The suicide index of the Rorschach also has received some empirical support as a helpful predictor (Eyman & Eyman, 1991). Some legal benefits also can be gleaned from psychological testing when used in such a way to "clarify the nature of the mental disorder and ... clarify, support, or modify initial clinical impressions" (VandeCreek & Knapp, 2000; p. 1346). However, psychological testing should never be used to replace clinical interviewing (VandeCreek & Knapp, 2000) or to supersede clinical experience and judgment.

The use of psychological testing also may be beneficial beyond the initial goal calculating a standardized score to better assess suicide risk. For example, asking patients to complete measures with clear face validity (e.g., BDI) and following through with a candid discussion and review of their individual items responses can provide a wealth of clinical information. This process also can help patients begin to acknowledge responsibility for their own actions, and foster open communication and trust in the patient-therapist relationship, and demonstrate that the therapist can tolerate a detailed discussion of suicide. The use of a formal, psychological "test" or instrument also can force some patients to better accept that their suicidal ideation is legitimate and serious. It is almost as though the formality and concreteness of the procedure increases the salience of the patient (and therapist's) reactions.

SUICIDE NOTES

Another pervasive myth is that people who commit suicide leave detailed suicide notes or messages that provide valuable clues about what led up to the suicide, and shed insight into the victim's underlying emotional state. Studies of actual completed suicides, however, reveal that only 20–30% of suicide victims leave a note or other message (c.f., Black, 1993; Hendin, 1995; Jamison, 1999; Rudestam, 1977), and that their interpretation is often equivocal, at best. It remains unclear whether the content of suicide notes provide any meaningful insight into the victim's mental state at the time of death.

What we do know about the content of suicide notes is that there are virtually no demographic or personal characteristics that can be used to predict who will leave a note and who will not. For example, Black's (1993) seminal study of actual suicide notes revealed no significantly significant differences between victims who left notes versus those who did not by their age, sex, martial status, socio-economic status, job status, or cause of death. Another consistent finding in the research is that people who are asked to imagine that they are suicidal tend to generate notes that are significantly different than those written by people who, in fact, did commit suicide (Black, 1993).

Specifically, the notes created by individuals asked to vividly imagine that they were suicidal were significantly shorter in length, and more likely to describe feelings of sadness and depression than the notes made by people who actually committed suicide. Actual suicide notes also are more likely to provide specific, detailed information about instructions for settling final affairs (e.g., 175 stock certificates for International Paper can be found on the top shelf of the hallway closet; I want Jason to have my marble collection), make greater mention of religious ideas (e.g., May God forgive me), and date the note (Black, 1993). Some notes even warn rescuers about the potential dangers of attempting to recover or resuscitate their bodies. Jamison (1999) described a suicide note written by someone who clearly acknowledged the impact of their act upon others. The note simply stated, "Be careful. Cyanide gas is in this bathroom" (p. 77).

In general, actual suicide notes seem surprisingly devoid of psychotic thought processes, and provide significantly more instructions and details about final affairs (e.g., delivery of possessions, the location of important legal documents, who should care for children or pets, instructions for burial) than people might normally expect. This sometimes analytical focus is consistent with stories from many patients who survive serious suicide attempts. One woman, resuscitated by paramedics after a nearly fatal drug overdose, described her thoughts before her suicide attempt. "At the time, it made complete sense—absolute, total sense. I wasn't irrational or emotional! I knew I wanted to die, and I didn't think I could make it through another day [with this severe depression]. That was my decision, and I was happy about it. I didn't think it was wrong or immoral. It was just something I had to do... But, I also wanted to make sure that my children would be taken care of." It is plausible that once deeply distressed individuals commit to a specific suicide plan, they consciously or unconsciously dampen their normal affective responses (e.g., fear or guilt about leaving their children behind), which would normally prompt them to abort the attempt. Unfortunately, such emotional detachment and numbing also lends itself to a poorer prognosis in psychotherapy (Hendin, 1995).

It also remains critical to note that these studies' findings about suicide notes are based on arithmetic averages. Actual suicide notes vary significantly in their specificity, length, and tone. Some notes clearly are intended to be cruel and biting, as a way to exact final control or revenge upon those they intend to leave behind. Although the majority of suicide notes do not place blame for the act upon friends or family members (e.g., I know you only meant the best for me), but instead convey a desperate wish for release from unrelenting pain and suffering (Jamison, 1999), traditional psychoanalytic theory suggests that the authors of these notes actually meant the opposite of what they wrote. Thus, a patient who writes, "I know you did everything you could for me. Please know that it isn't your fault" could have his message interpreted to mean, "You didn't do everything you could to help me. I want you to know that your lack of love and concern allowed me to kill myself." And, because these individuals have obviously died, it becomes impossible to ascertain their true intent or meaning. Although the following statement is clearly overly simplistic, it remains essential for therapists to focus upon the communications of our patients—while they are still alive.

VARIOUS CLINICAL SCENARIOS

It is difficult to talk globally about the assessment of patient suicidality. Focusing primarily upon a patient's personality characteristics, mental status, family background, demographic characteristics, cultural influences, social supports, and environmental stressors only provides a portion of the information needed to make appropriate clinical decisions and treatment plans. The conditions under which therapists work with suicidal patients, as well as the nature of the patient-therapist relationship, significantly influence any clinical assessment of the patient's situation.

A number of patient-therapist scenarios may be present when a patient's treatment focuses upon aspects of suicide. Some of these scenarios include:

1. telephone contact in which a patient call into a suicide "hot-line"
2. an initial session with a patient in outpatient treatment who reports suicidal ideation
3. an initial session with a patient in outpatient treatment who has recently made a suicidal attempt

4. inpatient treatment with a patient who is recovering from a serious suicide attempt
5. inpatient treatment with a patient who was involuntarily admitted because they were considered an imminent danger to themselves
6. in the midst of on-going out patient treatment, if a patient expresses suicidal ideation (either during a session or via an emergency telephone call or message)
7. in the midst of on-going outpatient treatment, if a patient attempts or commits suicide
8. providing back-up or emergency coverage for another clinician's patient
9. wrap around services (mobile crisis intervention unit)
10. telephone or hot-line centers

RISK MANAGEMENT

When discussing the clinical management of suicidal patients it is necessary first to address the contradictions inherent in term itself. The use of "clinical management" suggests that therapists have the ability and influence to exert control over our patients' thoughts, feelings, environment, and even their actions. This intent to exercise control over patient behavior (identified by some as manipulation; Hendin, 1995) appears in significant opposition to a primary goal in psychotherapy, in which patients are provided with the insight and skills required to take control over their own lives. From a pragmatic perspective, however, a primary task in crisis intervention is to provide structured, active interventions to avoid imminent death or injury. For example, a patient who is actively psychotic certainly requires a different type of care and support than one who is self-aware and articulate.

What remains true, despite the difficulties in negotiating the pull between a patient's free will (even that which calls them to hurt themselves) and a therapist's attempt to provide safety and stability, is that there will always be an element of risk in work with suicidal patients, no matter what kind of attempt is made to exert control over a patients behavior or environment. As stated plaintively by one clinical supervisor, "The only way you can even think you have control another person's behavior is to have a gun pointed at their head or have them under constant, 24 hour professional supervision ... We don't do that in therapy ... On some level, we always have to remember that patients ultimately will do what they want to do ... "

General Guidelines

A number of suggestions can be made regarding the clinical management of a suicidal patient. Some of these recommendations may be more useful for some patients than others. They are listed in no particular order. As with any clinical intervention, the relationship between the patient and therapist also must be taken into account. When faced with a suicidal patient, therapists can:

1. Remember that acute episodes (i.e., crises) are often time limited. Make specific goals to help a client make it through the most difficult times. It can be important for both patients and therapists to acknowledge that getting through a crisis often occurs only one day at a time.

2. Acknowledge that a lack of sleep (individuals with depression often report getting little or no sleep over 48 and even 72 hour periods) can significantly impair the judgment of even a non-suicidal person. Sometimes providing basic, instrumental assistance such as a consultation with a psychiatrist for a limited number (i.e., a non-lethal dose) of sleeping pills can help patients get through some of their worst moments. A few hours of sleep can provide patients with some inkling of hope or improvement, no matter how small or initially insignificant.

3. Discuss the actual consequences of suicide. Supply and encourage accurate reality testing, and help change a patient's focus from the immediate present to some point in the future. For example, "If you really kill yourself, we won't be able to work together anymore" or "If you kill yourself, you will not be able to see your children graduate from high school. They will be there, alone." Although some experts caution against using any relationship, and particularly the therapeutic relationship, to manipulate a patient into staying alive (akin to holding a patient emotionally hostage; Hendin, 1995), other experts consider the use of such relational leverage more than appropriate if it keeps a patient alive long enough to engage them in treatment (e.g., Linehan, Armstrong, Suarez, & Allmon, 1991).

4. Ask a patient who owns a gun or other weapon to allow a friend or family member to take it out of their possession, and place it in safe-keeping. Although it certainly is true that if a patient really wants to kill himself, he will find a way, the absence of available firearms makes it more difficult to engage in a fatal impulsive act. Sometimes a patient can be persuaded to call such a helpful friend or family from the therapist's office, and ask them to remove the weapon before they return home from their appointment.

5. Work in consort with a psychiatrist or other health care provider (sometimes a patient's family doctor or nurse practitioner) to help manage a patient's suicidal impulses. A trial of anti-depressant or anti-psychotic medication often can provide enough symptom relief for patients to think more clearly and acknowledge the possibility of change. This use of a team approach also bodes well in the unfortunate circumstance that if a patient does commit suicide, documented evidence exists to suggest that the therapist consulted with peers in order to make appropriate treatment decisions.

6. Identify at least one thing that a patient considers worth living for. When asking patients about their suicidal intent, many cite that their spouse, children, parents, or religious beliefs is the only thing keeping them from killing themselves. Again, although evoking a patient's sense of guilt or shame about abandoning someone or something can be perceived as manipulation (i.e., in which a patient chooses to remain alive only for the benefit of someone else), it also can be used in the short term as a way to keep patients alive and in treatment.

7. Talk with patients about the difference between suicidal thoughts and actions. Thinking about, or even being obsessed by suicidal thoughts, does not mean that actions must follow. It can be critical to remind patients that thoughts and actions are two separate entities, and that they have control over their own actions.

8. Consider carrying high-risk patients' phone numbers, addresses, and even license plate numbers (with code names or aliases to preserve confidentiality) on your person. One therapist reported that a patient called her at home one evening, and told her that he "couldn't take it anymore," and that he was going to take a bottle of pills at a distant recreation area and chase them with a bottle of rum. He said, "good-bye" and hung up before the therapist could initiate any conversation. In response, the therapist immediately called the police, and was able to give them detailed information about her patient, including a description of his car and license plate. The police found her patient in the park, unconscious, and delivered him to a hospital for medical treatment. The paramedics reported later that if the patient had been found even a few hours later, he might not have survived. Because the therapist had to drive more than an hour to reach her office (and the patient's file), she would have been unable to provide the police with this life saving information in time if she did not have immediate access.

9. Assist the patient in mobilizing at least one form of social support. Consider having a patient call a friend, family member, church, or other social agency from the therapist's office to plan some kind of

activity or set up an appointment. This allows patients to gain some sense of control over their situation, and at least may momentarily force them to assume some kind of external, interpersonal focus, rather than an exclusively internal, intrapsychic focus.

10. Engage the patient in a discussion of the possible suicide outcomes. Specifically, what if something "goes wrong" and they end up seriously injured, brain damaged, or in a vegetative state? Proponents of dialectical behavioral therapy (e.g., Linehan) suggest asking patient whether they really know for sure that committing suicide will make things better. For example, what if their religious beliefs are correct, and individuals who kill themselves are punished in the afterlife? What if when you die, you end up being forced to remember and perpetually experience the current terrible feelings you have right now? How do you know you won't end up barely alive, dying a slow painful death, only to be hooked up permanently to breathing machines? Although these types of questions may appear extreme, audacious, and even controversial, they are designed to foster reality testing and force patients to consider other, non-lethal means of dulling their pain

11. Many experts urge the therapists of suicidal patients to boost patient-therapist contact, by increasing the frequency of sessions to two or three times a week (e.g., VandeCreek & Knapp, 2000). However, other experts suggest that increasing the frequency of sessions only conveys the implicit message to patients that they cannot handle their problems on their own (Hendin, 1995). Increased contact, perceived as care and attention, may even positively reinforce the presence of suicidal behavior (Linehan et al., 1991). Despite these differing opinions regarding increasing the number of therapy sessions, most all experts agree that increasing patient contact by allowing, and sometimes even encouraging patient to call their therapists outside of regularly scheduled therapy sessions (within limits, however) can be beneficial. Sometimes encouraging a patient to call his therapist's answering machine to "just listen and hear my voice" can increase perceptions of emotional support and help provide object constancy.

12. Engage in strategies to increase the strength of the patient's observing ego. For example, ask them to begin to identify what precedes their suicidal thoughts or impulses. Is it being alone, shooting drugs, drinking heavily, seeing an ex-lover, or reviewing their finances? Encourage them to develop a plan to avoid those antecedents, and to develop a plan for coping if and when they do feel suicidal. Help patients come up with some specific helping behaviors, such as calling their therapist, calling a sponsor, going for a walk, writing in a journal, going for coffee with a friend, reading a good book, or volunteering with others.

Contracting for Safety

A commonly identified (Hendin, 1995) but sometimes controversial intervention in work with suicidal patients is to make a contract for safety. Contracts can take the form of oral or written statements which statement that the patient will not attempt to kill herself before some specific time (e.g., before our next appointment) or before making a call for help (e.g., to their therapist, an emergency room, or other support person). Ideally, patients will craft their own statements, typically during a therapy session, and both the therapist and patient can sign the document. One copy can be placed in the patient's chart for documentation, and another held by the patient, even on their person. General social psychological principles suggest that because we are so conditioned by strong social conventions (and often social prohibitions) to honor one's word or promise, signing a document or giving verbal ascent increases compliance with their commitment to seek help or support before commencing any suicidal acts.

Empirical studies with community living adults and college students indicate that asking an individual to sign a document or give a promise increases their likelihood of following through on their actions (c.f., the classic social psychological study, Freedman and Fraser, 1966). However, many therapists point out that simply signing a piece of paper in no way confers an increased level of safety against *suicidal* impulses. Patients under the influence of drugs or alcohol may not even remember signing such a contract. Other patients may experience psychological reactance, in which they feel their free will has been compromised by some impersonal bureaucratic process, and they engage in suicidal behavior to reassert their free will or spite their therapist. Still other patients may be in such psychic pain and discomfort that while they recognize the importance of their contract for safety, and would prefer to honor their obligation, the sense of pain, loss, and irrational thinking leads them to believe that suicide is the only solution to their problem. And, although many therapists regard the use of no-suicide contracts with children as helpful (Davidson & Range, 2000), it remains unclear whether children, particularly those under the age of six, truly understand what the contract implies.

Some therapists even consider the act of asking patients to sign a contract for safety demeaning or insulting. The reasoning here is that the entire process of distilling suicidality down to "a few paragraphs with an official signature" is overly simplistic, and dismissive of the complex, powerful forces and conflicts underlying patients' suicidal thoughts and impulses. Other critics suggest that asking patients to sign a contract indicating that they are not suicidal will lead some patients to underestimate the extent of their suicidal intent, or become fearful about discussing specific suicidal urges or plans with their therapist if they arise later in treatment.

In response to some of these concerns, one approach to creating a no-harm contract is to incorporate the use of specific coping strategies into the contact itself (Sells, 2001). In other words, the contract does more than commit a patient to safety; it commits a patient to engage in proactive behaviors that serve to maximize coping and minimize suicidal impulses. For example, one patient included in her contact, "I will ask my brother to keep my shot gun and hand gun at his home, locked in his basement, until my therapist and I decide it is time to return them," "If I start to think about really wanting to hurt or kill myself, I agree to call my therapist to talk about it first...If she is not immediately available, I will call my brother, Tammi, or 911," and "If I start to feel sad or depressed, I agree to go for a walk, visit my niece, go to the coffee shop, or call my therapist instead of sitting alone in my house." Planning for contingencies, such as what to do if the therapist is temporarily unavailable, becomes central in such contracts (Sells, 1998). Although these statements may appear somewhat simplistic, they encourage patients to take responsibility for their own actions, while providing a clearly sanctioned opportunity to seek help and support from others.

Despite the controversial nature of making contracts for safety with suicidal patients, one clear benefit exists—although it may provide more long-term benefits for therapists than patients. The presence of a signed contract for safety in a patient's chart can provide clear, unequivocal documentation that a therapist made the attempt to assess and thwart a patient's suicidal activity. If a patient does commit suicide and a malpractice suit is filed, this type of documentation will likely only support the therapist's case that he engaged in appropriate, professional activity and demonstrated adequate levels of professional competence (Harris, 1995; Soisson et al., 1987). For better or worse, these types of legal issues have begun to permeate the practice of psychotherapy. We can only hope that our patients do not suffer from our choice of responses to these issues.

COPING WITH COUNTERTRANSFERENCE

Dealing with a suicidal patient can represent one of the most stressful aspects of a therapist's job (also see Chapter 8). The countertransference encountered in work with a suicidal patient can be intense, confusing, and even overwhelming at times. Commonly reported reactions to suicidal patients include fear, anxiety, disdain, anger, alarm, and fascination, as well as more generalized aspects of rescue fantasies. Therapists must learn to process their countertransferential reactions in order not to act upon them. For example, the strong urge to rescue a patient from their angst could lead to inappropriate boundary disturbances (e.g., seeing a patient at all hours of the night; taking multiple emergency phone calls within the hour; having lengthy phone sessions while on vacation) if not dealt with carefully. One of the best ways to understand and temper such countertransference is to enlist the support of colleagues, consultants, and supervisors. In fact, when working with suicidal patients within the context of Dialectical Behavioral Therapy, Linehan (Linehan & Kehrer, 1993) requires that therapists have weekly peer sessions to guarantee such support.

Countertransference Hate

Suicidal patients in particular also may evoke a somewhat unique countertransferential response from therapists. Maltsberger and Buie (1974) regarded this reaction, in which otherwise calm, collected, insightful therapists develop an almost overwhelming loathing for their patient, as countertransference hate. Left unchecked, this intense feeling of hatred, rage, and disgust can easily lead clinicians to abandon patients, refer unnecessarily, and even begin to deny the suicide risk posed by their patients. Countertransference hate also may not be recognized immediately, and may manifest itself in a variety of unhealthy ways both in and outside of the patient-therapist relationship.

Elizabeth. A student extern was assigned to Elizabeth, an elderly, divorced woman who sought therapy because she was "feeling like dog crap." In the course of two months, the intern developed a relationship with Elizabeth, despite a string of missed appointments, cancellations, and sometimes dismissive or abusive remarks on the part of her patient. (Elizabeth liked to say at least once during each session, "Well, I don't know if you would really understand this because you aren't really a doctor, and I really wish I could have had that other gentleman as a therapist, but ... ") It became evident that Elizabeth was suffering from borderline personality disorder, and that she was quite ambivalent about developing any kind of true intimacy within the therapeutic relationship. Yet, the student extern sought additional supervision, read various works by experts in the field, and steeled herself for each session. She was determined to somehow connect with

Elizabeth and help her to better manage her intense feelings of anger
and depression.

Two weeks before the student extern's winter break, Elizabeth
became increasingly agitated and angry. She screamed at her student
therapist, "Who the hell do you think you are going on vacation? I sure
would like it if I had enough money to go on some nice vacation somewhere!" Although the student extern had not revealed any specifics
about her holiday plans, Elizabeth obviously was projected her own
thoughts and desires onto her therapist. The following week, Elizabeth
expressed fears that she would commit suicide in her therapist's
absence. She also gave her therapist a box of after dinner mints saying,
"You know, I do like you...Merry Christmas." After assessing
Elizabeth's suicide risk, developing strategies for coping in her therapist's absence (including the emergency contact numbers of a covering
therapist), and processing the nature of her small gift, Elizabeth pronounced at the end of their session that she "guessed that it was OK for
[her student therapist] to go."

When Elizabeth left the office, her therapist sat dejectedly at her
desk. She felt that she was trying her best to help her patient, and was
worried that all of her outside work and effort had amounted to little.
She also began to doubt her abilities as a clinician, and even questioned
her place in graduate school. After a few minutes of brooding, the extern
opened the box of mints and began to eat them. Soon, she described
devouring the candy, eating them voraciously, but without enjoying it.
Halfway through the box, she felt a momentary hint of nausea, but continued eating. With only a few left in the box, she told herself, "What the
hell. I might as well finish these off so I don't have to take them home or
leave them here." She then described eating the rest of the mints, without "really noticing what [she] was doing." (The student was of normal
weight and had no history of binge eating or any eating disorder.)

Only later in supervision did the student extern realize that her
devouring of Elizabeth's candy represented her own desire to attack,
destroy, consume, and control her patient, including those veiled
threats of suicide on the eve of her much anticipated family vacation.
Throwing the mints out would have represented her dismissal of
Elizabeth, and would not have mirrored the symbolic need of her
therapist to somehow be accepted by her while still keeping her trou-
blesome behavior in check. In the supervisory session, the student
intern was able to give voice to her anger at Elizabeth for "being such
a difficult patient," and for "treating [her] like shit."

The extern learned that it was Ok to become angry at a patient's
behavior, and that it was more than appropriate to set limits regarding

the use of inappropriate language during sessions. The student extern also was asked to consider the varying level of competence one feels as a professional in training and in practice, and was given strategies for addressing Elizabeth's comments about "really wanting a different therapist" during their sessions. Thus, having a safe, supportive environment to identify, label, and discuss her countertransference hate, without being judged for it, allowed these feelings to dissipate and for the student extern to place renewed focus upon her work with Elizabeth.

INVOLUNTARY REPORTING AND COMMITTMENT

The Perceived Need for Constant Supervision

Myth: People who are suicidal should never be left alone; a friend or family member should be with them around the clock. Although there are exceptions to every rule, the general consensus is that if a patient is so acutely suicidal that she requires around-the-clock supervision, she should be hospitalized or involuntarily committed rather than placed under the supervision of untrained, interpersonally related friends and family members. This call for constant supervision tells the patient, in essence, "You can't take care of yourself, so we will do it for you." This type of 24-hour watch also promotes a patient's external, rather than an internal, locus of control, and quashes any sense of self-efficacy. A home-based, round-the-clock monitoring also places a significant, inappropriate responsibility upon friends and family members, who may (even inadvertently) do or say something to make a patient feel worse about himself and his situation. Also imagine the guilt forced upon a caregiver directed to "watch" a suicidal family member, who, after a few hours of supervision asks to go alone to the bathroom (e.g., I have to do some private stuff, you know, and that would be really gross. I'll be right out, OK) for only three minutes, and proceeds to fatally hang himself.

What is so striking about this apparently pervasive, and typically inappropriate directive for friends and family members to provide constant supervision is that many professionals have great difficulty in acknowledging the following statement as true: if somebody really wants to kill himself, he will find a way." Other variants of this statement include, "The only way you can make somebody do something (e.g., not commit suicide) is to put a gun to their head. Even then, you still might now get them to do what you really want." This type of statement is not meant to be cavalier, or dismissive of the requisite need for thorough clinical assessment and involuntary hospitalization, if necessary. It is important to note, however, that patients in locked inpatient units, under professional supervision, can and do kill themselves.

A Tenuous Illustration

The following passage (also referenced in Chapter 3) is drawn from a purported textbook in abnormal psychology and crisis intervention. Note the balance of power in the patient-therapist relationship, and the lack of appropriate patient-therapist boundaries.

> "Betty, a 19 year-old university student, came to see me unexpectedly... She was ... seriously thinking about taking [some pills] because she 'didn't want to live anymore' ... I then suggested that it might be helpful for her to have some friends help her. She said that she had friends here, including roommate, but she had tried to keep her grief from them. *I secured permission from her to telephone her roommate and to arrange for constant companionship until our next appointment* [emphasis added] ... The next day, Betty felt that the crisis was over and that we could begin to meet regularly to work her problem through without fear of suicide."

In the excerpt, Betty's roommate is assigned to provide her with constant companionship until her appointment the following day. Betty's roommate is probably a teenager as well, and certainly would not have the clinical training to make a formal, clinical assessment of Betty's situation. Also consider, does the therapist or Betty expect her roommate to voluntarily and eagerly cancel her classes, work, and other commitments to stay with Betty? Would the roommate provide supervision only under duress or extreme feelings of guilt? Does Betty even have a good relationship with her roommate? This type of responsibility is overwhelming for anyone, much less someone who has a tenuous relationship with the patient.

Continued Controversy

Significant controversy exists regarding the costs and benefits of involuntary hospitalization. Some experts pose the question, "Who is involuntary commitment really for?" with the belief that commitment of suicidal patients only makes therapists feel better, and that it does little or nothing to benefit patients themselves. Indeed, a number of statistics suggest that inpatient stays may not benefit all patients. For example, the risk of suicide appears to increase immediately after release from an inpatient setting. And, a number of patients do kill themselves while in hospital settings, even under purported one-on-one, 24-hour surveillance (Jamison, 1999). While one could assume that these deaths occur as a result of poorly trained and unmotivated staff, one could also assume that individuals who genuinely wish to kill themselves will find some way to do it, and cannot typically be stopped or deterred by other people.

However, the majority of patients do not commit suicide either during or immediately after a period of involuntary commitment. Despite admonitions that such hospitalizations may arise from a clinician's wish to be momentarily free of worry and responsibility for a patient, others may argue that it is better to be more conservative than liberal when dealing with a highly suicidal patient. In other words, therapists can always deal with a patient's anger later; it is more important that the patient remain alive.

TREATMENT AFTER A FAILED ATTEMPT

There also are times when a therapist must deal with a patient who attempted suicide either before entering or during treatment. Borrowing from general tenants of dialectical behavior therapy (Linehan & Kehrer, 1993) and family therapy (see Sells, 1998; 2001), forcing the patient to relive those final moments and to recount those final decisions can prove unpleasant enough (and insightful enough) to discourage future attempts. Thus, no matter how difficult, therapists must work through patient resistance.

Mr. M.

Mr. M was a 55 year-old Vietnam veteran admitted involuntarily to a VA hospital after making a suicide attempt. Mr. M was unemployed, and had lived in the basement bedroom of his older brother and sister-in-law's home for the past four months. The night before Mr. M's admission to the hospital, he was discovered in the downstairs family room, lying unconscious on the sofa, by his sister-in-law when she came home from work. Mr. M was revived in a local emergency room after his stomach was pumped and he was given appropriate medication. He reported that he had taken 35 aspiring and "a few" sleeping pills; his lab results confirmed that he had not taken any alcohol or recreational drugs during his attempt.

While in the inpatient psychiatric unit, Mr. M was belligerent and enraged that he was in the hospital against his will. He refused to discuss his suicide attempt, and would scream at his therapist, "You don't know what the fuck you are talking about! I'm here now...what the hell do we have to talk about [my suicide] attempt for?...That was in the past. I don't want to talk about it. I'm not going to do it again! I'm fine now...Why don't you do something to help me get out of here and get a real job, OK? That's what's going to help me...I don't want to waste my time talking about things in the past." Other members of the treatment team had no progress in getting Mr. M to disclose any details about his suicide attempt. Some staff members even expressed fears of him. Although Mr. M seemed to make acquaintances on the unit, it was clear that his only discussions with others involved only general complaints about the unit meals and scheduling. It was as though Mr. M had succeeded in using his anger and apparent logic to divert attention from his true, underlying problems.

Mr. M's therapist, however, made a conscious effort to keep her voice low and calm in the face of his tirades. When he began yelling, she would state, "Mr. M, I can't help you when you are shouting. I'll wait until you are finished and then you can tell me what is bothering you." She forced herself to stay calm, and told him that she didn't like asking him to talk about his suicide attempt either, but that talking about it was the only way that "in [her] professional judgment" they could understand what happened and move on to help him plan for the future. By calling upon her role as a professional rather than personalizing her insistence, Mr. M acquiesced.

Although an initial session involved discussion of tremendous hatred and contempt for his brother "who put me in this fucking place," little was said about his suicide attempt. After some additional prodding, a detailed story began to emerge. Mr. M had lost his job as a salesman, and had to move into his younger brother's home. He stayed in their finished basement, and had begun to search for jobs. Mr. M had taken a handful of sleeping pills and aspirin one afternoon, and lay down on the sofa in the lower level of the living room. When his sister-in-law came home from work she found him, couldn't rouse him, and called for an ambulance. His sister-in-law and brother then sought an involuntary commitment for him, against his will.

When asked what happened immediately before his attempt, and what led him to take pills (versus something else) and place himself somewhere where his sister-in-law would find him, even more details emerged. Apparently, things were going well with his extended family until his sister-in-law complained to his brother about the bathroom, and Mr. M's towels being "a mess." Apparently, Mr. M had external and internal hemorrhoids that started to bleed. (He suffered from hemorrhoids off and on since he was a young adult, and they did not appear to be related to any type of self-mutilation, stimulation, or consensual or nonconsensual anal sex.) Mr. M's brother demanded that he go to the doctor in order to remain in the house with them. And, his brother even accompanied Mr. M to the doctor, who indicated that surgery was the only way to permanently control the pain and bleeding.

Not wishing to have surgery while in the midst of a series of job interviews, Mr. M lied and told his brother that he would have the surgery sometime in the next few weeks. One week later, Mr. M's brother confronted him and told him that he spoke to the doctor, and that they went ahead and scheduled his surgery. Mr. M reluctantly went to the hospital, signed the necessary papers, and submitted to pre-op blood work. It was on the day before his scheduled surgery that Mr. M tried to kill himself, and left himself for dead in his brother's house.

On the face of things, Mr. M was quick to say that he was so "fucking mad" at his brother because he thought he could "make him" have surgery. Both patient and therapist also had a bit of a laugh about the brother's indirect attempt to "fuck him up the ass" via the surgery. It was more difficult for Mr. M to articulate, and admit, however, that he was really furious about his own willingness to give his brother to have so much control over his own life, and that he didn't feel enough worth as a human being to make his own decisions about his body, job, and health. In essence, Mr. M began to focus upon his own thoughts, feelings, and expectations rather than upon those of his brother. He also admitted ruefully that he might have left the bathroom "a little messy" one day in hopes of receiving some sympathy, and that his plans indeed backfired. In addition, Mr. M worked with his therapist to develop strategies to avoid falling into the same cyclical dynamics (c.f., Wachtel, 1977) with his brother and sister-in-law, in which he assumed a one-down position.

In a subsequent treatment team meeting with family members, invited by Mr. M, the therapist helped Mr. M maintain control of the meeting agenda. Plans were made for Mr. M to move into a local YMCA until he located a job, despite his brother's insistence that he couldn't take care of himself. Due to additional working through of his previous conflicts in therapy, Mr. M literally was able to use words, rather than indirect, self-destructive actions, to tell his brother that he was in charge of his own life. He also was able to ask if his brother and sister-in-law would be willing to have dinner with him once a week so that he would not feel so isolated. He also took responsibility for what he did during his suicide attempt, and apologized for any grief he caused them. Upon hearing this, his sister-in-law burst into tears and reached out to touch Mr. M's hand, while his brother thanked him quietly, and said that he had been feeling so guilty about what he had done himself. During his final day on the inpatient unit, Mr. M told his therapist, "Thank-you for not giving up on me."

THE IMPACT UPON THOSE LEFT BEHIND

In one of the more rigorous empirical studies of family members' responses to a suicide, Rudestam (1977) found that surviving family members reported a significant increase in a number of behavioral, emotional, and psychosomatic problems, which persisted more than 6 months after the death of their family member. The family members' complaints included feeling "deeply unhappy" or depressed, feeling numb or apathetic, being fearful about spending time alone, crying jags, loss of appetite, increased outbursts of anger, diminished interest in sex or sexual dysfunction, migraine headaches, colitis, increased alcohol consumption, insomnia, and social withdrawal. Contradicting many assumptions that family members of suicide victims attempt to "hide" the event or keep it a private, family affair, the vast majority of the survivors sought help from family members and friends, as well as the police and other authorities, when they first learned that their family member committed suicide.

Although the death of a family member has been identified as a risk factor for suicide (Hendin, 1995; Jamison, 1999), presumably because it breaks the typically strong social taboos against suicide, many empirical studies suggest that the majority of individuals who are left behind by a family member do learn to cope with the experience. Some family survivors cite improved relations among their remaining members, and even a reluctant sense of relief that their troubled family member "is finally at rest" (e.g., Rudestam, 1977). It certainly takes courage for family members to admit that they may also experience some sense of relief in the midst of their grief, especially if they perceived their loved one as perpetually unhappy or abusive in their personal relationships. Thus, it is vital to help survivors acknowledge any ambivalence they may feel about the suicide.

However, empirical studies suggest that those survivors who manifest the more extreme manifestations of grief and stress are those of parents who lost a child to suicide. See Chapter 8 for additional information regarding the impact of suicide upon psychotherapists and other mental health professionals, and suggestions for more effective coping.

7

Violence
What is This Person Going to Do?

*Patient violence can never be predicted with 100% accuracy.
However, a careful analysis of violent acts often (but not always)
reveals a series of identifiable precipitants, with potential opportunities for intervention.*

The recently released report from the APA's Task Force on Education
and Training in Clinical Emergencies and Crisis (2000) states plainly
that current professional education and training in behavioral emergencies, including the management of patient violence, is lacking and
even substandard. For example, national surveys of psychologists indicate that most practitioners received an average of only one hour of
clinical training on the management of patient violence (Guy, Brown,
& Poelstra, 1990) and that graduate training in sexual and physical
abuse received poor student ratings (Pope & Feldman-Summers, 1992).
These findings are particularly distressing because additional
national surveys indicate that nearly 90% of the psychologists reported
having significant fear that a patient would commit violence against a
third party, and that more than 60% reported having a patient who actually committed a violent attack against a third party while in treatment
(Pope & Tabachnick, 1993). Still other researchers suggest that therapists themselves often find themselves as the target of patient violence.
Data from additional national surveys indicate that up to 40% of psychologists were physically attacked by a patient at some point in their
practice (Guy et al., 1990), and that more than 80% of psychologists
received direct threats of patient violence (Tyron, 1986). In response to

such high levels of violence within the context of psychotherapy, practitioners would appear to benefit significantly from high quality instruction on the management of patient violence and aggression.

DEFINITIONS AND ORIGINS

The investigation of patient violence itself is complex. However, a review of basic definitions can help put some aspects of this phenomenon in perspective. Fromm (1996) stated that violence represents only one subtype of aggression, which, at its essence, is a requisite force for human survival. Specifically, Fromm identified three specific types of aggression:

- benign
- pseudo
- malignant

Benign aggression can be thought of as assertive behavior, in which an individual engages in specific behavior that causes no, or limited, negative consequences for others in order to procure basic requirements for survival including food, water, shelter, and in our society, money. Pseudo aggression represents a role-play of behavior that, outside of its specific context (e.g., participation in contact sports; wrestling between father and son; playing practical jokes), would otherwise be considered dangerous or inappropriate in most social settings. Fromm reasoned that psuedo aggression allows individuals to model or practice behavior that they hopefully will not need to employ in daily life, to establish some degree of social status or pecking order, and to release psychological and physical tension and stress.

In contrast, malignant aggression or *violence* is defined by its apparent lack of purpose; its only goal is to cause harm or distress to others in the absence of any material benefit. Patient violence often includes malignant aggression directed toward family members, spouses, and children, as well as employers, government representatives, primary therapists, and staff members. Some individuals may engage in malignant aggression in order to achieve, or attempt to achieve, some degree of psychological pleasure or release, at the clear expense of another human being. Individuals who engage in violent behavior may or may not recognize, acknowledge, or empathize with the plight of their victim. A lack of empathy for one's intended victim is common among patients with antisocial personality disorder or those in the midst of a psychotic episode.

FACTORS THAT PROMOTE VIOLENCE

Although one cannot easily identify all inter and intrapersonal factors that promote violence, a wealth of informative empirical studies and case reports allow therapists to get a basic understanding of some critical features. The following issues all appear to contribute to malignant aggression—otherwise referred to here as patient violence or aggression. These factors include:

1. Social learning. Seminal research by Bandura (e.g., including the Bobo doll study which showed that children are likely to mimic violent behavior in their play after viewing an attractive, adult model; Bandura, Ross, & Ross, 1961), coupled with more recent findings from the APA and AMA (Commission on Violence and Youth, 1993), suggest that many individuals, and particularly children, tend to mimic the violent behavior of other people, including violent individuals on television. A number of factors tend to exacerbate this effect. For a variety of reasons, the media tends to report upon significantly more violent, than altruistic, behavior. Various empirical studies suggest that a greater number of hours spent watching television news coverage is positively linked with increasing, and often distorted, perceptions of violence and danger (Gerbner, 1994), and even physiological desensitization when witnessing future violence (Drabman & Thomas, 1974). The slang commonly used to describe violence in our culture (e.g., road rage; air rage; going postal) appears to be well accepted in our daily lexicon, almost as though it is to be expected. And, the incidence of domestic violence continues to increase; estimates suggest that more than four million women a year will experience such violence first-hand (Berry, 1996).

2. Organicity. A significant factor in the incidence of violent behavior is associated with physical or chemical changes in brain function. For example, a number of medical conditions cause functional changes in the brain that are linked to a decrease in impulse control, executive function, the ability to interpret of other's emotions, and self-awareness. Some of these conditions include seizure disorders, brain tumors, Huntington's chorea, Alzheimer's disease, vascular dementia, malnutrition, urinary tract infections (primarily among elderly adults; e.g., Hillman, 2000), and closed head trauma, including concussions.

3. Situational factors, including the real or perceived experience of loss, rejection, or disrespect. Particularly in relation to workplace violence, rejection from superiors, co-workers, and customers can become especially disturbing and inflammatory. Fears of loss, particularly of job security, raises, promotions, also cause many individuals to experience

a disciplinary action, lay-off, or job termination as a significant narcissistic injury. Because such a job related loss may consciously or unconsciously remind individuals of prior, unresolved losses, a disproportionate amount of distress, anger, and rage may result. Individuals who feel that their rights have been violated or that they have been subject to a lack of respect also may project their anger onto an employer or coworker (e.g., I'll show them they can't do this to me…If they can screw me, I can screw them…I may be going out, but I'm not going out alone"; Miller, 1996; p. 161) and react with a show of violence that cannot be dismissed or ignored (Albrect, 1996).

4. Alterations in mental status. Significant changes in sensation and perception can also lead to an increase in violent behavior. Individuals who manifest psychotic features including delusions, hallucinations, paranoia, and dissociation can be particularly dangerous. A number of mental disorders including bipolar disorder (formerly referred to as manic depression), schizophrenia, substance abuse, and major depression (particularly among elderly adults; see Hillman, 2000) are often associated with significant chronic, episodic, or transient disturbances in reality testing. Interactions and side effects among various prescription and over-the-counter drugs can also lead to significant alterations in perception and mental status.

5. Personality disorders. By definition, a number of Cluster B personality disorders, including antisocial, narcissistic, and borderline disorders, are associated with erratic behavior that often disregards the rights or safety of others (APA, 1994). Although the genesis of personality disorders remains unclear, it is likely that a number of environmental, socio-cultural, and organic factors contribute.

6. Anxiety. Individuals with anxiety disorders, including PTSD, panic disorder, phobic disorder, and dissociative identity disorder, tend to have extreme emotional and physical responses to stress. As noted in Chapter 4, the natural fight or flight response in humans is associated with a series of chemical changes within brain and throughout the body that can reduce sensations of painful stimuli and prepare one's body for the use of explosive bodily movements. Extreme states of anxiety or panic, including those often experienced during dissociative states, also can precipitate violent behavior.

MYTHS ABOUT PATIENT VIOLENCE

It is critical that mental health providers help patients, as well as members of the general public, dispel a variety of myths about patient violence. Some of these myths will be discussed here briefly, and with clinical anecdotes offered for illustration.

Myth #1: You never really know when someone is going to become violent. Most people just lose it one day and "snap!" Contrary to popular belief, the majority of patient (and workplace) violence appears to occur in response to a number of precipitating factors. Consider yourself the last time you got really angry in response to a small, every day event. The relatively insignificant event that may have elicited a disproportionate amount of anger (e.g., having the neighbor's dog go to the bathroom in your yard; forgetting to return an important phone call; misplacing the car keys) often represents the cumulative effect of unresolved anger, anxiety, fear, and frustration in response to other, previous events or personal problems, often including a series of difficult or trying incidents throughout the day or week. Thus, especially in a structured setting, clinicians sometimes can gather enough information via patient interviews or observation from team members (e.g., "Mr. J spent three hours waiting at the cardiac clinic for his appointment, which was ultimately canceled. I think he is very upset...) to intercede before physical violence occurs.

Myth #2: Men continue to be significantly more violent than women; women are at limited risk for serving as the perpetrator of violence. According to recent crime statistics, men and boys do engage in greater numbers of violent behavior, leading to conviction and incarceration. However, particularly among younger age groups, participation in violent acts by women is increasing significantly. A number of factors may account for this dramatic increase in female assailants. Substance abuse, increasing among women and girls, can often precipitate violent behavior. Women and girls also tend to bear the brunt of most domestic abuse; they are intimately familiar with violence. Gangs in both urban and suburban areas now have male and female members who must often perform initiation rites that require physical assault and even murder. In addition, a number of mainstream movies and television shows (e.g., *Thelma and Louise*, *Buffy the Vampire Slayer*) feature female leads who engage in a variety of assertive, aggressive, and violent behavior. In sum, women are surrounded by violence more than ever.

Myth #3: Elderly people aren't dangerous; they're too old and sick, and they probably don't have the strength or energy to hurt anyone anyway. Before exploring this myth that purports that older adults, including those who were violent in their youth, somehow burn out or mellow with age, please consider the following poem authored by a patient in an inpatient forensic unit.

> *TITLE = how many arms have held you*
> How many arms have held you?
> How many lips have touched your's
> Darling please don't tell me
> I really don't want to know
> how many years will go bye?
> Before we will meet again
> Darling I love you
> But this is goodbye—I know
> How long will I remember?
> Your many charms and your cute ways
> How long will I remember
> the times you didn't care
> I will always Remember and Wonder
> How you could have been that way
> But I *will* forget those times
> And always remember the times I thought you cared
> I do not want your pictures
> If I can not have you
> So Goodbye my wonderful Darling
> I will always love you

by XXXXXXXXXXXXXX

When asked to analyze this poem, presented anonymously as part of a class exercise, many college undergraduates hypothesized that the author is an adolescent, developmentally immature, and uneducated (e.g., the incorrect use of "your's charms and cute ways"). Others hypothesized that the author is a male, pining over a break up with an unfaithful girlfriend. Still others ventured that the author engaged in violent behavior against his "wonderful Darling," and that he may have even killed her.

Thus, most students were surprised to learn that the author of this poem was an 83 year-old man engaged in treatment in a forensic inpatient unit for murdering his wife with a tire iron after 60 years of marriage. The author, "Daniel," was 78 years old when he bludgeoned his wife to death with a tire iron as she lay sleeping in bed. From accounts of other family members, Daniel had become increasingly paranoid that his wife was having an affair. He had begun to follow her when she went on errands and attended functions at the local senior center. Although Daniel did not have a history of violent behavior per se, he was a middleweight boxer during his 20's and early 30's. He also worked at a large industrial production plant, and continued to lift weights and engage in daily three-mile runs after his retirement.

A series of psychological tests and evaluations suggested that Daniel was not suffering from dementia, schizophrenia, or substance abuse. He had no sensory impairments, such as hearing or vision loss, that often precede increasing levels of paranoia among elderly adults. He did not show any neuropsychological deficits sometimes associated with boxing (i.e., head injuries). All independent accounts, including reports from police investigators, suggest that Daniel's wife was never involved in an affair. There also were no reports of domestic abuse, and Daniel had no previous criminal record. He drank one or two cans of beer a week, and never appeared to engage in any drinking binges. He was in excellent physical health for a man of his age.

In treatment, Daniel was an active participant in group therapy, as long as the topic does not involve anything about him. Although he became angry and defensive when asked to talk about his reasons for incarceration, Daniel liked to write in his journal, and read selected poems during group sessions. Daniel originally was placed in a medium security prison after he was convicted of second-degree murder, but he was brutalized and beaten by younger inmates. The court then placed him in a psychiatric facility. In sum, this plaintive poem demonstrates that community-living older adults are not devoid of aggressive impulses or violence.

Myth #4: Patients with schizophrenia represent the most violent patients in mental institutions. Most research findings regarding the incidence of patient violence in institutional settings consistently identify elderly adults in long term care (i.e., nursing home residents) as the most violent patient population in institutional settings. An analysis of documented violent incidents at a regional VA medical center (Hillman, 2002), for example, indicates that the 50% of both the patient to patient, and patient to staff assaults took place in extended care units. Half of the staff to patient assaults took place while staff members performed some aspect of primary care (e.g., activities of daily living; ADLs), 25% were associated with significant changes in patient mental status (primarily paranoid delusions and hallucinations), and the remaining 25% were associated with limit setting behavior by staff members. Thirty-five percent of the assaults involved weapons, which typically included environmentally available items such as food trays and chairs. The units with the lowest proportion of patient to patient, and staff to patient assaults were the outpatient counseling and inpatient PTSD units. Those with an intermediate proportion of assaults were the inpatient substance abuse and acute psychiatric units.

A number of reasons may account for this potentially unexpected, large number of violent assaults in nursing home settings. Many older adults in institutional settings are cognitively impaired. They may not understand what a staff member is trying to do when helping them take medicine, bathe, ambulate, or eat. (To reduce the risk of patient distress, staff members can tell their patients with dementia how and why they are going to touch them, before they do so; Hillman, 2000.) Elderly adults with dementia may not typically recognize social prohibitions against hitting, biting, and kicking. (Very young children and psychotic patients can also pose a threat of serious injury to staff members for similar reasons.) Long-term care settings are often understaffed and fraught with high staff turnover; such inconsistencies in staffing can make it difficult for cognitively impaired patients to develop any kind of relationship with their caregivers. Other elderly adults in nursing home settings may be frustrated and about their loss of previous abilities and perceived freedoms, and have limited outlets for its expression. In sum, it is vital to recognize that patient violence does not discriminate by age, sex, psychiatric diagnosis, religion, education, or SES.

IDENTIFYING PREDICTORS OF VIOLENCE

As noted previously, patient violence is never 100% predictable. However, a number of factors have been identified as possible predictors of violence. Although the following sections read somewhat like a laundry list, this type of checklist can help provide a more objective assessment of the risk for patient violence, as well as for general review and training purposes. It also is important to note that the presence of any or even all of these warning signs provides no guarantee that a patient is in danger of becoming imminently violent. Similarly, patients who display none of these signs or indicators may engage in violent activity.

Social History Indicators

Potential precipitants of patient violence based upon their social history and aspects of their current situation include:

1. Past history of violent behavior. Consistent with general social psychological findings, past behavior is typically the best predictor of future behavior. (It also is interesting to note that among a sample of psychiatric inpatients, the presence of any prior violent activity, and

not just recent violent activity, was associated with aggressive inpatient behavior; McNeil & Binder, 1995.) A therapist can simply ask a patient, "What is the most violent thing you have ever done?" It also is helpful to identify the conditions surrounding prior violent actions by establishing when, where, and how they were violent, as well as the intended victim. For example, one therapist felt very anxious about interviewing a convicted murder. When he revealed that he had been violent only toward other men who were police offers, while he was under the influence of alcohol, his therapist was still cautious and somewhat guarded, but she also felt a bit less anxious.

2. Past use of drugs or alcohol (including certain prescription and over-the-counter medications such as Valium, Xanax, and alcohol rich cough syrups).

3. Past use of drugs or alcohol.

4. Arrival from a violent incident involving either the patient or another individual as an intended victim.

5. Ownership of weapons. It also is important to ask patients if they have any weapons with them—right now.

6. Criminal and court records. Because patients may not be reliable reporters for a variety of reasons, criminal records can provide important insight into a patient's past violent activity.

7. A poor driving record, including DUIs, reckless driving, and even manslaughter. To illustrate, one patient admitted to his therapist that he killed his ex-girlfriend's boyfriend. When asked how he did it, he answered simply, "Well, I just ran him over [with my car]. It was pretty easy."

8. Conflicts about one's sexual identity. Homophobia can foster inappropriate behavior toward others, including violent behavior.

9. Unusual or inconsistent work history. Individuals who have recently been fired or laid off, reprimanded, or denied raises or promotion may be at risk for violence. Patients with a sporadic work history may have difficulty with following rules or a schedule, which also poses a potential risk for violence.

10. Social isolation. Self-imposed social isolation may suggest that a patient is severely depressed or that they cannot tolerate a lot of stimulation or interpersonal contact.

11. Medical problems. Chronic pain, high medical bills, depression and anger over a diagnosis (e.g., rage over transmission of the HIV virus from a spouse), and changes in adaptive function can increase the propensity for violence.

12. Service in the military, police, or corrections. Although it is critical to note that membership in the armed forces or the police force

does not necessarily target individuals for risk of violence, some individuals seek out such service because it allows them to discharge already present aggressive or violent impulses, which may sometimes emerge in appropriate behavior. By the nature of the work they perform, these individuals have ready access to a variety of firearms and other weapons. Individuals in these professionals also receive relatively little pay in comparison to the dangerousness of the work they perform. They may also suffer from PTSD or other stress related disorders. Asking patients about their discharge or retirement from service (e.g., were they honorably or dishonorably discharged) can also be helpful.

13. History of physical, sexual, or emotional abuse as a child or adult. Many survivors of abuse suffer serious psychological trauma as a result. The impact may include the formation of PTSD, a lack of trust in many relationships, intense anger and resentment, and even representation in a new cycle of violence.

14. The presence of scars, tattoos, and body piercing. Although this statement may not be considered politically correct, the presence of literal body mutilation may reflect a variety of inter and intrapersonal issues. More specifically, individuals may receive scars from participation in street fights or organized combat. Tattoos also may indicate membership in military units or street gangs.

15. Special bonds or membership in groups formally associated with violence. Street gangs represent a primary example of a group of individuals who engage in coercive tactics to recruit and retain members, and encourage a high tolerance for pain and combat.

16. Developmental problems. Asking patients how they liked school can provide some vital information regarding potential bullying, expulsions, or the presence of undiagnosed learning disorders such as dyslexia or ADHD. Students with learning disorders may have grown up believing that they were "stupid, dumb, or lazy" and incapable of effecting change without the use of physical violence or aggression.

17. Rejection. Rejection by a significant other, peers, authority figures, or employers can provide a catalyst for violent behavior and perceived retribution.

18. Patient feels afraid or trapped. Particularly in institutional settings, patients may feel that they have limited control over what may happen to them, and fear for their own safety. For example, patients may be afraid of "becoming a walking zombie" by use of prescription medication, being seen naked by other patients and staff in public spaces or bathrooms, and losing their confidentiality, freedom, and even their identity.

19. The presence of grief. In response to a personal loss, anger often represents a significant component.

20. Poor language skills or a general inability to communicate. If patients have difficulty articulating their feelings into words, actions may literally be all they have left.

Therapists also tend to overestimate and underestimate certain factors as predictors of future violence and aggression among their patients. For example, a number of therapists were significantly more likely to overestimate the potential risk for violence between versus female, and nonwhite versus white psychiatric inpatients. Recent reports of aggressive behavior before admission to a psychiatric inpatient facility also led clinicians to underestimate those patients' risks for violence when compared to patients who engaged in violent acts long before their admission (McNeil & Binder, 1995).

Mental Status Indicators

Various alterations in a patient's mental status may pose a significant risk for violent behavior. (See Chapter 3 for a comprehensive review of the mental status exam.) Some of the most vital indicators to assess and *clearly document* include:

1. Homicidal ideation, intent, and plan. When performing any clinical assessment, it is important to ask patients if they ever think about physically injuring or killing someone. Each aspect (i.e., ideation, intent, plan) must be noted in the Thought Content section. The use of patient quotes also is recommended. For example: + Homicidal ideation (Pt. reports thinking about killing her ex-husband obsessively; "I just think about killing him all day, like I just can't get it out of my mind even if I try.) +Homicidal plan (Pt. indicates that she has a loaded shotgun under her bed at home); −Homicidal intent (Pt. reports that she is "afraid of going to jail and not being able to see my kids").

2. A/V hallucinations, delusions, or paranoid ideation. The presence of impaired reality testing can pose a significant threat for violence, and should be extensively documented. Descriptions of specific content and frequency should be identified, typically including commentary with the patient's own words. For example: +auditory hallucinations (pt. reports persistent command hallucinations; "the voices tell me to kill the lady at the subway booth because she is Mary Magdeline... They tell me to do it all day, and even when I try to go to sleep".

3. Dissociative symptoms. Depersonalization and derealization also pose a significant, potential risk. For example: +depersonalization

("I don't feel like myself; I feel outside of myself, like I am just going through the motion like a robot; someone else seems to be pulling my strings").

4. Impulse control. If a patient has limited or poor impulse control, it becomes vital to document the areas in which the patient has diminished control, and provide specific details when possible. For example: patient reports poor impulse control over his sexual impulses, especially when drinking or engaging in elicit drug use.

5. Vegetative symptoms. A constellation of specific vegetative symptoms also poses a risk for danger. For example, problems with, or changes in: sleep (insomnia early, morning, late), energy, psychomotor activity (i.e., agitation, shaking), somatic symptoms (e.g., headache, diarrhea, frequent urination, facial flushing, sweating, dizziness, increased respiration, cool extremities).

6. General descriptors/behavioral observations. Other potential indicators for patient violence include a tone of voice that is either very soft or very loud, extreme eye contact (i.e., staring or averting gaze), a lack of spontaneous conversation, clenched fists, stomping, pacing, and issuing ultimatums. Patients who have difficulty in establishing an initial therapeutic alliance and working collaboratively with their therapists also are more likely to engage in patient violence (Beauford, McNeil, & Binder, 1997).

RISK MANAGEMENT

A number of critical legal issues exist regarding the determination of a patient's potential for violence. Consider the situation in which a patient announces, "Yep. When I get out of here [an inpatient facility] I am going to settle some shit with my ex-boyfriend...I can't believe he turned me in and he got off scot-free. I'm going to make him pay for this...I still have my 22 [caliber gun] stashed in my kitchen drawer. There's no way he could have found it. I'm going to fucking kill him, and I really mean it this time." It appears that this patient presents with positive homicidal ideation, intent, and plan, coupled with a specific, identifiable target for that violence.

When a patient presents such imminent danger to an identifiable victim, practitioners often must consider their prescribed duty to warn or protect that potential victim. Unfortunately, no one set of rules can be used to easily guide therapists' actions; individual states' (as well as individual Canadian provinces') laws and statutes often differ significantly from one another. Thus, as noted in the APA ethical standards

(APA, 1992), it remains essential for a therapist to become familiar with the laws and provisions in one's own state or province. In addition, ignorance of one's state laws and guidelines cannot be used as protection against ethical or legal violations (VandeCreek & Knapp, 2000).

Tarasoff and the Duty to Protect

Most practitioners are familiar with the case of "Tarasoff" (1976), in which a college student at U.C. Berkeley, Projenit Poddar, sought treatment at a counseling center after becoming depressed when a fellow student, Tatiana Tarasoff, spurned his romantic advances. Projenit confided in his therapist about his plans to kill Tatiana when she returned to campus in the fall, and his therapist responded with a failed attempt at involuntary hospitalization. (When police were called to implement the psychiatric commitment, they did not follow through.) Projenit also refused to attend any more therapy sessions after his therapist attempted to place him in the hospital involuntarily. When Tatiana returned to Berkeley in the fall, she had no idea that Projenit was plotting to kill her. A few weeks later, Projenit did kill Tatiana, and her parents then raised a wrongful death suit against the University, various members of the Counseling Center, and the local police. When the Tarasoff case went to the California Supreme Court, the court ruled that Projenit's therapist was at fault for not warning his intended victim. In effect, the court ruled that mental health practitioners have "a duty to [warn and] protect identifiable targets from imminent danger coming from their patients" (VandeCreek & Knapp, 2000: p. 1337).

Because the Tarasoff statute has not been adopted by all states, as noted previously, practitioners must become aware of their own state's unique variants on this protective theme. For example, current statutes in Vermont suggest that imminent threats of property damage also may elicit a therapist's duty to warn if that property damage could easily involve a loss of life (e.g., arson). Still other states' statutes (e.g., Florida; Virginia) have ruled against a therapist's duty to protect, effectively stating that a therapist has no legal duty to control the behavior of her patients. And still other states have no readily identifiable statutes related to Tarasoff (i.e., the duty to protect and warn.) Unfortunately, recent studies suggest that therapists may not follow duty-to-protect statutes in accordance with specified laws (e.g., McNeil, Binder, & Fulton, 1998). Thus, experts suggest that, particularly in those states in which no clear guidelines are available, practitioners should err on the side of caution and warn third parties about imminent danger. In only rare cases have therapists been found liable for making an honest attempt to protect a third party from imminent patient violence (VandeCreek & Knapp, 2000).

General Guidelines

Other experts note that making the appropriate ethical and legal decision to warn a third party of imminent patient violence alone does not exonerate therapists from legal liability. (One way to avoid additional complications in one's duty to warn is to inform patients at the beginning of treatment, as a matter of consent, that it is the therapist's obligation to report or prevent patient acts that are intended to harm another—so that patients do not feel tricked or betrayed if a discussion of future, violent actions does ensue.) A variety of additional factors, including treatment planning, implementation, and documentation are critical in providing a legally acceptable standard of care. Fortunately, a number of forensic experts present comprehensive yet concise guidelines for appropriate risk management (e.g., VandeCreek & Knapp, 2000). Therapists are advised to follow a step-wise process in order to satisfy Tarasoff related responsibilities (see Appelbaum, 1985).

Table 2 presents general guidelines that can be used to engage such a step-wise process and provide "minimally accepted standards of care." Therapists also should recognize that the justice system does not

TABLE 2. Risk Management Guidelines for Patient Violence

1. Become knowledgeable of state and federal laws, statutes, and regulations as they pertain to patient confidentiality and the duty to protect.
2. Conduct a thorough evaluation of patient dangerousness.
   a. interview the patient directly
   b. request and obtain past psychological, medical, and criminal records
   c. interview the patient's significant others, if warranted
3. If a risk of imminent danger exists, develop an appropriate and reasonable treatment plan.
   a. develop a plan consistent with acceptable professional standards
   b. consider the potential of traditional mental health treatment (e.g., inpatient hospitalization) as opposed to the automatic assumption that a warning has to be made (if not required by law)?
   c. Seek clinical consultation if needed
4. Implement the treatment plan appropriately.
   a. modify the treatment plan as circumstances change
   b. notify third parties without the patient's consent if necessary to reduce the likelihood violence.
   c. provide appropriate follow-up
   d. document all activities

Note. From VandeCreek and Knapp (2000). Adapted with permission by John Wiley & Sons, Inc.

expect mental health providers to predict patient violence with 100% accuracy! Rather, therapists are required only to demonstrate acceptable (versus substandard) professional judgment when making those decisions (Litwack, Kirschner, & Wack, 1993).

The first step is for a therapist to assess the *imminent danger of patient violence*. Legal statutes suggest that, at a minimum, therapists are required to interview the patient directly, and be sure to ask specific questions about the presence of previous violent behavior and current homicidal ideation, intent, and plans. In addition, various statutes indicate that therapists also are required to request and receive past patient records, which may include psychological, medical, and criminal records. In addition, various statutes suggest that therapists are required (in the interest of demonstrating appropriate standards of professional care) to interview the patient's significant others when threats of violence emerge. Studies have shown that approximately half of all targeted individuals for patient violence are adult family members (McNeil, Binder, & Fulton, 1998). Despite the need to undertake these aforementioned measures, however Tarasoff statutes do not require therapists to "interrogate their clients [or] conduct independent investigations (p. 1337)" in order to determine the identity of an intended victim (VandeCreek & Knapp, 2000).

The second step in the process is to formulate an appropriate and reasonable treatment plan. The goal of that treatment plan would be to diffuse or reduce the likelihood of violence (Appelbaum, 1985; VandeCreek & Knapp, 2000). As noted by various forensic experts (VandeCreek & Knapp, 2000), protecting an identified target from harm might be accomplished by engaging in *one or more* of the following activities, where permitted by state law:

- warning the intended victim (required in states with duty-to-protect statutes)
- notifying someone who will notify the intended victim
- notifying the police
- undertake voluntary or involuntary hospitalization for the patient
- engaging the patient in a structured environment (e.g., a partial hospitalization program)
- increasing the frequency and intensity of outpatient therapy
- including the person targeted for violence in psychotherapy, especially if the targeted individual and patient are related.

Because no empirical evidence is available to suggest that warning a potential target of violence about a threat is no more effective in preventing violence than inpatient hospitalization, the initiation of psychotropic medication, or traditional psychotherapy, therapists who feel that informing the victim may actually inflame the potential for violence (in states which do not have formal duty to protect statutes) may consider hospitalizing the patient or intensifying treatment (e.g., Monahan, 1993).

Many therapists are less familiar with the legal obligations and statutes related to the third step of the process, *implementing the treatment plan.* Therapists who use appropriate professional standards when assessing patient violence and developing a treatment plan still may be liable if they do not engage the treatment plan properly (i.e., as intended; in a reasonable manner). For example, a therapist who warns an intended victim about a patient's intent to harm them may encounter a potential target who vehemently denies or minimizes their risk of danger. In such a situation, sending a certified letter to the individual targeted for violence can be helpful in conveying that message more directly, as well as in demonstrating to the court, if necessary, that the intended victim was warned clearly and sufficiently (VandeCreek & Knapp, 2000).

When a patient is admitted for voluntary or involuntary hospitalization in response to threats of imminent violence, the therapist's responsibility does not end when his patient crosses the threshold into the inpatient unit. The patient's therapist is expected to provide all relevant hospital staff with clear, direct, and specific information about the patient's threat of violence, including the overall seriousness of the threat (VandeCreek & Knapp, 2000). Additionally, therapists must continually assess a patient's potential for violence regardless of the immediate intervention selected, and update treatment plans and subsequent interventions as needed. Clear and timely documentation including the use of patient quotes to illustrate the presence of homicidal ideation, intent, or plan, and a review of the therapist's decision making process (including a brief rationale of why one treatment option was selected whereas another was rejected; Beck & Schouten, 2000) also remains essential, and can be employed using the SOAP model (Weed, 1971; see Chapter 3).

From a more clinical, as opposed to legal, perspective, implementing the treatment plan does not occur in a vacuum. It appears that the best outcomes, in which patients do not follow through on plans to inflict harm upon their intended victims, are more likely to occur when patients and therapists work collaboratively, and share specific information about any third party notification. Certainly, many patients do not want their therapist to warn their intended target of violence, and as a result become angry, reticent, avoidant, or even terminate the therapeutic relationship. Studies suggest, however, that therapists who inform patients about their legal obligation as a mental health provider, and attempt to obtain consent from their patient before issuing third party warnings are significantly more likely to keep a patient in treatment, even if that patient initially becomes angry (Binder & McNeil, 1996). For those patients who do not consent to a third party notification or warning, asking them to sit (with the therapist) while phone calls are made and letters are written can help patients feel that they are not victim to secretive or factious treatment interventions (e.g., Beck, 1982; Sells, 2001; VandeCreek & Knapp, 2000), or "being talked about behind their backs."

In addition to issuing warnings (if deemed necessary), therapists and patients should work together to identify precipitating factors of violence, which may include drug or alcohol use, fights with a spouse over financial matters, visits to a club where a previous lover can often be seen with a new love interest, or any number of things. Therapists and patient also should work together to identify alternative behaviors to violence, and develop concrete plans for implementing those socially acceptable coping behaviors during particular times of stress. Just as with threats of patient suicide, therapists also can help patients recognize the realistic outcomes of their behavior, which may include jail time, disdain from friends and family members, fines, lawsuits, a permanent record, an inability to obtain work in various jobs, fears about being punished for one's actions via religious beliefs, ruining the lives of innocent others in addition to the intended victim, nightmares, concerns about retribution, and feelings of guilt and shame.

CLINICAL INTUITION: FACT OR FICTION

Another tool for assessing the potential risk for patient violence is clinical intuition. It may be described as a gut feeling or even as a variant of projective identification. Some clinicians dismiss this ability outright, whereas others suggest that psychotherapy is as much an art as it is a science. However, recent insights from social and neuropsychology (e.g., Lieberman, 2000; Whalen, Rauch, Etcoff, McInerney, Lee, & Jenike, 1998) suggest that clinical intuition may represent an actual, if not always accurate, phenomenon in some specific cases.

Consider the following. Researchers conclude generally that an individual's first impression of a person or project can be distilled into a simple linear equation: Interpersonal impact = verbal communication + vocal communication + non-verbal communication (c.f., Mahl,

1987). In other words, people's first impressions are not just based
upon what someone says, but upon how they say it, and how they look
while they are saying it. A host of empirical studies confirm that many
of evaluations we make about people are based upon non-verbal cues
such as height, weight, attractiveness, clothing, and even a male or
female surname (e.g., Zuckerman, Miyake, & Elkin, 1995).

More importantly, however, many of these studies suggest that the
vast majority of individuals who make such differential ratings are
not even aware (i.e., conscious) of the factors that influenced their
judgment (e.g., Phelps, O'Connor, Cunningham, Funayama, Gatenby,
Gore, & Banaji, 2000). To add to this conundrum of unconscious influence, our emphasis upon nonverbal and vocal cues also is likely to
increase with one's level of anxiety and stress. Thus, the more anxious
a patient or therapist becomes, the less likely either is to focus upon the
content of what is being said. Patients in extreme distress may not even
be able to process the meaning of words.

Neuropsychological Support

Although some neuropsychologists posit that brain function is not
as localized as once believed, most agree that structures in the frontal
lobes and prefrontal cortex are generally responsible for man's ability
to plan, imagine, empathize, perceive danger, and perceive emotions
(Damasio, 1994). Recent empirical studies suggest specifically that the
amygdala (Whalen et al., 1998), the insula (particularly in the right
hemisphere), and other limbic structures (Damasio, 1994) may help
account for the "gut feelings" we experience when asked to view a disturbing picture (Damasio, 1994), attempt to determine if someone is
being truthful (Whalen et al., 1998), and ponder ethical and moral
dilemmas (Green, Sommerville, Mystrom, Darley, & Cohen, 2001).

One explanation for the presence of clinical intuition is that the
right temporal lobe of the brain recognizes various kinds of non-verbal
and vocal cues during interpersonal interactions, while the left brain
typically focuses conscious attention upon the logical arguments and
sequences typically associated with language. Because the right
hemisphere itself is not typically capable of language production (see
Springer & Deutsch, 1993 for a review of split-brain research), it may
attempt to convey this important piece of clinically relevant information using what it has available—somatic changes (e.g., Damasio, 1994;
Phelps et al., 2000; Whalen et al., 1998). Thus, a therapist may experience this somatic "message" from the right hemisphere's insula, amygdala, and prefrontal cortex as a strange sensation, a funny feeling,

generalized anxiety, fleeting nausea, or even "the raising of hairs" on the back of one's neck. (It also is possible that the controversial notion of projective identification may be manifestation of such right hemispheric activation in response to a patient's non-verbal and vocal cues.) In sum, clinicians who get some kind of "gut feeling" in work with a patient may do well to at least explore the reasons why their various right hemispheric brain structures are presenting such a quiet signal of alarm.

Randy. A psychology intern was asked to provide neuropsychological testing for a 45 year-old, single white army veteran. When Mr. X (who preferred to be addressed as "Randy") arrived for his appointment, his diminutive stature and frail appearance struck the examiner as surprising for someone in military service. Randy said that he had been an investment counselor, but that he had been laid off, and that he had lived with his mother for the past seven years. He said that he "just couldn't get it together," and described a history of alcohol and amphetamine abuse. Randy also reported that he did not have a girlfriend right now because he wanted to focus on "getting better."

Randy was quite cooperative during the testing. He engaged in spontaneous conversation that focused primarily upon concerns about his test performance, and made apologies for not "going faster." He also thanked the examiner repeatedly for making sure his appointment was on time. Randy's speech was somewhat rapid, and his hands often shook when he was asked to assemble puzzle pieces or manipulate objects.

Despite Randy's innocuous clinical presentation and cooperative nature, the examiner began to experience some disconcerting thoughts and feelings. She began to worry about whether her colleague was next door in her office, or out on a coffee or lunch break. Her heart started to race as they finished the testing protocol, despite admonitions to herself to "settle down" because she was "just imagining things" and "feeling kind of creepy" without other people being around in the older building.

Three weeks later, the psychiatrist on Randy's unit reported in an intern meeting that Randy was in some serious legal trouble. Randy's mother had become increasingly annoyed with her son's behavior; he had put a large padlock on his bedroom door, and would not allow her any access or explain the reason for the lock. He also failed to contribute financially for his room and board, and expected his mother to cook and clean for him. After seeking counseling herself, Randy's mother told him that he would have to move out and "begin to take responsibility for himself as an adult." Randy became angry, and broke some dishes on the kitchen floor. He spent the next two weeks sleeping on the porch, begging his mother to let him return to the house.

When Randy's mother formally evicted him from the premises, the police had to be called to remove him from the premises. Upon her request, they removed the padlock from Randy's bedroom door, and found a collection of more than 13 illegally modified semi-automatic guns with silencers, and a large number of hollow tip or exploding (i.e., "cop killing") bullets. The police also confiscated more than 300 pornographic videos including a large number of sado-masochistic and snuff films. Although Randy had not engaged in any violent behavior, nor did he profess any homicidal intent, the circumstances surrounding his eviction from his mother's home certainly are suspicious. More important to a discussion of patient violence, the intern on this case gained a greater sense of confidence in her clinical instincts and intuition.

Relationship to Therapist Safety

This psychology intern also recognized the need to be honest with herself about her level of comfort with certain patients. She also was empowered to insist upon performing patient evaluations only if another staff member were present in the wing of her office building. (She often was the only therapist on the floor, but her supervisor had stated, "Well, if these patients can get permission to leave their own units, they can't be all that dangerous!) Thus, all clinicians, including those who are quite experienced as well those in training, should feel comfortable in following their own instincts, particularly if it enhances their own sense of personal safety. Clinicians should not need the benefit of a police report or other "proof" to legitimize their intuition, or to generate the feeling of entitlement needed to ask for safe working conditions. Yet, it also is important to note that limited empirical evidence is available to suggest that clinical intuition has any formal "success rate;" care must be taken to view intuition in consort with other known, empirically validated predictors of patient violence.

Other matters for therapists to consider in fostering a safe work environment include the use of prewired "panic buttons" and alarm systems in private or group settings, taking advantage of self-defense classes and training offered at work or in the community (without developing a false sense of mastery), working in teams, and becoming familiar with all therapists and staff members. One therapist described being in session with a patient when he suddenly grabbed her, threw her to the floor, and began to tear at her clothes. Even though it was after hours, the janitor on duty heard her screams, recognized her voice, and came immediately to her aid. Upon later discussion, the janitor very honestly admitted that if he were not familiar with the therapist's voice (and presumably in a respectful, collegial relationship with her), he may have hesitated before deciding to investigate.

VIOLENCE PREVENTION

It always is preferable to prevent violence rather than respond to it. Prevention in any mental health setting is essential. Unfortunately, many staff members in inpatient settings (including mental health professionals) are unaware that many of their own behaviors foster patient distress and increase the potential for violence.

- Staff members who walk around a unit, jangling their keys, only remind patients that they have control over their access to the outside world and as well as to a variety of privileges.
- Not following through on promises of patient privileges also can incite patient frustration and violence. For example, patients may become extremely, and often justifiably, frustrated when staff members make false promises to let them take a cigarette break "a little later," that "the doctor will be here any minute," or that they "will probably go home tomorrow." Although such frustration certainly does not excuse any violent behavior, such empty promises by staff members can inflame many patients who already have limited impulse control to violence.
- In contrast, ignoring inappropriate patient behavior (i.e., not setting limits), in an attempt to appease certain patients or avoid patient-staff conflict, can also engender patient violence. In many cases, patients' behavior often escalates until they meet with resistance. It is as though patients need and want structure and limits, coupled with staff members who are, or who at least appear to be, confident enough to enforce those limits.
- Patient violence often can be averted via a clear discussion of boundaries and limits in the therapeutic relationship. When a patient discusses their prior violent activities, therapists can simply state that violent behavior, in any shape or form, in unacceptable in a working, therapeutic relationship.
- Therapists can enlist their patient in a structured discussion about acknowledging and discussing any problems or concerns in the relationship *before* they escalate to violence. In other

words, a therapist can tell his patient, "if you become upset or angry, even a little bit, I expect you to tell me about it so that we can work on the problem together before it starts to feel like it is getting out of control."

Therapists also can be honest with patients if they need additional supervision, (e.g., in a forensic setting) or choose to keep an office door open during sessions or assessments, stating, "I also need to feel safe in order to do my job properly. But, we can certainly talk about what it is like for you when I have to do that [set these kind of limits or engage in such preventive measures.]" Such clear messages let patients know that firm limits exist within the context of the therapeutic relationship, but that their therapist is willing and able to discuss a variety of topics with them, including aggressive urges and interpersonal conflict. Patients also benefit from clear articulations that their therapist is able and willing to assert her own needs for personal safety.

WHEN PATIENT VIOLENCE IS IMMINENT: GUIDES TO INTERVENTION

In some instances, despite a host of preventive measures, patient violence may seem imminent (e.g., an actively psychotic patient believes that her therapist is possessed by the devil and must be killed). Fortunately, a number of tactics can be employed in an attempt to deflect, or at least respond effectively, to patient violence. A number of behavioral management techniques available for use in a variety of clinical settings will be discussed. Many of these interventions are applicable in unit or other institutional settings. It also is important to acknowledge that a therapeutic response to patient aggression will be quite different if the event occurs outside of a structured, or even semi-structured, setting. For example, therapists who expect to experience patient violence in an uncontrolled, unstructured, or unfamiliar setting (e.g., a patient's home, neighborhood, or workplace), as is typical in wrap around services and mobile crisis intervention, are advised to act defensively and remove themselves from the immediate environment. Therapists cannot treat a patient if they themselves are injured or in danger.

Nonverbal Communications

1. Assemble a security team. Seek help or get advice from other professionals and staff members. In even simpler terms, don't try to be a hero.

2. Monitor your own physiological response to stress. Acknowledge changes in breathing, heart rate, and perception. Stop for a moment and breathe deeply and evenly.
3. Focus upon a specific plan.
4. If at all possible, obtain a detailed patient history.
5. Remove all potential weapons from the immediate area. Also consider that tables, chairs, food trays, pencils, hangers, and glass from [broken] windows often serve as weapons for patients, as well as more traditional weapons such as guns and knives.
6. Get the person who has the best rapport with the patient to approach them. Note that this individual may be a licensed mental health provider, a nurse, staff aid, receptionist, or cleaning person. Using an authoritarian figure (e.g., a staff administrator) to make initial contact typically is not helpful.
7. Approach the person slowly at a 45 degree angle. As evidenced in animal models, approaching an anxious organism directly can be perceived as a direct challenge to fight.
8. Never turn your back on a potentially violent patient.
9. Stay between the patient and the door, but do not block their exit or make them feel cornered.
10. Stand far enough away from the patient so that you are out of their immediate reach (i.e., at arms length), but not so far away that you need to talk loudly. Standing too far away can project an impression of significant fear, and may give patients the sense that they are almost expected to be violent.
11. Keep your posture open and non-confrontational. For example, stand with your knees slightly bent, and your feet a shoulder width apart. Also keep your hands open at waist level. This non-verbal communication suggests that you (literally) are not hiding anything or being deceitful. Self-defense experts also recommend this "T-stance" because it allows for easy shifting of body weight for escape or defensive body movements.
12. Move evenly and slowly. Do not make any sudden movements.
13. Make the situation private. Remove all bystanders to avoid engaging additional potential assailants and victims, and to remove social demands for patients to follow through on any threats made in front of other patients. Removing bystanders also tends to decrease the heightened arousal associated with an audience (for both patients and staff members) and can allow patients to save face.

14. Relate to patients at eye level. If a patient is standing, talk to them while standing. If a patient is sitting, sit across from them while talking. In non-verbal terms, patients should regard any communication as emanating from someone of equal, rather than superior or inferior, status.

15. Maintain eye contact but do not stare. Such persistent eye contact can be interpreted non-verbally as a direct threat.

16. Remove watches, pagers, rings, nametags, earrings, necklaces, ties, bracelets, and high heels. These items could be used as weapons, or allow a patient to grab onto you.

17. Observe universal health precautions to avoid potential contact with HIV, hepatitis, and other infectious diseases (e.g., put Band-Aids on small cuts and scratches).

18. Keep track of all personal materials including matches, pens, and pencils.

19. Remove sources of outside stimulation, including radios, TVs, and bright lights. In some institutional settings, unbalanced florescent lights may emit a consistent, buzzing sound. Sometimes simply turning off the overhead lights (during daylight hours, of course) can alleviate a significant source of patient stress or irritation.

20. Do not touch the patient unless absolutely necessary. Any violation of personal boundaries can be misinterpreted as a violent act.

21. Be aware of your own feelings, which may include anger, fear, and excitement. Note that any emotional response to a stressful situation is entirely normal.

Verbal and Vocal Considerations

1. Even under normal conditions, most people respond more to someone's tone of voice than to their actual message (e.g., Mahl, 1987). Thus, when patients are agitated or upset, speak in a low, slow, soft tone. Studies also show that people attribute greater power and authority to individuals who talk in a soft voice; they project the impression that what they are saying is so important that others will become quiet in order to listen.

2. Introduce yourself. Tell the patient your name and function.

3. Use the patient's name. Specifically, ask them how they would like to be called or addressed. This procedure is twofold. First, it shows the patient that they are acknowledged as

an individual, second, it helps focus their attention and increases a sense of personal accountability.

4. Attempt to understand why a patient is violent (e.g., identify the precipitating factors.) Asking a patient directly, "Can you tell me what is making you so angry and upset?" or "Alice, you look angry to me. Can you tell me what is going on?" is often helpful. For example, a male patient who was overturning chairs and tables in a unit lounge responded that he was furious that he could not climax through masturbation due to side effects from his antipsychotic medication (see Hillman, 1999). Scheduling an appointment with his psychiatrist for later in the day promptly ended his violent behavior.

5. Tell them you are there to help; "I am here because I want to help you. Is there anything I can do for you?"

6. Listen without interrupting.

7. Use reflective listening, but be careful not to patronize a patient by appearing to only parrot their statements.

8. Apologize if necessary (e.g., "I'm sorry that no one was there for your appointment; I'm sorry that the nurses didn't get the correct information that you have increased privileges during the last shift change").

9. Avoid analyzing their motivation.

10. Avoid laughter. Although this point is rather obvious, some individuals do engage in nervous laughter.

11. Don't ramble on.

12. Do not give advice (e.g., If I were you I would ...). Instead, give options or make suggestions: "In my professional opinion, I think between [X, Y, and Z], a good option would be to ..." and "As your therapist, I can only advise you about a good choice of action. What you do is completely up to you." In other words, do not personalize the advice, or make a patient think that they are doing something to please someone else, which may engender psychological reactance.

13. Focus on the here-and-now. For example, statements such as, "OK, here he goes again" or "You did this last week, you know?" generally are not helpful.

14. Do not talk about the patient to other staff members or patients as if they were not there. It is perceived as insulting and degrading. It also suggests to a patient that they have limited control over their own actions.

15. If a patient tells you, "I think I am going to lose control right about now" or "I'm going to choke the shit out of you if you

don't get out of my room" these threats must be taken seriously. If no serious consequences are apparent, it is best to terminate contact temporarily and reevaluate the situation.

16. Make requests first, then commands or demands. When asking patients to do something, use their name and engage in normal social conventions (e.g., say "please.")

17. Only make a demand if you have the ability to back it up, typically with the support of an on-site emergency response team. As one clinical supervisor liked to state, "Don't let your mouth write checks that your body can't cash." Sometimes a collection of emergency support personnel allows patients to recognize the seriousness of their situation. Also remember that patients probably know if and when their therapist or a response team member is "bluffing."

18. If a patient is doing something inappropriate, or will not comply with a specific request, state exactly what they are doing and why it is appropriate.

19. Offer specific alternatives to violence. These may include:
    a. gross motor movement (swimming, walking, playing individual sports)
    b. providing quiet seclusion (remove irritating stimulation)
    c. meeting any reasonable demands
    d. just sitting quietly with another staff member
    e. food choices such as a milkshake, crackers, or a cool drink

20. Without giving an ultimatum, offer choices and limits (e.g., The decision is up to you … you can go to your room or talk this out, and you will keep all of your privileges, or you can continue to throw chairs here in the lounge and have your smoking privileges revoked.

21. If possible, give the patient time to calm down (e.g., I'll give you 20 minutes to think over what you would like to do. It's your choice to make.) However, be careful that the amount of time given for consideration is not too short or too long, in order to avoid frustration as well as boredom.

A Last Resort: Physical Intervention

If a patient will not comply with requests or demands to engage in safe, appropriate behavior, it is important to enforce appropriate limits and consequences, but not in a spirit of anger, punishment, or revenge. Many therapists elect to call emergency support teams to provide physical support so that they themselves do not have to physically exert control over a patient, and risk acting out in response to heightened emotions.

It also is critical to note that physical intervention represents a *last resort* in the management of patient violence. In most cases, the first attempt to minimize violent behavior is to ask a patient to move themselves, under their own power, into a quiet seclusion room for a specified period of time, often in order to "help them calm down and think about what they think might help make the situation better." If this approach fails, staff may inform that patient that because they chose to continue to engage in their violent behavior, staff members will approach you to take you to the seclusion room. Any time a staff member who attempts to restrain or move a patient should have institutional training and approval.

If a patient continues to engage in violent or self-injurious behavior in a quiet setting or seclusion room, staff members may choose to inform them that "if you are having this much difficulty controlling yourself right now, we will have to use restraints to prevent you from hurting yourself. We are doing this to help *you* regain better control over yourself and what you are doing." Patients should be treated with respect at all times, and told calmly and specifically about what is going to happen via any physical contact. Informing patients about the specific plan for the use of physical restraint is often helpful, even, and sometimes especially, if patients appear unresponsive or psychotic.

A common mistake made by staff members and therapists who must resort to the use of physical restraints is that they may inadvertently take both the sense of emotional and physical control away from the patient. For example, one training manual used in a community-based center suggested the use of statements such as "If you can't handle yourself right now, we will help you to do that," which could be misconstrued easily by patients as "If you can't handle yourself right now, we will do it *for you*." Staff members who may not receive advanced training in the use of restraints or psychological intervention may also make such inappropriate statements. Although this focus upon semantics may seem obsessive, conveying to patients a sense of dignity, control, self-efficacy, and expectations for calm, rational behavior is critical during potentially violent situations.

Every state has general guidelines for the use of physical restraints. Their use is considered a last resort, and most states and institutions require constant staff monitoring, physician approval within 15 or 30 minutes, and additional requests for the use of restraints after an initial hour-long period. (It also is helpful for staff members to relay this information to patients to help keep them informed about the procedure, and to give them some sense of predictability and control.) Thus, therapists should become familiar with the specific requirements of their clinical setting and their state.

As an absolute last resort, sedation may be used to prevent patients from harming themselves or others. The use of prescription medication to sedate patients, including those who are not posing an immediate threat to self or other, is criticized widely, particularly in geriatric settings. Some reports describe psychiatric units in which "unruly" or loud patients receive medication to help them "sleep" or calm down. Although this may certainly reduce the number of behavioral problems for staff members and ostensibly create a calmer atmosphere on the unit, the involuntary use of sedatives remains antithetical to the basic premise of therapy, in which patients are helped to gain insight into and control over their own actions.

However, some situations do exist in which the use of sedatives appears to be appropriate. For example, one 310-pound patient, "Brian," diagnosed with paranoid schizophrenia, was brought into an acute inpatient psychiatric unit in four point restraints. Previously, he had been living in a local group home, and had attacked three residents and the director of the facility with a steak knife. Staff members at the group home reasoned that Brain had not been compliant with his medication regimen, and had become actively psychotic, with intense paranoid delusions. Upon admission to a local ER, Brian bit a nurse with such force on her arm that he crushed both bones in her wrist and caused extensive nerve damage. Brain would not release his grip on her arm, even when a new nursing assistant hit him on the head with a gas canister (which is absolutely inappropriate in any setting). He only loosened his grip when he received more than 100 mg of Haldol. Subsequently, Brian responded well to medication and group therapy. He agreed to receive monthly IM injections to increase his medication compliance.

SUMMARY

In sum, therapists must be cognizant of the risks of patient violence. It is imperative for practitioners to become familiar with state and federal laws regarding patient confidentiality as well as any legal statutes regarding the duty to protect potential victims. Documentation of patient mental status and social history appears critical in making and supporting competent professional decisions. Recent scientific evidence suggests that one's clinical intuition may serve as a very real indicator of a patient's potential for violence. Preventing violence is clearly superior to responding to patient violence. Institutional factors and conditions that arouse patient frustration and aggression also need to be examined. At all times, an emphasis should be placed upon the patient's ability to regain control of themselves and their own actions. The use of physical restraints should be used as a last resort, but may be essential if others (including the patient herself) are in imminent physical danger and previous attempts to deescalate the situation without the use of force have failed. As in most other aspects of crisis intervention, therapists can only help their patients if they themselves remain safe.

8

Helping Therapists Cope
Patient Suicide and Burnout

Two of the most significant occupational hazards for mental health professionals are patient suicide and burnout. Recent statistics suggest that throughout their career, therapists have a one in four chance of having a patient in treatment actually kill themselves.

Although work in mental health can serve as one of the most personally rewarding of professions, it also can be relatively low in pay, and fraught with the potential for violence. Clinical work also can, at certain times and in certain settings, require long evening and weekend hours, excessive attention to insurance companies' paperwork, 24 hour availability for patient emergencies, an acceptance of slow or sporadic progress (e.g., consider a patient suffering from paranoid schizophrenia who is not compliant with her anti-psychotic medication), long periods of intense mental concentration, legal consultations, and the management of profound countertransference. Therapists also must consider the very real possibility that a patient under their care may attempt or successfully commit suicide.

WHEN A PATIENT COMMITS SUICIDE

Patient suicide is one of the primary occupational hazards for mental health providers. A series of epidemiological studies suggest that mental health practitioners are at relatively high risk for having a patient commit suicide (Chemtob, Bauer, Hamada, & Pelowski, 1989). A survey of more than 350 psychologists revealed that 22% had a patient who completed suicide while in treatment. A search for personal and professional characteristics that could be used differentiate between the therapists who had a patient commit suicide versus those that did not revealed some clear, but surprising, findings (Chemtob et al., 1989). First, the researchers found that therapist age, sex, and years in practice were unrelated to the experience of patient suicide. In contrast, one singular factor had significant predictive power in assessing which therapists had a patient kill herself: level of training. Therapists with lower levels of formal education and training were significantly more likely to have a patient commit suicide than their colleagues with more advanced degrees.

Specifically, therapists with post-doctoral training had a 10% rate of patient suicide, Ph.D. level therapists had a 26% rate, and Masters level therapists had a 32% rate of patient suicide. Translated into odds ratios, therapists in general can expect a 1 in 5 chance that they will have a patient kill himself. In comparison, Post-doctoral therapists have only 1 in 10 odds, Ph.D.s have approximately 1 in 4 odds, and Masters level therapists have nearly a 1 in 3 chance of experiencing a patient suicide. Of course, it is easy to make the assumption that increased levels of training and education bestow superior clinical skills in assessment and therapy, and effectively serve to prevent patient suicide. However, because this finding represents only an observed, one must also consider that this difference in training and education is actually liked to another, separate factor that is related to suicide risk.

Another likely hypothesis is that therapists with post doctoral or doctoral degrees are more likely to be in private practice (including psychoanalysis), which may afford them the luxury of working with a specific patient population. Established therapists may choose to avoid work with actively psychotic, personality disordered, or non-psychologically minded people in crisis, and refer these patients elsewhere. For someone with advanced training in psychoanalysis, most of the patients they will see in their practice are typically well educated, articulate, with an ability to pay for treatment despite the typical limitations of managed care and many private insurance carriers. These patient characteristics, including adequate financial resources and the ability to engage in higher level thought processes, can all serve to mediate the impact of any psychological trauma and crisis. Although certainly not representative of all therapists with advanced training, one analyst remarked upon his ability to "take only wealthy clients, who could be identified on even their worst days as members of the 'worried well.'"

In contrast, Master level therapists are more likely to work in social service agencies, walk-in clinics, and long-term care (i.e., institutional) settings with patients who are more likely to be chronically mentally ill, homeless, without social support systems, personality disordered, or court referred. Masters level therapists often see patients who do not have the financial resources to see a therapist in private practice. Thus, their patients must often cope with additional environmental stressors such as concerns about physical safety, substandard housing, and poverty. Therapists in these types of (valuable and essential) settings may be treating a number of patients who are actively suicidal, or in crisis, at any one time. The emotional stress associated with such high risk cases can only add to the difficulties associated with working in lower paying, crowded, often undervalued clinics. Thus, it appears appropriate to conclude that even though lower levels of professional training or associated with increased suicide risk among patients, some critical intervening factors related to their patients themselves (e.g., serious psychopathology; lack of financial resources; extreme environmental stressors; societal devaluation; lack of social support) may actually account for a large proportion of this suicide risk.

Virtually no empirical data is available to examine the numbers of bachelor's level therapists who lose a patient to suicide. Due to changes in legislation that will probably increase demand for "wrap-around" and "mobile" community services, more bachelor level workers will be working with seriously disturbed patients. Based upon previous findings, one can only extrapolate that these therapists with only minimal levels of training will experience unprecedented rates of patient suicide due to the nature of their patient population. Sadly, these individuals also are likely to receive the least amount of training on how to handle crisis, and how to cope with the death of a patient.

The only good news in these research findings, however, appears to be that more than 75% of all licensed therapists can expect to complete their careers without losing a patient to suicide (e.g., Chemtob et al., 1989). The findings of these aforementioned studies, coupled with a thoughtful analysis of their results, suggest that mental health professionals need to focus upon patient characteristics as a risk factor in treatment. Yet, it also seems requisite for training programs, particularly Masters and bachelors level programs, to provide information about crisis intervention, and to provide them with the coping skills necessary to manage this increasingly common occupational hazard. Current estimates suggest that less than half of all graduate programs in clinical psychology even offer formal training in suicide (Bongar & Harmatz, 1991).

The dearth of training in dealing with patient suicide may only become more problematic as greater numbers of our population continue to age, and experience painful and debilitating chronic or terminal illnesses. Many individuals may view suicide or euthanasia as a rational, effective solution to their medical problem. It also remains unclear what any therapist should do in that situation, particularly if she is professionally opposed to suicide, but more personally accepting of her patient's decision. (Also see Chapter 9.) Although assisting a patient in suicide is clearly unacceptable, significant questions remain about whether or not a therapist should deter or discourage patients from pursuing euthanasia or similar courses of action. For better or worse, after extensive peer, professional, and legal consultation, each therapist must decide for himself what to do.

The Impact upon Therapists

Chemtob et al. (1989) found that nearly half of all therapists who lost a patient to suicide experienced a number of somatic and psychological symptoms, many of which are remarkably similar to those present in individuals suffering from Post-Traumatic Stress Disorder. Additional responses by many of these therapists included:

1. increased focus upon legal aspects of treatment
2. increased tendencies to hospitalize patients
3. refusals to accept suicidal or severely mental ill individuals as patients
4. increased focus upon potential suicide "clues"
5. the production of less detailed and specific patient records
6. impaired relationships with peers (outside of the profession), colleagues, and family members
7. increased consultation with colleagues
8. ruminative thoughts about death
9. loss of self-esteem
10. dreams or nightmares about suicide
11. pervasive guilt
12. excessive anger or irritability
13. emotional numbing
14. social withdrawal

Interestingly, some of these changes cannot automatically be deemed negative. An increased focus upon the legal issues involved in treatment (e.g., having detailed knowledge of the statutes and precedents in one's state) and increased consultations with colleagues cannot automatically be considered inappropriate or negative. From a legal standpoint, however, one of the more problematic behaviors reported by Chemtob et al. (1989) as relatively common among therapists who lost a patient to suicide is a tendency to provide abbreviated, limited documentation in subsequent patient sessions. Although some practitioners may content, "they [prosecuting attorneys] can only hang me if I give them enough rope," the presence of fragmented, minimal, or otherwise substandard progress notes is more likely to provide additional support for the prosecution's case (e.g., "Because there is no specific information here about my client's suicidal ideation, intent, or plan... We can infer that this means that Dr. X did not properly assess her patient... Otherwise, this vital information would be included and fully documented").

Shelly. The common denominator in therapists' responses to patient suicide, however, appears to be increased self-doubt and unpleasant, ruminative thoughts. Some therapists even engage in excessive "self-punishment" an attempt to assuage their often unfounded, but somewhat natural, feelings of guilt. Consider the case of Shelly, an experienced social worker in an inpatient psychiatric unit. During the month of November, Shelly had two patients commit suicide within a two-week period. And, despite clear protestations from her unit supervisor and hospital lawyer, Shelly *insisted* on holding group debriefing and support sessions for her dead patients' friends and family members. Shelly's supervisor wanted to protect her from inappropriate, affectively charged responses from her patients' family members. Shelly's supervisor also was concerned about Shelly's own mental health, stating, "Someone else can do it; I can do it... Right now we need to have you take care of yourself... you need to deal with this, too." In contrast (but of similar importance), the hospital's legal counsel expressed concerns the disclosure of specific treatment details could be used against Shelly or the hospital in future litigation.

During one of the family sessions that Shelly held, a number of family members were openly hostile with Shelly. One lamented, "Why couldn't you do anything?... How could you let this happen! What kind of doctor are you!" Another said, "I hope your mother goes for help someplace and no one does anything for her. Then see how you feel about it." These kind of emotional outbursts are quite understandable, but Shelly herself was in no position to help these family members appropriately process these issues and intense emotions. On a number of levels, Shelly also knew that these family meetings would be antagonistic, affectively charged, and disconcerting. It is as though Shelly's guilt about her patients' suicides was so intense that she consciously or unconsciously arranged to literally be punished by their families.

It also is notable that both of Shelly's patients committed suicide a few days after they were discharged from the inpatient unit, against Shelly's treatment recommendations. Her patients' insurance companies recently failed to renew their contracts with the hospital, and would only agree to pay for a limited amount of inpatient care. Extremely upset and concerned about her patients' impending discharge, Shelly made numerous, direct attempts to arrange for extend treatment coverage. She spent much of her time during lunch breaks making phone calls to the insurance companies, and sending letters and faxes to various parties including the hospital and legal contacts. When the insurance companies flatly denied her requests, Shelly did everything she could to provide continuity of care for her patients, including the recommendation for weekly outpatient visits with both psychiatrists and psychologists. Shelly's patients' fixed, monthly income made it impossible for them to pay for their own recommended inpatient care.

When asked about the insurance company's role in the death of her patients, Shelly replied flatly, "I could have called [to attempt to overturn their decision] one more time... Those people were counting on me, and I just gave up on them." It took more than three weeks, with constant support and encouragement from her co-workers and supervisors to even consider her patients' suicides as multidetermined events, and to begin to acknowledge the (clear) role that the insurance company played in overruling her own clinical judgment. Shelly also came to learn that her self-imposed guilt was not effective in vindicating her patients' deaths. Six months after the death of her patients, Shelly began a professional campaign in which therapists, hospital administrators, and patient family members were encouraged to make complaints about limited insurance coverage.

Mary. Therapists who lose a patient to suicide also may ascribe to the myth that "good therapists never allow a patient die." This pervasive myth is a natural corollary of the faulty belief that therapists can use their advanced clinical skills and clear sense of purpose to effectively control the behavior of others. For such therapists, the death of a patient to suicide can foster significant changes in one's personal and professional self-image. However, these changes will result optimally in the development of a more realistic, honest self-appraisal.

Mary, a 76 year-old woman living in a community based nursing home, took over her family's business in the production of corrugated paper products when her father died suddenly of a heart attack at age 51, Mary was a strong, self-assured, articulate woman. She described her transition to company president as "rocky and interesting." Mary said that a number of her employees didn't want to listen to "a skirt," but that she showed them she could do any job in the plant as well as they could, and she was fair, and she was willing to listen. The company flourished, and Mary sold the company to a smaller competitor when she retired at age 67.

After retirement, Mary bought a dog, Cliff, and stayed busy doing volunteer work at a local hospital. Mary had never married, and from her reports, she was "never interested in a husband or boyfriend." Mary had been one of four children, and at age 76, she was the only remaining sibling alive. She loved her home, nestled out in the country, and did all of her own yard work and house maintenance. Mary said that she was better with a lug wrench than a saucepan. Then, one day Mary woke up and found that her leg side "seemed sluggish" and her voice "didn't sound right." When she had trouble getting into the kitchen, she called 911 from the floor of her bedroom. Upon arrival at the hospital, the staff determined that Mary had a major stroke.

After two months of intensive physical and occupational therapy, Mary moved into the nursing home. The move was intended to be temporary. After two months in the nursing home, Mary began withdrawn, and no longer participated in any of the planned (or spontaneous) activities in the center. She cried easily, stopped combing her hair, and stopped using her walker and reverted to her wheelchair, which she had significant difficulty in moving. Upon the recommendation of the nursing home's social worker, Mary began a trial of psychotherapy, and was seen by a psychiatrist for a trial of anti-depressant medication.

In therapy, Mary was slow to develop a trusting relationship with her therapist. Over time, she began to discuss her disgust that she could no longer take care of herself. She was angry that someone else had to help her get dressed, and to even move about. She expressed clear suicidal ideation, "I wish I could just die and get this over with...I'm not good to anyone like this anyway," but no specific plan or intent. When asked what was keeping her from committing suicide, she responded, "I am Catholic. Always have been and always will be. I just can't do it. The result [going to hell] would be even worse...So, I'm stuck here."

In another month, Mary was back to using her walker. She was significantly less tearful and she developed a fledgling friendship with another resident down the hall. Then, when Mary was trying to go to the bathroom by herself, without the aid of her grab bar, she fell and broke her hip. She had to return to her wheelchair, and her depression regained its previous intensity. In one session, Mary broke down and told her therapist that she decided to sell her house, and eventually move into a local assisted living apartment complex upon her discharge from the nursing home. Although Mary said that she always thought she would have to give up her home sometime," she was most upset about giving away her dog. (Her niece had been taking care of her dog, but she lived in an apartment herself and could not take him in.) She tried to convince the nursing home administrator to let her bring Cliff as a therapy dog or mascot, but the administrator responded that they could not have dogs full time on the premises due to the increased liability risk. Mary reasoned that at least Cliff would be taken care of by someone, rather than cooped up alone for so much of the day, just waiting for her. Her biggest lament was that she couldn't take care of Cliff anymore.

Mary met the middle-aged couple who agreed to take Cliff in. She liked them very much, and her niece assured her that they gave their other two dogs lots of exercise and attention. In therapy, Mary was helped to mourn her loss, and to express her feelings of fear and helplessness. Over time, between her antidepressant medication, her work in therapy, and her work in physical therapy, Mary's mood brightened. She gained 10 of the 15 pounds she had lost in the past few months. She began to tend to her hair and personal hygiene with greater care, and even purchased new clothes on some sponsored trips to local department stores. She played cards once a week with a group of women on her floor, and had lunch with some of them during the week.

In therapy, Mary reported feeling much better. She said that although she missed Cliff terribly, she was determined to get back her "fighting spirit" and "do the best that I can with what I got [her physical limitations.]" Mary denied the presence of any suicidal ideation, stating, "God will see me through now ... And, I have some things [and friends] to keep busy." Her psychiatrist and physical therapist were thrilled with Mary's progress. They were delighted about her situation; many of their patients never have the opportunity to leave the nursing home. All of the treatment team members concurred that Mary was no longer at significant risk for suicide, and that nothing more could be done to keep Mary in the nursing home for psychological treatment. Thus, after spending a total of seven months in the nursing home, Mary was discharged with her major depression in remission, and moved into her own, new apartment.

Mary had agreed to consider outpatient therapy, at least once a week, in her discharge planning. Although she would need to take a cab or public transportation to make her appointments, she felt fairly confident that she could manage the trip. When Mary's therapist had no heard from her in two weeks, she called Mary to find out how she was doing. Mary reported, "Oh, I'm sorry I haven't come over there yet...I think I'm doing all right. I talk on the phone to my Rummy 500 friends, and I met a lady I kind of like down the way. I like that. And, there is a social worker here. She said that I could see her if I wanted, so that I didn't have to travel and worry about my walker and things." Mary's therapist wished that they could have continued their work together, but was pleased that Mary was considering other options for outpatient treatment that would better address some of her difficulties with transportation.

Mary's Therapist.   Approximately five months later, Mary's therapist, Stephanie, was writing up progress notes in the staff lounge. The physician assistant on Mary's case saw her sitting there, and stopped to talk. He said evenly, "Have you heard yet?" Stephanie looked up at him and asked what he was referring to. The PA responded, "I thought you might have heard already. They found Mary yesterday; she killed herself. She jumped from the 5th floor of her apartment complex around three in the afternoon. The doors to the patio were supposed to be locked (it was during the wintertime)...Somehow she found it, or got it, open."

Stephanie's first internal response to Mary's suicide was anger and rage. She thought to herself, "Jesus Christ! Who found her? I mean, what if some young kid found her, lying there on the ground while coming home from school? Didn't she think about the fact that someone else, like a kid, could be affected by this!" While Stephanie sat silently with her thoughts, the PA added, "You know, Steph, we did the best we could. The family agrees. They thought she was so much better when she left the nursing home. We all did. They aren't blaming anyone, and as far as we can tell, they aren't pressing any charges or filing a lawsuit. Hmm. That might be tough anyway, since she had been discharged for a few months...Mary's niece also told me that Mary's youngest brother hung himself when they were kids. I guess that helped set the stage, too." Stephanie turned to look at the psychiatrist and said, "Thanks for telling me...I'm glad I got to hear it from you first instead of someone else."

In the next moment, Stephanie felt incredibly guilty about how she could possess such negative feelings about Mary. It is interesting to note that Stephanie was so distressed by her patient's suicide that she could not recognize the issues underlying her first thoughts upon hearing about Mary's death. Apparently, Stephanie unconsciously viewed thought of herself as an innocent "school girl" (i.e., a fledgling professional) who had something horrible happen that was completely unexpected, and beyond her immediate control. It is as thought Stephanie wanted to be angry with what Mary did, and also somehow acknowledge that she had made the best attempt possible to prevent any such suicidal attempt.

Over the next few days, Stephanie continued to berate herself, "My god! Mary must have gotten so depressed again. She must have felt so hopeless and alone ... Why didn't she call me, just to touch base or let me know that she needed me?" Stephanie continued to lament her inability to foster such a strong therapeutic alliance that Mary would call her in the midst of a severe depression, and she began to blame herself for Mary's death. Stephanie recounted, "I thought that if I had just asked for more specific information about all of her brothers and sisters [all 10 of them], and how they all died and when, she might be alive right now ... I started thinking that I was a complete failure as a therapist and as a human being ... I even started to think that maybe I should be the one who's dead, and entertained some fleeting thoughts of suicide, myself."

Stephanie even berated herself for not making "house calls" to see Mary, despite the extreme distances involved, and the fact that Stephanie was not paid or permitted to make home visits for both legal and professional reasons. Stephanie still couldn't accept her presumed lapse in clinical judgment, despite the full agreement of all professionals on Mary's treatment team that she was no longer suicidal, and cleared for discharge. Stephanie described feeling sick to her stomach for days, and reported having a series of nightmares in which Mary's house was washed away in a flood, and Mary was left sitting on an outcropping a few feet away, crying.

Stephanie also felt embarrassed and ashamed. She worried that her colleagues thought that she was as poor of a clinician as she now perceived herself. Despite fears that one of her peers would think her incompetent, Stephanie brought up the discussion of patient suicide with a practicing classmate from graduate school. Stephanie's classmate said, "Wow. Sounds like a tough one. Not fun." When Stephanie tentatively asked, "Do you mind if I ask you if you ever had anything like this happen?" her colleague responded immediately, "Oh, yeah.

You aren't alone there, I'm afraid." The two of them then made a lunch date.

During their meeting, Stephanie's colleague reported, "Well, not like this would make you feel better, but I thought it might be good for you to see." She pulled a wrinkled piece of paper from her briefcase. She slid it across the table and said, "Take a look at that." It was a suicide note written by one of her patients, who killed herself about three years ago. It read, "Dear Dr. P., I am so sorry to do this. I know how hard you worked to help me. I'm sorry that I'm not getting better. I just have to do this. I left a note for my mom, and told her that it wasn't her fault, either. Good luck, M."

Stephanie's colleague continued, "She was 28 years-old. Stepped right in front of a commuter train. She was just released, too ... She also left a note for her social worker, pretty much the same as this one. It took me a long time to come to grips with this, and sometimes I don't know if I've dealt with it as well as I think I have ... Maybe I'm fooling myself, but I know I did everything that I knew how to do. And, I think some of what she said in her note might really be true. I mean, maybe she blamed me for some of it, but maybe she wanted to let me know that I shouldn't suffer that much, too." The two psychologists also discussed the classic warning sign of suicide, in which a patient suddenly seems better or more energetic, within the context that aside from stating concerns about suicide and talking about their intent or plan, no one can commit patients for "feeling better."

Stephanie respected her colleague and their discussion. Their time together, coupled with her own work in psychotherapy, allowed Stephanie to cope better with Mary's suicide. She began to acknowledge that it was up to Mary to continue in outpatient treatment after her release (Stephanie had made numerous attempts to make referrals), and that it was up to Mary to jump from that balcony or not. Stephanie continued in clinical practice, felt that she was able to learn from the experience, began to experience a renewed sense of competence, and enjoyed her work.

Revisiting the Case. A few years later, Stephanie described sitting at home, reviewing a textbook for a course in Personality Psychology. She was preparing to give a lecture for a colleague who needed to miss class unexpectedly for a funeral. Stephanie was reading a biographical sketch on the famous existentialist, Binswanger, that discussed his work with a young woman suffering from major depression and various obsessions. Three days after release from the hospital, Binswanger's patient killed herself (May, Angel, & Ellenberger, 1958).

Stephanie recalls with clarity literally snorting to herself, "Yeah, some great clinician this guy was. He must have been *great* in therapy. I guess he had no clue what he was doing." Suddenly, with a growing sense of horror, Stephanie recounted, "Oh, my god. This is me. That's what happened to me ... I might as well be talking about myself... So I guess that makes me a pretty shitty therapist ... How the hell do I know what I'm doing?!" So, even years after apparently coming to terms with her feelings about Mary's suicide, Stephanie still clung to the pervasive myth that "good therapists don't let patients kill themselves." She noted, "It kind of scared me how I responded so negatively to this description. It was absolutely automatic... even after knowing what happened to me and to other therapists I respect and trust."

After experiencing renewed feelings of guilt and self-doubt during the next few weeks, Stephanie decided to reenter therapy to help reconcile these conflicting self-views and underlying conflicts. Consistent with the work of various therapists, who believed that parents did not have to be, and even should not be "perfect" in order to raise a healthy, secure child (e.g., Winnicott, 1971), she began to truly internalize the belief that she was a "good-enough" therapist. Stephanie began to accept herself as a therapist—who was only human.

Coping Strategies for Therapists

A number of concrete suggestions can be offered to therapists who experience the suicide of a patient. The first step, which ideally would occur before the unexpected event occurs, is education about the likelihood of patient suicide. Many therapists have never received information about this critical occupational hazard, much less even seriously considered what steps they should take immediately after the event, if it should ever occur. For many therapists, the suicide of a patient affects them as much as the death of a family member. Just as we tell our patients that they are entitled to help and support after a traumatic event, therapists would be well advised to listen to their own advice. Some suggestions for coping, culled from discussions with psychologists who have experienced a patient suicide and (sadly but necessarily) from legal experts, include:

1. Be prepared to experience an onslaught of emotions, from shock, despair, disbelief, sadness, anguish, anger, terror, fear, or emotional numbing.
2. Obtain as much factual information as possible about the suicide. This procedure is important for a number of reasons. First,

gathering the facts can help avoid denial about the experience. Second, it can prevent introspective rumination on part of the therapist and the development of fantasies about what occurred.

3. It is important to remember, however, that gathering information from family and friends of the patient (as well as family and friends of the therapist herself) can be far from objective. Sadly, in acknowledgement of the pervasive risk of litigation in our society, discussions of any kind with the surviving family members, even those that are well intentioned and designed to help comfort the survivors, can significantly compromise the therapist's legal position. Thus, the best way to gather objective information without additional concerns is to talk to the police or the coroner's office.

4. When seeking information about the suicide, do not implicate yourself in the suicide. Remember that your emotional state is highly charged, and that you may not be in full command of your emotions or completely aware of the facts behind the situation. One solution to this problem is to have a clinic or other outside agency collect the information.

5. Acknowledge the traumatic nature of the situation, and seek help and support. Although it is unfortunate, many peers and family members who are not mental health professionals may find it difficult to relate to the situation, and they may themselves ascribe to the pervasive myth that "good therapists" can exert total control over people's behavior. Seeking help from a fellow professional, either in consultation or in therapy, can be quite helpful.

6. Remind yourself that you are not alone. As noted, more than 1 out of 5 therapists will experience the loss of a patient to suicide. You deserve to have understanding and sympathy, and to receive protection as a professional.

7. Consider following the practical advice that therapists often give to their patients in time of crisis. For example, avoid alcoholic beverages and other drugs. Allow yourself sufficient time for sleep and rest, and try to exercise and eat right.

8. If working in a clinic or hospital setting, allow the clinic to talk to lawyers about the specifics, and handle the collection of chart and progress notes. Also ask them to contact the consulting psychiatrist.

9. Remember that feelings of guilt do not automatically imply causality or blame. If thoughts and guilt over the suicide become ruminative, consider professional support.

10. Although somewhat controversial, many therapists recommend returning to work as soon as possible, even on a part-time basis. Seeing clients again can help the survivor by providing them with adherence to their routine, and (hopefully) by avoiding the development of diffuse, generalized doubts regarding professional competence.

11. Acknowledge the natural tendency to become more conservative in work with your patients, reported in empirical studies as a common response to patient suicide (e.g., Chemtob et al., 1989). If a therapist has patients who are actively suicidal, and it becomes easy to question whether clinical decisions are based upon an objective assessment or upon fears and doubts, consider referrals to other professionals. It is acceptable for professionals to receive professional support.

12. Be alert to indirect or unconscious manifestations of guilt. For example, an increase in the number of severity of "accidental" bruises, cuts, or falls, the loss of car keys when in a dangerous area, getting stuck in a rain storm without appropriate cover. Suicidal ideation is common.

13. Recognize and accept feelings of ambivalence over the incident. Acknowledging a sense of relief over some aspect of a patient's suicide does not negative other, simultaneous feelings of sadness, grief, or frustration.

14. Consider that even a cursory resolution of the event may take a few months. Self-forgiveness is critical, along with an acknowledgement of the limitations of professional power.

15. Some therapists describe coming to terms with a patient's suicide when they are able to learn, or "take something valuable" away from the experience. For example, one therapist learned to take detailed histories about any suicide attempts made by her patients' family, friends, and neighbors. Another therapist incorporates information about coping with patient suicide in his lectures to students so that, unlike him, they can be better prepared if a patient does commit suicide.

THERAPIST BURNOUT

Burnout is another serious occupational hazard for mental health practitioners. Freudenberger first coined the term in 1974. He defined burnout as a "syndrome of physical and emotional exhaustion, involving the development of negative self-concept, negative job attitudes, and loss of concern and feeling for clients." Freudenberger conceptualized his notions about burnout while working with clients and supervising staff members at a "free clinic" in the 1960's. Freudenberger became frustrated with staffing the clinic because the vast majority of his volunteers left the center after one year, or even sooner. From his discussions with these volunteers, and his own observations about the prevailing "mental health environment," Freudenberger (1974) reasoned that this high turn-over was a reflection of his volunteers' intense involvement with clients, and their perceived need to "give constantly" to others in acute stress.

Although many therapists describe a sense of deep personal and professional fulfillment in their work, it remains clear that in our culture, the overwhelming majority of people who seek out mental health practitioners are in crisis, actively depressed, anxious, or otherwise having problems in coping. Other patients who do not voluntarily seek help, but who are required to participate in treatment (e.g., via court orders; involuntary hospitalization) are often seriously mentally ill or highly antagonistic. In sum, the vast majority of patients seen in psychotherapy are suffering in some way, shape, or form. Although a significant number of patients show improvement in their symptoms, quality of relationships, and their perceptions of their life situation, others show limited progress or remain seriously ill or distressed. One must consider the impact of being surrounded by individuals whose lives are in turmoil, pain, or strife upon a therapist. It makes sense that patients, by definition, require something from their therapists. As noted by Freudenberger (1974), problems appear to arise when therapists cannot properly modulate the amount, and type, of help given.

Symptoms and Warning Signs

1. limiting or reducing the time spent with clients
2. making an excessive number of referrals
3. referring to clients in dehumanized, technical ways, or using sick humor in reference to clients and their problems
4. increased emotional lability
5. turning excessively to other staff members for help in coping with emotional or physical problems, or with professional responsibilities
6. developing uncharacteristically rigid ways of thinking or displaying an inability to adapt to change
7. holding cynical attitudes about clients' inability to change
8. minimizing time spent at work (e.g., facetiously calling in sick, arriving perpetually late)

   9. spending excessive amounts of time at work, but getting less
      and less work done
  10. feeling that facts about patients seem to blur together, until
      they all seem "alike"
  11. increased use of drugs or alcohol
  12. acting out (e.g., forgetting about or missing appointments, for-
      getting to return phone calls, forgetting to arrange consults or
      follow-up on referrals)
  13. disturbances in one's family or social life due to work related
      stressors
  14. increasingly prevalent or severe psychosomatic symptoms
      such as headaches, GI distress, muscle aches, dizziness, and
      fatigue
  15. taking unnecessary risks at work
  16. increasing social isolation at work and at home
  17. difficulties in maintaining personal and professional boundaries

   Also see items from Figley's (1995) self-test for compassion
fatigue in Table 3.

Myths that Foster Burnout

   As noted, a variety of factors (e.g., low pay; long hours; consistent
exposure to intrapsychic trauma) appear to contribute to professional
burnout. However, some factors appear more amenable to therapist
control, and subject to intervention. Specifically, the pervasive myths
that many clinicians ascribe to regarding the things that mental health
providers can, and should, be able to do are endemic in the development of burnout. An examination of these myths can be useful in terms

TABLE 3. Sample Items from Figley's Self-Test for Therapist Burnout

---

15. I have thought that there is no one to talk with about highly stressful experiences.
28. I have wished that I could avoid working with some therapy clients.
31. I have felt weak, tired, rundown as a result of my work as a therapist.
34. I feel little compassion toward most of my co-workers.
35. I find I am working more for the money than for personal fulfillment.
36. I find it difficult separating my personal life from my work life.
37. I have a sense of worthlessness/disillusionment/resentment associated with my
    work.
38. I have thoughts that I am a "failure" as a psychotherapist.

Note. From the Compassion Fatigue Self-Test (Figley, 1995), which has a total of 40 items. The items presented here are scored such that higher numbers indicate greater levels of fatigue. Reprinted with permission.

of psychoeducation, and can help in prevention. Some of these myths include (also see Chapter 2):

1. *If I am a good therapist, I can help or save everyone.* Such rescue fantasies literally can cripple otherwise competent therapists. Just as a therapist would advise a patient, "It is simply not possible to be liked by everyone or to like everyone you interact with," therapists must keep in mind that they may not have the best chemistry or working relationships with all patients. Some patients may benefit from a referral to a specialist, or to a therapist with a different approach or personality. Still other patients may already have predetermined plans to commit suicide or engage in violent behavior, and no therapist could prevent or predict their behavior.

2. *Because I am so aware of my own issues as a therapist, it is OK if I stretch the patient-therapist boundaries once in a while.* The desire to violate patient-therapist boundaries can be strong, particularly in the face of certain types of psychopathology (e.g., dependent and histrionic personality disorder). For example, one student intern relayed the story that while conducting intelligence and personality testing with an outpatient volunteer at their college counseling center, he felt so sorry for his patient (who cried openly and stated that she had no one to talk to or eat lunch with during their break between tests) that he began to accompany her to the cafeteria. Fortunately, his testing partner called him aside and "reminded him" of a previous engagement. Later discussion of the incident with his clinical supervisor proved beneficial, in that the intern could then recognize the significant influence with which his patient attempted to recreate a familiar, although inappropriate, relationship.

Primary Prevention

A number of specific recommendations can be offered to help mental health professionals avoid the development of burnout. Although some of these suggestions may seem rather simplistic, and even egregiously obvious, the simple act of identifying and articulating them may help therapists internalize an increasing sense of entitlement for the fulfillment of their own, even basic, needs. The following suggestions are applicable for all mental health practitioners, across a variety of settings.

1. Join or start a peer supervision group. Working in isolation can be stressful, and having input about clinical issues, as well as the ability to socialize with other colleagues, can provide both instrumental

and emotional support. Some therapists join groups based upon their work with a specific patient population (e.g., long-term care; addictions), their theoretical orientation (e.g., cognitive-behavioral; interpersonal therapy), their alma mater, or their overall geographic proximity to one another.

Although not described in the literature, future consideration may be given to holding such groups via telecommunication or internet technology, pending the ability to provide a secure transmission among members for confidentiality. Peer supervision groups often meet weekly, bi-weekly, or once a month for one to three hours. Because gaining different perspectives on similar issues is a key benefit of peer support, care should be taken to recruit members from at least two different practices, agencies, or at least departments. Local psychological associations may have a listing of already established groups, or access to members who would be interested in joining such a group.

2. Vary participation in professional activities as much as possible, even within a single workday. Consider any combination of individual and group therapy, testing and assessment, clinical interviewing, consultation, chart review, process notes, couples and family therapy, team meetings, teaching, skills training, and supervision of trainees and interns. Consider working with different patient populations from time to time.

3. Join professional organizations, whether they are national, regional, or local. Some organizations offer opportunities for networking and continuing education. Participation in community projects, directly related to the use of clinical skills or not, can also provide an enhanced sense of accomplishment and personal and professional fulfillment.

4. Develop a routine that allows for a smooth, clear transition from work to home. Having a planned, predetermined ritual can help place some literal and figurative distance (and perspective) from the events of the workday. Time spent alone is best to allow for greater introspection, and sense of control. A myriad of options for such a transitional period include healthy activities like a short walk, a brief period of exercise, listening to favorite music, gardening, yoga, stretching, playing an instrument, meditating, spending time with a pet, enjoying a cup of coffee, and light reading. Sometimes even sitting quietly in the car listening to a favorite music station (even in the garage, with the engine off, of course), can provide a moment of respite for therapists who return home to immediately begin their second full time job as a parent or caregiver. Developing a sense of entitlement for these few moments of self-reflection and relaxation is almost as important as the activity involved in the ritual itself.

Although obvious, alcohol and drugs should not be part of one's regular work to home transition. One therapist described the moment that she knew she had to make some changes in her personal and professional life. Anne noted, "I had been working at an inner city clinic. It was my first job out of school, and I had to get my hours in for supervision. The place was like a "Medicaid factory," I was assigned to literally take busloads of kids to a pool to go swimming, or on some "field trip." It wasn't therapy in any way, shape, or form. And, what the hell was I supposed to do—see my patients in a swimsuit? But the agency sure got to claim a lot of patient visits... And it seemed like every other patient I had was suicidal. I mean, really suicidal, not, 'I think about killing myself sometimes,' but 'I have a loaded revolver in my locker at school and I think about shooting myself after school in the locker room.'

My fiancé didn't understand what I was so upset about. He would say, 'Hey, you went to school for all of this. You took out all of those student loans that we'll be paying off... You're a doctor now, and you're doing what you always wanted to do. What's the problem?' I felt out of control, and my co-workers already seemed to have checked-out. They just did whatever they were supposed to, and didn't seem to really care. I started not wanting to get up and go in to work. Even coming home after work to see my fiancé and cat didn't seem to help anymore. So, I started getting into the routine of greeting the cat for a few minutes, and then starting dinner for Patrick and me. While I was getting it ready, I put out some fruit, cheese and crackers, and some wine. Patrick loved it, and thought I was this great cook; he loved what he thought was extra attention. In three months time, I realized that I was having two or three glasses of wine before dinner, without thinking about it. And, it didn't have any kind of relaxing effect on me anymore; it was just something I did. And, I realized that was what my mom did, when I was growing up ... I knew that I had to figure out something else to do...I decided that I was going to look for another job, because I deserved it, no matter how much or how little experience I had."

5. Develop or sustain existing hobbies and outside interests. That does not mean reading professional journals "just for fun" or attending interesting continuing education seminars. Participation in hobbies and other activities allows therapists to occupy multiple roles, which often provides a sense of stability and resilience in times of stress and crisis (e.g., Well, I was a shitty therapist for today, but damn can I cook a great meal."). Participation in outside activities also allows for interaction with people outside of the profession, who may provide a proverbial "breath of fresh air" in a sometimes narrowed focus upon clinical practice.

6. During a work day, take frequent breaks. Get out of a chair, get out of the office, go out for lunch, or take food to another part of the building or to a bench outside. Be sure to eat something decent for lunch (or dinner or whatever). Drink lots of fluids; have a water bottle or drink on hand. Spend time talking with friends about things other than work, either in person or on the phone during breaks or at lunch. Unless one has a significant preference for it, try not to schedule patients back-to-back. Allow time in the day for variety and change.

7. Take regular vacations. If you work in a hospital, business, or clinic setting, use all of your vacation days. If you are in private practice, consider the impact of at least two weeks of vacation time (i.e., the decrease in expected income; the effort required to provide coverage) upon your overall business plan. This advance planning helps avoid the temptation to cancel vacations in order to either "make a financial killing this year" or "make ends meet."

8. If you are truly sick, cancel your appointments, see a physician, and recuperate comfortably at home. Despite sometimes overwhelming fears about abandoning patients, remember that a therapist who cannot take care of herself certainly is in no position to take care of others. And, therapists can be expected to model good self care for the benefit of themselves and their patients (e.g., Munroe, 1999). Have a back-up plan for emergency visits or referrals to a colleague in case you are ill.

Jonathan. Therapists often overlook the physical consequences sometimes associated with coming to work with an illness. One psychologist recounted ruefully, "Yeah, I was kind of like "Father Teresa." I wanted to be a miracle worker...I was working with a bunch of kids at this center downtown. They were really young, around 8 to 10 years old. And, this one kid and I were starting to connect, and really make some progress with certain things. This kid's dad died the year before, and his mom was seriously depressed. I felt like this little guy was just starting to trust me, and to allow himself to actually look forward to our sessions."

He continued, "So, one day I woke up and felt like someone hit me all over with a sledge hammer. I had a raging fever, and I was afraid to even try to eat anything for breakfast. What I really wanted to do was call in sick, pull up the covers, and stay in bed all day. But, I went in to work because I just had to see that kid. I thought that I couldn't abandon him like that, and basically force him to relive the loss with his father all over again. He needed to know that someone would be there for him if they said they would be. For better or worse, I thought I was that important to that kid. And, maybe right then I was, I don't know.

Anyway, when it was time for our next appointment, I get a call from the kid's mom. He came down with the flu two days after our last session, and he got so dehydrated that she had to take him to the ER to get an IV. Boy, did I feel like shit, But, I really learned something from that one. Even though it can be really, really hard, it's better to talk something out later in therapy [i.e., a patient feeling angry and abandoned] than do try to do it from the ER or a hospital bed."

9. Use a team approach.
10. Hold realistic expectations about patient's progress in therapy.
11. Engage in periodic social functions with co-workers ... with an emphasis upon periodic!
12. Avoid negative people at work.
13. Set appropriate boundaries at work.
14. Ask for a raise. Recognize your value as a professional who is entitled to make a living.
15. Insist upon a safe work environment (i.e., one that addresses risks for violence and provides adequate patient-staff ratios).
16. Trust your own instincts!

Non-Traditional Approaches: Informed Consent

Because therapists may work with survivors of traumatic events on a daily basis, it becomes important to acknowledge the possible impact of this exposure. Similar to many of the theories behind Critical Incident Stress Management (see Chapter 10), in which emergency service workers such as police officers, fire fighters, and paramedics may be affectively overwhelmed after a particularly traumatic event or rescue, therapists should be aware of the critical need to process and manage their own countertransferential responses to patients. Some experts (Munroe, 1999) have even suggested that therapists in clinics, hospitals, and group practices sign formal consent forms, in which they acknowledge the difficulties inherent in work with trauma survivors, and affirm their ethical obligation for appropriate self-care. The Appendix at the end of this chapter provides a model of such consent. Beyond the obvious, potential legal benefits for various reasons, the use of such consent forms could be particularly helpful among trainees and interns to reinforce the need for therapists to take good care of themselves as well as their patients.

CONCLUSIONS

Patient suicide and therapist burnout are two of the most serious occupational hazard that therapists face. Fortunately, psychoeducation appears to provide some help in either preventing the occurrence of these problems (in the case of burn-out), or at least in easing the nature of their resolution (in the case of patient suicide). It probably is most important for therapists to recognize that they cannot, despite all of their clinical training, skills, and acumen, control the behavior of other people. Therapists also cannot predict their own emotional responses to their patients' problems and behaviors, particularly if they instigate suicidal or homicidal behavior. Therapists must be willing to ask for, *and accept*, help, social support, peer consultation, and legal support when necessary. We must remember that unless we can help ourselves, we cannot expect to help others. We must "come first."

APPENDIX

Informed Consent Form for Trauma Therapists

I, _____, have been informed by the staff at _____, that this program works with survivors of trauma, and that I therefore will inevitably be exposed to the effects of secondary trauma. I have been informed that these effects can have beneficial or detrimental results; if dealt with openly, such responses can be viewed as parallels to the clients' trauma responses and as such, are valuable clinical information; if denied or ignored these same responses can lead to an altered world view which may impede my clinical judgment and interfere with my personal life. I have been informed that my age, experience, or professional training may not provide adequate protection from secondary trauma. I have been informed that the staff expects each member, including myself, to work to understand and act on how this work affects each staff member in the delivery of services to our clients. I have been informed that the staff believes all of its actions and interactions related to secondary trauma are considered models for our clients and that each member of the staff is expected to recognize an ethical obligation to model good self care.   _____ ____
                                                                    Signature   Date

Note. Reprinted with permission from Munroe (1999), Ethical issues associated with secondary trauma in therapist. In B. H. Stamm (Ed.), *Secondary traumatic stress* (pp. 215). Lutherville, MD: Sidran Press. Hillman also recommends the inclusion of a clinical supervisor or administrator's signature.

9

Death and Dying, Partner Abuse, and Other Subtypes of Trauma

Although every trauma has similar elements, a general under-standing of some various subtypes of trauma can be helpful in assuaging survivors' distress, and assisting them in a return to pre-vious levels of functioning.

LOSS AND IMPENDING LOSS

Virtually any crisis, by definition, includes some element of loss or unexpected change. And, it is highly unusual for any individual to state that they have not experienced some kind of traumatic loss in their lifetime. Common occurrences include the death of friends and family members, the loss of a job, prized possessions, or property, sep-aration from loved ones, the diagnosis of a chronic or terminal illness, divorce, a loss of independence, a loss of personal body boundaries through sexual assault or abuse, a loss of opportunity (e.g., infertility), and death of a beloved pet, among others.

Please also note that not all specific subtypes of trauma and loss will be presented here in any comprehensive fashion (it is beyond the scope of this text). The choice to include certain topics here for discussion is not to ascribe greater meaning or importance to one type of loss versus another. Various topics (e.g., domestic abuse; elder abuse; use of ecstasy) were selected for inclusion based only upon the emergence of recent research findings, theoretical perspectives, or risk management concerns.

Early Perspectives on Grief

Lindemann was one the first researchers to scientifically examine the psychological and physiological impact of grief and loss. In his now classic work, *Symptomatology and Management of Acute Grief*, published in 1944, Lindemann asserted, "acute grief [resulting from a traumatic loss] is a definite syndrome with psychological and somatic symptoms" (p. 7). He based his suppositions upon a series of clinical interviews and laboratory tests performed with more than 100 survivors and bereaved family members of victims from the infamous Cocoanut Grove nightclub fire in Boston. Lindemann (1944) observed that in comparison to his participants who experienced the death of a family member in a more traditional hospital setting, who typically resolved most of their intense grief reactions after four to six weeks, the survivors and bereaved family members of victims from the Cocoanut Grove fire displayed distinctly different symptoms for a significantly longer period of time.

Specifically, Lindemann found that the interviewees associated with the Cocoanut Grove fire (i.e., who experienced an serious, unexpected, traumatic loss) often displayed:

- no grief reaction until weeks or months after the traumatic event. (Lindemann thus coined the term "delayed grief reaction.")
- dramatic changes in their normal personality, including anger, aggression, and a "furious hostility against specific persons" (p. 15).
- the emergence of characteristics associated with their deceased family member, including hobbies, mannerisms, and even heart conditions. (This adoption of characteristics probably represent an attempt to internalize the dead person as a self-object.)
- physical problems such as colitis, rheumatoid arthritis, and asthma.
- social isolation.
- a tendency to give away valued resources or make "foolish" business deals, primarily as a means of assuaging guilt through self punitive behavior.
- "agitated depression," which typically included insomnia, feelings of self-hate and loathing, feelings of worthlessness.
- suicidal ideation and attempts.

Lindemann's directives for treatment are generally consistent with contemporary approaches to trauma. Unlike most health professionals at that time, Lindemann posited that extreme grief and stress reactions would be ameliorated best by *actively discussing the loss*, when patients were ready. He encouraged an interdisciplinary approach, in which social workers and pastoral figures would work collaboratively with mental health practitioners, including psychiatrists. He also cautioned against ascribing solely to religious dogma, which may distort survivors' beliefs about the nature of the trauma or their reaction to it. Vital topics for discussion included the change in the quality of one's relationships after a trauma, as well as the actual events surrounding a trauma. Lindemann especially emphasized the need to seek out positive interpersonal relationships in order to engender social support.

DEATH AND DYING

Another researcher, Elizabeth Kubler-Ross, helped shape American culture's perception of death and dying in the 1970's. Kubler-Ross (1969) examined the qualitiative responses of individuals dying from various terminal illnesses, and reported that their responses to impending death varied dramatically, but that they tended to follow a sequence of denial, anger, bargaining, depression, to acceptance. Although recent research findings suggest that not all individuals experience each of these stages, and that not all individuals move through these stages in any particular order (e.g., Schneider, 1984), Kubler-Ross's work has helped make the general topic of death and dying more acceptable in every day conversation. She also has alerted both professionals and laypersons that death is a multidimensional construct, with a wide variety of interpersonal responses.

Cross-Cultural Perspectives

A variety of cultures respond to death and dying quite differently than that of mainstream America. For example, the vast majority of people in Mexico formally celebrate "the Day of the Dead." This celebration typically takes place over a period of two to four days, and typically involves family oriented events. People use oversized marigolds, representing the flower of death, liberally to decorate homes and gravesites. Skeletons are often depicted in paintings and in small papier-mâché' models, and often feature what many Americans might consider bizarre but humorous representations of those skeletons doing a myriad of things including drinking tequila, dancing, cooking, and working as politicians, laborers, and dentists. In nearly every store, sugar candies are sold in the shape of skulls and skeletons, and are shared among adults and children alike. Some candy makers pride themselves on making realistic looking skulls that are personalized with the (living) recipients' names in red or blue icing. It is as though the message is to say, "Well, death is bound to find us all someday, so we might as well take it in stride and enjoy life while we can."

The culmination of the celebration takes place during nighttime, when family members gather at the gravesites of loved ones. Most families bring blankets, makeshift tents, small fire pits, and prepare the favorite food and drink of the ones departed. Most people hold a small party and even sleep overnight at the graves for one to two nights, "hoping patiently" that their loved ones will return.

Although the Day of the Dead is largely celebratory, it also is expected that individuals will experience a variety of emotions when asked to think about their departed loved ones, including everything from anger, sadness, joy, forgiveness, relief, and longing, to hope. Any expression of emotion is valued, and no one is expected to act in a certain way. The social nature of this annual event also makes issues related to death and dying a familiar, social affair rather than an isolated, individualizing experience. Attention to loved ones' previous likes and dislikes also allows survivors to reminisce about their dead relatives and friends in a socially acceptable way. Such a celebration would be considered almost unthinkable in most American cities and towns; many clinicians would consider a wish to sleep at a gravesite a sign of potentially serious psychopathology.

Ethical and Legal Issues

Recent controversies regarding death and dying typically involve the very meaning and definition of life itself. Complicated legal, moral, and ethical dilemmas exist regarding the definition of life as: consciousness; the ability to engage in self-directed activity; the ability to consume solid food; greater periods of consciousness than unconsciousness; the presence of a heart beat; minimal electrical activity in the brain; or electrical activity in the brain's cortex versus the brain stem. Current expenditures for Medicare and Medicaid top millions of dollars a year, in large part due to the increased cost of medical care in long-term health care facilities (e.g., nursing homes) and related costs associated with respirators, dialysis treatments, round the clock nursing care, and intravenous feedings. Many patients often must face the impending death of a loved one (or even themselves) within the context of a complicated institution of medicine.

In work with individuals facing issues of death and dying, particularly in cases involving life support and euthanasia, therapists should become familiar with current state and local laws regarding living wills, power of attorneys, durable power of attorneys, Medicaid and Medicare regulations, assisted suicide, hospice care, and the use of narcotics and other controlled substances as comfort measures. It also is important to note that in some instances, a living will signed by an individual will not be honored if the patient is transported to a hospital via an ambulance. In other cases, individual doctors may choose not to honor a living will.

As in other situations involving communication between a patient and family member and a medical professional, therapists can be vital in helping those individuals communicate honestly, openly, directly, and assertively. And, things can only get more complicated if an injured or dying person has different religious beliefs or ideas about long-term care and life support when compared to other family members. It can be quite challenging to provide open lines of communication between friends and family members, as well. Therapists must be careful to serve as a conduit for their patient's own wishes, and not project their own feelings, thoughts, and issues about death and dying upon them.

Professional and personal boundaries. In some instances, it also can be difficult for therapists to determine what motivates individuals' decisions about death and dying. Consider an elderly couple, Mr. and Mrs. P, who have been married for 51 years. When Mr. P received a diagnosis of terminal pancreatic cancer, he drafted a living will according to the current laws in his state. He wished to avoid the use of any heroic measures in maintaining his life, including the use of feeding tubes and antibiotics. He also signed various papers giving his wife a power of attorney. Three years later, Mr. P lay in a bed in a nursing home, gaunt and generally unconscious. He also appeared to be in a lot of discomfort evidenced by bodily contortions and guttural noises, and received high doses of morphine and other narcotics. His weight continued to drop, and his moments of lucidity diminished until they basically stopped; Mr. P now appeared to be in a vegetative state.

During the last six months of her husband's illness, Mrs. P participated in a local spousal support group. During a recent meeting, Mrs. P reported that her husband's physician estimated that he would die within three weeks. She also indicated that even though his living will stated that he was to be provided only with comfort measures, she insisted that the doctor initiate tube feeding. She explained to the group members, "I can't live without him ... I can't say good-bye to him yet ... It's so terrible, but I want him to be with me as long as possible." She showed little remorse in ignoring her husband's prior directives, "No one knows what they really want when they are trying to think about dying, anyway." The vast majority of the individuals in the support group also supported Mrs. P in her decision. Only one other support group member questions Mrs. P's refusal to support her husband's living will, and she was quickly silenced by other group members (e.g., "Oh, let her do what she wants; she's got to live with her husband's illness, too.)

The support group leader, a psychology intern, felt almost personally betrayed when hearing about Mrs. P's decision. She interpreted Mrs. P's decision to have her husband placed on life support as a literal form of retribution that Mrs. P decided to take upon a previously abusive and domineering husband. (Mrs. P had revealed in earlier meetings their marriage was marked by periods of emotional instability and abuse.) Although these urges appeared to be suppressed from awareness, it was as though Mrs. P now wished to assume the role of aggressor, and make her husband experience an ultimate form of submission. The intern also had a difficult time addressing this issue because she felt that her interaction with Mrs. P was limited by her membership in a support group, and not a consensual, therapeutic relationship. She felt that she had no ethical right to challenge Mrs. P and lead her to closely examine her decision making.

Although he never regained consciousness, Mr. P lived for another seven months, and Mrs. P felt satisfied with her decision. Probably no one could determine the best outcome for this scenario, and the Psychology intern eventually came to accept the ambiguity of the situation, as well as her inability to engage Mrs. P in a therapeutic, insight-oriented process.

REPRODUCTIVE CRISES

In conjunction with increased professional interest in the intersection of women's physical and mental health, members of the general public have become increasingly aware of reproductive crises such as infertility, miscarriage, postpartum depression, and postpartum psychosis. Fertility clinics and specialists are now available in large and medium size cities (despite long waiting lists), and some psychologists and psychotherapists have developed niche practices in response to the mental health needs of these patients. Thus, some general information about infertility will be presented in this following section, along with practical approaches to assessment and treatment.

Infertility

Recent estimates suggest that between 10 and 20 percent of all couples attempting to conceive a child will have difficulty doing so. Infertility specialists define infertility as the inability to conceive after one year of "regular" sexual intercourse (an obviously vague term) in the absence of contraceptives. Most women seeking the help of a fertility doctor are past the age of 25, and some patients have expressed considerable anxiety and concern that "I don't have a year to sit around and just wait and 'see' if I'm going to get pregnant ... I'm almost 35 ... " Therapists may be able to aid these patients in having open, honest discussions with their physicians about the merits of waiting to do an intervention, or forging ahead with various treatments.

Many female patients who take fertility drugs, including both oral and injectable forms, are generally unaware of the significant, clinical side effects that may result. Many of these drugs may produce anxiety, depression, weight gain, and excessive hair growth, among other unpleasant symptoms. At a time in their lives when they may already feel most vulnerable (e.g., "I feel like I am defective ... a mutant"), these patients, as well as their physicians, may be unaware of the "double difficulties" imposed upon them by the very medication designed to help them.

Still other women describe the extent to which fertility treatments begin to consume their sense of self, as well as their daily routine. One patient stated, "Yeah. You know, my husband gets up, goes to work, does his thing, comes home, eats dinner, drinks a beer or whatever, and can put all of this shit out of mind for a while if he wants to. I don't have that choice. First thing in the morning I'm taking my temperature, checking my [cervical] mucus, preparing my shot ... Then I have these dizzy spells during the day from my meds, and then I have do pretty much to do the same thing all over again at night ... And the next day I can't wear the pair of pants I want because I'm getting fatter. And I can't even have a beer even if I want one, because I wouldn't want to hurt the baby—not like I'm really even able to have one; so that's just *great*! It's like I can't escape, even if I want to. I have just become this walking 'bag' of fertility drugs ... And my husband doesn't understand why I am so 'preoccupied.'" Couples therapy often is critical in allowing each partner to better understand the realities and perspectives of the other.

Men who have difficulties with conception face another series of stressors. Although it flies in the face of common sense, many fertility specialists themselves do not even ask male patients to submit to a sperm analysis until their female partner has had numerous, and sometimes even invasive, fertility tests. One woman stated, "Yeah. So I go to the hospital to get this dye pumped into my fallopian tubes—it didn't feel that great—and they found nothing [no blockage or scar tissue.] Then after all of that the doctor gets around to asking [my husband] to donate a [sperm] sample for testing. Why the fuck didn't we do that right away? I mean, maybe it is him." It is as though even trained medical specialists do not want to subject men to what they perceive as a humiliating (i.e., castrating) experience, and often inadvertently prolong a couple's diagnosis or treatment.

Even worse, men certainly are not socialized to discuss this issue with other men or women, and have virtually no available social support. One man stated, "I'm from this huge Italian family, and I'm supposed to tell everyone that I'm 'shooting blanks.' Right. That's going to go over real well ... I just wish my wife would tell everyone that it is 'her.'" Many couples seek therapy because the male partner does not want to discuss his experience of infertility (including possible solutions or options for surrogates or adoption) whereas his female partner may want to address the situation aggressively.

Regardless of the physiological difficulties discovered for either partner, it becomes critical that therapists allow each party to express their feelings, but also take care not to place blame on one partner or another. Of course, it remains vital for partners to be able to express their fears openly and honestly to get to that point. For example, one woman told her partner, with tears streaming down her face, "If you want to leave me to have babies with someone else, I can understand that. Just do it now, and be honest with me."

Upon hearing her most base concerns, her partner was helped to respond honestly. He spoke to her about his sadness and regret about not having biological children of his own, but added that this would not compare to how he would feel without his life partner or "soul mate." Later, this woman remarked, "If you [the therapist] had just told us that everything would be fine, and that we could just love each other and make it through this, that kind of nice-nice bullshit, like the kind that your friends try to tell you to do, wouldn't have let us really get into it, and start to get passed it. I mean, I needed to hear him say that he was upset, too. Just brushing it under the rug wouldn't have helped at all."

In addition to the challenging emotional issues related to infertility, couples often face challenging financial limitations and decisions.

Few insurance carriers provide coverage for fertility treatment, and those that do often maintain high deductibles and strict spending caps. One patient noted, "It got to the point when we had to decide whether we were going to buy a house or try getting pregnant again ... It's hard to know when to stop trying when your financial hopes and plans for the future start to go down the drain, too." Some individuals resort to illegal practices such as purchasing other women's unused fertility drugs at a discount through the internet or other underground auctions. Individuals from a lower socioeconomic status may rightly experience discrimination in seeking effective fertility treatment, and often must cope with the implicit declaration that "only the middle-class and wealthy" can get help to have children.

RISKY BEHAVIOR AND ALTERED MENTAL STATUS

Assisting individuals in crisis can be quite challenging when individuals in the midst of danger or crisis does not perceive themselves at risk. In other words, it is significantly more difficult for clinicians to treat ego syntonic, maladaptive symptoms and behavior than ego dystonic symptoms and behavior. What supercedes treatment of any addictive type problem is the need to address patient safety (e.g., particularly in the case of a drug interaction or psychotic episode) and the level of patient insight. It is difficult, if not impossible, to treat a patient for high-risk behavior if they themselves feel that their behavior is not a problem.

Although some specific information will be provided about various subtypes of high-risk behavior and instances of altered mental status, an in depth discussion of all of these topics is beyond the scope of this text. Thus, an effort will be made to focus on a few focal issues and report upon recent research findings. For example, recent advances in neuropsychology suggest that addictive behavior, including gambling, may be driven by some degree of brain dysfunction, particularly in the frontal lobes and limbic system (Damascio, 1994).

MDMA/Ecstasy

A virtual cultural phenomenon among adolescents in industrialized nations (Szostak-Pierce, 1999) is that of raves, all night (and sometimes one or two day long) parties that typically feature loud techno music, crowded conditions, glow in the dark toys and pacifiers, and the presence of 3,4-methylenedioxymethamphetamine (MDMA or

Ecstacy). Most of these parties take place in bars or warehouses in the early hours of the morning, after bar owners are no longer allowed to sell alcohol, and individuals under the age of 21 are allowed to enter. Sometimes large companies sponsor raves, and sell soda or sports drinks at reduced prices. Some parents and guardians may be lulled into a false sense of security about such raves because they assume that corporate endorsements legitimize these typically "underage" parties and preclude the use of illegal drugs or other dangerous substances.

Also known as XTC, X, E, Adam, Clarity, Lover's Speed, Cadillac, Love Pill, Lollipop, Smile, Snowball, and California Sunrise, one oral dose of Ecstacy in tablet or capsule form is purported to bring users an increased sense of empathy and love for others (McDowell & Kleber, 1994), increased energy and stamina, a sense of peace, release from anxiety, heightened sensory awareness (of lights and sounds), and a decreased need for sleep, food, and drink. Many users of Ecstacy also experience involuntary teeth and mouth clenching; many rave goers buy infant pacifiers to suck on during parties to avoid painful and sometimes disfiguring bites to their lips and tongues. Adverse effects of Ecstacy, observed among both short and long-term abusers, include psychomotor agitation, hypertension, hyperthermia (high body temperature), renal failure, heart attack, stroke, seizure, and long-term psychological effects such as memory impairment, paranoia, panic attacks, serotonin deregulation, and depression (Croft, Klugman, Baldweg, Gruzelier, 2001). The environmental conditions present at most raves, including loud noise (Morton, Hickey, & Dean, 2001), crowded conditions, and high temperatures may exacerbate these effects (Green, Cross, & Goodwin, 1995).

Therapists must be aware of the increasing use of Ecstacy in both suburban and rural areas, among adolescents of both low and high socioeconomic status. Many teens feel that Ecstacy is not a "problem" or "hard drug" because it is taken in pill form, and its cost is relatively low, at $5.00–$30.00 a dose. One user noted, "Well, I guess I didn't think it was that bad. I mean, just listen to the name. I thought I was going for a good time, not like I was doing something harsh or 'bad' like crack, acid, weed, or dope … those just even sound bad." Many pills and capsules also contain contaminants such as heavy metals or other illicit drugs.

Therapists also should be aware of the dominant subculture and underlying psychological neediness often associated with Ecstacy use. Some proponents feel strongly that "Ecstacy [breaks] social inhibitions while engendering an *emphatic imperative* that [fosters] new levels of emotional bonding" (Rushkoff, 2001, emphasis added, p. 350). Parents and primary physicians also can benefit from increased education about this emergent drug and its implicit but hollow promise of social support and connection.

Inhalants

Another type of substance abuse that has become increasingly popular, particularly among young children, is that of sniffing or "huff-ing." Although previously recognized as a problem of epidemic pro-portions among impoverished children in Mexico and South America (Jansen, Richter, Griesel, & Joubert, 1990; Moiron, 1974), recent surveys suggest that huffing is now a significant problem for many children in the Unites States. The majority of children who inhale substances for recreational drug use in the US are White, and have their first experi-ence by age 13. Although inhalant use technically refers to three dif-ferent classes of compounds: volatile hydrocarbons (e.g., toluene, rubber cement, gasoline) which depress the central nervous system and cause a relaxed or "mellow high;" volatile nitrites (e.g., amyl nitrate, "poppers," "rush") which dilate blood vessels and increase heart rate; and anesthetic gases (e.g., nitrous oxide) which minimize sensation/perception and impair consciousness, their use will be discussed somewhat globally here.

The substances inhaled or huffed most frequently by children include gasoline (by more than half of all sampled users), freon, lighter fluid, glues, and nitrous oxide (McGarvey, Clavet, Mason, & Waite, 1999). However, many children (as well as teenagers and some adults) employ a variety of inexpensive, easily obtainable substances to get high. They may turn to correction fluid, nail polish remover, magic markers, dry-erase markers, paint thinner, carburetor cleaners, and vir-tually anything in aerosol form including whipped cream, spray on leather cleaner, deodorant, hairspray, cooking spray, spray paint, and air freshener. Most people "huff" by placing a volatile substance in a plastic or paper bag, and then putting that bag over their mouth or their entire head. Others saturate rag with chemicals and hold it to their mouth and nose, or sniff certain gasses such as nitrous oxide directly from tiny, pressurized cylinders (i.e., "whippets").

Some abusers, of adhesives in particular, show a pink rash or a whitish ring around their cheeks, nose, and mouth. Whippet users may display mouth sores or cuts; when gas is expelled from the metal cylin-der, the temperature drops precipitously and can actually freeze the user's lips or tongue to the container. One user explained, "It was so disgusting... there was blood everywhere. I told her not to hold [the whippet] so close to her face ... [then] she freaked and pulled it off ... it seemed like half of her lip came with it ... we were so stoned that we didn't even clean it up ... the camp counselors were asking about it the next day." For most users, there are few obvious signs of inhalant abuse other than a chemical-type smell on one's clothing or a noticeable hoarding of certain products (e.g., cleaners, magic markers).

Unfortunately, most children who use inhalants are unaware of their serious, long-term effects. Huffing is associated with short term memory loss, visual scanning problems, slurred or stuttering speech, diminished attention and concentration, ataxic gait, cerebral atrophy, enlarged ventricles in the frontal and temporal lobes, abnormal brain waves, resting tremor, hearing loss, hallucinations, catatonia, and disruption of cardiac rhythms (Jansen et al., 1990; Moiron, 1974). Huffing also is associated with cardiac arrest and suffocation (depending upon the method used to inhale the substance). Education about huffing is requisite for parents, teachers, physicians, therapists, and community members, as well as for children as young as five and six years of age. Public policy makers and educators also cannot overlook the role of poverty, poor decision-making skills, and peer influences (e.g., Ives, 1994) when designing effective prevention, assessment, and treatment programs.

DOMESTIC ABUSE

The term domestic abuse can be applied to a wide range of traumatic situations and behaviors experienced among individuals. Examples include child abuse (e.g., physical, sexual, and emotional abuse), domestic abuse (including violence in married, cohabitating, dating, heterosexual, and gay and lesbian relationships), sexual assault (by a significant other, acquaintance, or stranger), and elder abuse. The intent of this section is not to provide a comprehensive overview of such interpersonal abuse, but to provide some clinically relevant information regarding recent empirical investigations and treatment approaches in response to these horrific events. One overarching issue in any form of interpersonal abuse is that of patient safety. The physical well being of the intended victim must initially become the therapist's *number one* priority.

Child Abuse

Although a comprehensive discussion of child abuse is clearly beyond the scope of this chapter, an attempt will be made to provide some general updates regarding repressed or "lost" memories, and general guidelines for therapeutic risk management. Most clinicians and researchers agree that child abuse is a terribly serious issue, and that it is often associated with increased anxiety, depression, PTSD, sexual dysfunction, dissociative disorders, substance abuse, and susceptibility of suicide in adulthood (e.g., Beitchman, Zucker, Hood, daCosta, Ackman, & Cassavia, 1992). (There is no controversy, however, that therapists in all states are mandated to report child abuse to the appropriate child protective service agency; practitioners should familiarize themselves with all related state laws and requirements.) Some researchers even suggest that child abuse may represent a causal factor in the development of schizophrenia, above and beyond that of the dissociative features often linked to traumatic stress (Read, 1997).

What remains controversial in relation to child abuse is the validity of so-called repressed or "recovered" memories. Some experts believe that the majority of recovered memories are colored significantly by therapeutic suggestion, leading questions, and overall errors in memory storage and retrieval (e.g., Loftus, 1993), whereas others purport that some survivors *do* forget and then recall abusive incidents years later (e.g., APA, 1994). Regardless, many lay persons, as well as therapists themselves (Knapp & VandeCreek, 1996) falsely ascribe to the myth that memory is like an "internal videotape" of life events, which can be "replayed" with considerable accuracy after hypnosis or some other type of age regression. Empirical research suggests that, despite the validity of repressed memories on the whole, many memories can be distorted easily by the intentional or accidental leading questions of others (Leippe, Romanczyk, & Manion, 1991; Widom & Morris, 1997), including police officers, psychotherapists, and support group leaders.

Thus, the legal implications associated with the recovery of abusive memories within the context of therapy are great. Some recommendations for risk management include: (See Knapp and VandeCreek, 1996, for an extensive review.)

- Obtain informed consent, in writing, if a patient wishes to actively retrieve lost memories. Therapists must tell patients about the significant limitations of hypnotherapy and age regression (which generally have no demonstrated effectiveness in retrieving accurate memories, Nash, 1987), as well as the general inability of material culled during such interventions to be used in court.
- Sessions involving recollections of abuse should be documented thoroughly, often with the use of audio or videotapes. If a lawsuit

of some variety ensues, this verbatim account may allow a therapist to demonstrate that he did not ask leading questions or "implant" false memories.

- Therapists should be honest with their patients about how they perceive the accuracy of their recovered memories. Although it would be ideal for therapists to focus only upon the feelings and beliefs of their patients, some patients may choose to make drastic decisions to sue family members or sever family ties based upon recovered memories. In such instances, a therapist can reinforce that while she believes that the patient experienced the event as real, the courts and other organized groups *may not* recognize those memories as valid, particularly in the absence of corroborative evidence.
- Document sessions clearly, and include "what" was done as well as "why" it was done. Professional consultations (also highly recommended) should be placed in the patient's chart, and include statements about the specific questions and answers discussed during those meetings.
- Advise patients to avoid confrontations with alleged abusers *while in the midst* of acute symptoms, distress, or the emergence of "new" memories or information.

In sum, practitioners need to be aware of the high incidence of child abuse in our country (and our culture's propensity to deny the prevalence of this abuse; Herman, 1997; Widom & Morris, 1997), as well as the limitations and risks associated with recovered memories and any related court proceedings. Therapists also need to remember that the ultimate goal in treatment remains the reduction or amelioration of patients' subjective stress and maladaptive symptoms, regardless of their origin.

Partner Abuse

Domestic abuse continues to be a significant, often misunderstood social problem. Estimates suggest that nearly one in three women who visit a hospital emergency room is the victim of domestic abuse, and that nearly one in five women requiring emergency surgery do so in response to serious injuries received from an abusive partner (Guth & Pachter, 2000). And, many women face a heightened risk of abuse when pregnant (Berry, 1996). Yet, the emotional costs of domestic abuse surely supercede the annual, multimillion-dollar societal costs of lost time at work, decreases in overall productivity, and emergency medical care.

Domestic abuse occurs among gay and lesbian, as well as hetero-sexual, couples. Domestic violence also occurs among teenagers and elderly adults, and among well educated, financially secure individuals as well as individuals from a lower SES. Although significantly less common, men as well as women can become the victim of domestic abuse. In addition, public service messages, prevention programs, or other outreach programs do generally not target individuals from such "unexpected" groups. Regardless of their background, many victims of domestic abuse are either unaware of their treatment and legal options, or too embarrassed or afraid to seek help from others. It also is important to remember that no shelters for battered women existed until after 1970 (Berry, 1996).

Many laypersons have difficulty understanding why someone "keeps going back to" an abusive partner or fails to get out of an emotionally or physically abusive relationship. Current perspectives on domestic abuse are predicated on an understanding of operant conditioning as well as general theories about typical responses to captivity (c.f. Herman, 1997). The typical cycle of abuse, apologies, and exaggerated efforts at reconciliation (i.e., the Honeymoon period; Walker, 1984), clearly represents intermittent or variable reinforcement. Variable reinforcement itself is known to account for much of the addictive pull of gambling, and intermittent abuse has been associated with more frequent psychological ambivalence and distress among victims of domestic abuse (Dutton & Painter, 1993).

When subject to captivity and abuse, individuals who had no previous relationship with their captors often have been found to develop a unique emotional response to them. Often referred to as the Stockholm syndrome, hostages and other captives may become protective of their abusers, and even begin to rationalize and support their inappropriate behavior (Herman, 1997). Although members of the general public may be somewhat understanding of the mental anguish forced upon a hostage, most laypersons have limited sympathy for a spouse or significant other who may live in virtual captivity, under the virtual control of their abuser, in their own home.

Regardless of the reasons for domestic abuse, all treatment objectives must focus first upon patient safety. The statistics show that women are most likely to be killed by an abuser immediately after they leave the relationship. Thus, significant care should be taken to plan an escape carefully, and to consider a variety of factors including the presence of emergency shelters, legal advocates, social support, job opportunities, and money. In other words, therapists should not simply encourage a victim of domestic abuse to leave their partner without having a specific plan in place. Therapists also should be aware that most women make more than three to six attempts to leave the relationship before they are able to make a complete, permanent break (Walker, 1979).

A variety of concrete suggestions can be offered in order to help our clients who may be in danger or who are currently living with an abuser. Although this compendium is not all inclusive, some helpful suggestions include (also see Berry, 1996).

1. Get information about abuse, and programs for help!
2. Go ahead and call local hotlines and crisis lines and shelter to plan ahead!
3. Pack a bag with emergency supplies such as change of clothing, money, toothbrush, telephone numbers, food, copies of important documents (e.g., children's school records, social security cards, marriage certificates, birth certificates, immunizations, titles to property or cars, bank account numbers, tax returns, medical records, paycheck stubs, leases, documents from any public assistance programs)! Consider hiding the bag with a trusted friend or family member.
4. Keep your car in good repair! Keep the tank at least half full. Park in the driveway for easy and quick exits. Get a car phone. Drive with the doors locked. Don't take the same route to work every day. Have a lock on your gas cap. Check the front and passenger areas before entering your car.
5. Tell trustworthy friends and relatives what is going on, and that when You are ready, you may want their help
6. Consider carefully whether you want to use a gun, pepper spray, etc. (can often be used against you)
7. Talk to a legal advisor about restraining/stalking orders. Can often get free legal aid
8. Talk to you kids about what is happening. Not to scare them, to prepare them. They may already have noticed either the violence, or your change in moods due to fear.
9. Get a detailed safety plan- in your wallet- keep phone numbers of friends, shelters, police, keys to a friend's house, extra keys to the car and house, someone who can loan you money in an emergency
10. Learn new job skills (domestic abuse if have to live independently)
11. Go to a support group. Make new friends (don't tell abuser if very possessive)

12. Learn the signs of coming violence! Work on sharpening your observational skills... is it drinking, yelled at at work, sulk more than usual, tone of voice...
13. Write down these clues to abuser's behavior (if stranger or stalked, too) document every threat or harrassing incident. Record telephone conversations (literally and write them down), note the date, time, etc.
14. Get an unlisted phone number and caller ID
15. Remove knives and scissors from countertops.
16. If phone lines or electricity cut (means security system off), have flashlights handy!
17. Unload any guns in the house and put ammunition somewhere else.
18. Rehearse a quick departure—also think about how you will feel, who you will go to first.
19. Ask anyone at door to identify himself. Ask for Id
20. Have a wide angle peep hole and window
21. Have porch or outside lights at a height that makes them hard to reach. Put in extra outside lighting. TRIM and illuminate shrubbery—no taller than 3 feet, keep away from front of door
22. Make sure dead bolts on all outside doors. If ANY keys missing, change locks. Change locks often anyway. Keep all other doors and windows locked. Install locks on outside gates.
23. Keep the fuse box locked. Keep flashlights and spare batteries on hand.
24. Don't open or accept strange packages
25. Get an automatic timer for your lights
26. Vary your travel route from home to work, as well as other often traveled locations
27. Share with family, doormen, co-workers picture of person who is threatening, or stalking you! OR about dangerous patient!
28. Make sure no one at your work releases personal information about you!
29. For abused person, get PO Box number for listings on bills and checks, job applications, driver's license (personal investigator or agencies can help with this, too).
30. Upper floor apartments and offices are considered safer than ground floor ones.
31. If in danger, go to nearest populated area (e.g., mall, police station)

A persistent myth among laypersons is that most domestic abuse takes place in low income, inner city settings. For better or worse, domestic abuse takes place among wealthy and poor individuals, among individuals of high and low levels of education, across various ethnic and religious groups, and in rural and suburban as well as urban areas. More importantly, such misconceptions, coupled with environmental issues and a general lack of nearby support services, typically make getting medical care in response to physical abuse particularly challenging in rural environments. Most treatment centers, police stations, hospitals, lawyers' offices, and shelters are located in urban areas.

Some women develop effective modes of communication and help-seeking behavior in the midst of such challenging conditions, however. For example, two abused women who lived in a sparsely populated rural area made a secretive arrangement in which each woman could turn off one particular porch light in the event that they had been beaten and needed some help. (In this case, the women's husbands would not allow them to visit the local doctor or call an ambulance after a beating.) Upon seeing this signal, one neighbor could travel the half-mile between homes and "just stop in" ostensibly to deliver to fresh baked goods or recently harvested vegetables. The brief visit also would allow for a few minutes of makeshift medical care. Of course, it would be ideal for these women to enact specific and effective plans to leave their abusive relationship, but it is always a start for an abused individual to seek immediate help in response to physical needs!

Typically Overlooked Targets: Adolescents, Gays, and Lesbians

Mental health providers and other related professions (e.g., school counselors) appear to have limited knowledge about the high levels of partner abuse among individuals who are dating, including boys and girls as young as 12 (Burcky, Reuterman, & Kopsky, 1988), same-sex couples, and women who physically and emotionally abuse their male partners (Bogal-Allbritten & Allbritten, 1985). Dating violence also has begun to reach epidemic proportions, particularly among adolescents. Various estimates suggest that between 10 and 40% of all high school students have been abused emotionally or physically by a romantic partner (Avery et al., 1997). Even more striking, interviews with nearly one in four adolescent targets of dating violence describe those episodes of violence as acts of love or affection (Henton, Cate, Koval, Lloyd, & Christopher, 1983).

Gay and lesbian individuals who experience partner violence face additional hurtles in their ability to seek and receive appropriate help and services. Pervasive stereotypes and myths still fuel many members of society's inappropriate, hostile and negative attitudes toward gays and lesbians. (Practitioners must continue to be aware that many gays and lesbians, as well as bisexual and transgender individuals, suffer discrimination and abuse from complete strangers as well as known individuals, due only to their membership in a marginalized minority group.) Few shelters cater to, or even accommodate, same-sex survivors of abuse. For example, gay men in abusive relationships are unlikely to seek help from battered women centers, and typically describe those services as unhelpful (Merrill & Wolfe, 2000).

In addition, men who suffer abuse within the context of a heterosexual relationship suffer from similar, inappropriate societal attitudes and stereotypes. Many men who have been physically or emotionally abused by a romantic partner often are too ashamed or embarrassed to admit that they have been abused "by a woman" or are led to falsely believe that they should just "take it like a man" (West, 1998). In sum, mental health practitioners must make a concerted effort to consider the unique context, as well as societal press, upon such typically overlooked victims of partner abuse.

Elder Abuse

Although many therapists appear cognizant of clinical situations that may represent child abuse, significantly fewer professionals appear cognizant of the increasing prevalence of elder abuse (Welfel, Danzinger, & Santoro, 2000). Conservative estimates suggest that more than one and a half million older adults, or about one out of every 20 older adults in this country, experience some type of serious mental, physical, or financial abuse. More than half of the victims of elder abuse are middle-class, white women, who are more than 75 years of age. In addition, more than 60 percent of all maltreated elderly adults are abused by their own family members. Most assailants are adult children, with the majority of abusers being daughters (Tatara, 1995). Various risk factors associated with elder abuse (for the elderly person being abused) include cognitive impairment, physical disability, an inability to perform activities of daily living (ADLs), behavioral problems (e.g., screaming; throwing food; wandering), living with an adult child, social isolation, a low socio-economic status (Choi & Mayer, 2000; Tatara, 1995), clinical depression (Dyer, Pavlik, Murphy, & Hyman, 2000), and a history of family violence and emotional abuse.

However, the best predictors of elder abuse are a caregiver's characteristics (Reis & Nahmiash, 1998). Caregivers with behavior problems (e.g., angry outbursts), mental illness, substance abuse (Choi & Mayer, 2000), marital problems, financial dependency upon an elder, unrealistic expectations for caregiving, and inexperience with caregiving are significantly more likely to engage in abusive behavior (Schiamberg & Gans, 2000). Caregivers abused by a parent during childhood are significantly more likely to abuse their own, elderly parent than children raised in a family without violence (Reis & Nahmiash, 1998).

Various experts posit that while one out of three child abuse cases is reported, only one out of every eight elder abuse cases is reported (Tatara, 1995; 1999). A factor that likely contributes to this notable discrepancy is that many states do not place the same legal demands upon health care providers regarding elder abuse as child abuse. For example, a number of states (e.g., Pennsylvania) do not have laws that mandate psychologists to report suspected elder abuse; such reporting is only voluntary. Still other states do not even regard certain forms of elder abuse as an actual crime. To compound the problem further, various Congressional committees, including the Health and Long-Term Care Subcommittee of Aging, are no longer in existence (Tatara, 1995). In sum, deficits in the reporting of elder abuse probably can be attributed to three primary factors: (1) differences in legal requirements; (2) stereotypes that elderly adults offer little to society, and that they do not deserve help; and (3) a general lack of information about elder abuse and its warning signs among professionals as well as laypersons.

The remainder of this section will be devoted to a discussion of some specific types of elder abuse, warning signs of abuse (c.f., Reis & Nahmiash, 1998), and general suggestions for intervention. The most commonly reported forms of elder abuse, from most to least common (Tatara, 1995) include:

- *Self-Neglect.* Self-neglect or self-abuse can be defined as not providing oneself with basic necessities or care, thus threatening one's own personal health or safety. The vast majority of these cases arise from an elder's mental impairment or illness, coupled with social isolation.
- *Caregiver Neglect.* In these cases, a caregiver willfully or inadvertently fails to fulfill a duty to provide care, including attention to both physical and mental health. Active neglect also is sometimes referred to as "granny dumping," in which caregivers take an elder to a hospital ER and abandon them there. Passive neglect is just as damaging to an elder, and may result from

a caregiver's lack of knowledge, mental illness, or physical infirmity. Warning signs of neglect (caregiver or self-induced) among elders become obvious, and include body odor, overgrown toe and finger nails, skin abrasions and sores, constant calling out for food or drink, infrequent changes in clothing, dirty clothing, missing socks or shoes, the presence of urine, feces, or old food, limited social interaction, disrepair in the home, infestation with insects or other pests, a lack of heating or cooling, being tied to furniture, and a lack of needed hearing or walking aids.

- *Financial Exploitation.* The unauthorized use or misuse of funds, properly, or any resources of an older person by caregivers has become increasingly common. Although more difficult to detect, common warning signs include sudden back account closings or withdrawals, radical changes in an older person's will, an elder who is unaware of their income or assets, stolen or missing property, selling of an elder's house without their permission, unnecessarily executed powers of attorney, missing social security checks, elder unaware of reasons for caregiver's visits to bankers or attorneys, no receipts available for bank withdrawals, caregiver lives with elder without paying rent or utilities, caregiver well dressed while elder is poorly dressed, caregiver generally uncooperative with service providers, and will not allow the elder to be interviewed alone.
- *Psychological Abuse.* It is likely that this type of abuse, in which a caregiver willfully inflicts mental or emotional anguish by humiliation, intimidation, and verbal or nonverbal conduct is dramatically underreported to state agencies. Warning signs among caregivers include talking of the elder as a burden, threatening an elder with acts of violence, confinement, institutionalization, abandonment, or eviction, talking about the elder's death, cursing treating the elder like a child, and speaking with others as if the elder were not there.
- *Physical Abuse.* Acts of intentional physical force that result in bodily injury, pain, or impairment can sometimes be difficult to differentiate from accidental injuries sustained during falls or extended bed rest. However, various warning signs may include fractures (e.g., particularly bilateral injuries of the upper arms), improperly healed fractures, retinal hemorrhages or detachments (from vigorous shaking), internal injuries (e.g., hematomas from striking or punching), joint dislocations, burns of any kind, open or weeping bed sores, and bruising in the shape of a hand, cord, or other restraining device.

Sexual Abuse. Defined as non-consensual sexual contact of any kind with an elder adult, sexual abuse is probably another highly underreported form of elder abuse. Social stigmas, fear, and shame may prevent elders from seeking help, whereas other elders may be unable to understand or convey to others what has happened to them. Warning signs include the presence of sexually transmitted diseases (including oral diseases such as gonorrhea), the presence of semen or other bodily fluids on clothing or other personal care items, and bruising around the genitals.

The role of mental health professionals in the detection, reporting (Welfel et al., 2000), and subsequent treatment (Choi & Mayer, 2000) of elder abuse is paramount. As in other crises involving human abuse, patient safety takes first priority in any clinical intervention. Although it can become easy for clinicians to become angry and frustrated with neglectful and abusive caregivers, some of the most effective interventions in the prevention of elder abuse focus upon providing caregivers with social support (c.f., Reis & Nahmiash, 1998), offering caregiving education, and developing realistic expectations about caregiving. Many local chapters of various national organizations (e.g., the Alzheimer's Association of America) offer support groups for caregivers. Referrals to appropriate agencies also can help provide caregivers with instrumental assistance such as part-time home care aids, the delivery of at least one meal a day via Meals on Wheels, low cost or subsidized transportation for an elder to visit a community or clinic day program, and sometimes even financial assistance.

Clinicians also must become aware of their own biases and beliefs regarding long-term care among older adults. Cultural issues regarding the treatment of elder abuse (see Tatara, 1999) must be evaluated and addressed in any treatment plan. Although many caregivers consider institutionalization of their elderly parent as a last resort, clinicians also must remember that placement in a nursing home or other long-term care facility may significantly benefit an elderly adult and a caregiver, particularly if the caregiver has a significant number of risk factors for abuse (e.g., mental illness, limited finances). Even a temporary respite in nursing home care can allow for emotionally and physically burdened caregivers the opportunity to recharge and reach a more healthy state of equilibrium.

10

Violence in Social Settings
The Workplace, School, and Community

The vast majority of school systems and government agencies (including the FBI, emergency response services, and the United Nations) employ some type of critical incident stress debriefing after a traumatic event occurs. And, due to increases in work related and school related violence, the need for such rapid responses to trauma appears great. However, despite the widespread use of such protocols, the scientific community can offer only limited empirical support for their use.

WORK PLACE VIOLENCE

The economic costs of work related violence are staggering. U.S. businesses alone lose more than four billion dollars a year due to work related violence, and some experts estimate that each individual episode of work related violence costs employers more than $250,000 in lost productivity, worker compensation claims, lawsuits, and additional litigation (Albrecht, 1997). Thus, many mental health professionals are being called upon to consult with employers in order to prevent the incidence of work related violence and aggression (Miller, 1999; VandeCreek & Knapp, 2000) for financial as well as humanitarian reasons. Three primary foci of consultation include:

- preventing current employees from becoming the victim of work related violence
- assessing job applicants' for their own potential for violence

- managing the behavior of current employees who appear in danger of engaging in work place violence

The need for such forensic consultation also can be expected to provide some therapists with burgeoning practice opportunities (Fletcher, Brakel, & Cavanaugh, 2000) in Employee Assistance Programs (EAPs) or as an independent contractor. Before discussing the clinical aspects of violence prediction and prevention, however, an examination of epidemiological trends regarding the actual type and frequency of workplace violence is necessary.

Although portrayals of media violence in the popular media suggest that disgruntled co-workers account for the vast majority of work related deaths (Beck & Schouten, 2000), homicide represents only the second leading cause of death in the workplace. The number one cause of death at work is due to automobile, truck, or other transportation related accidents. In addition, approximately 95% of all employees killed on the job are not murdered by co-workers, but by customers, patients, significant others, and strangers. And, the overwhelming majority of work related homicides take place during a robbery or break-in. In other words, only five percent of all work related homicides are due to employee-to-employee violence. Although clinicians certainly should not underestimate the impact of employee-to-employee homicide, the popular myth that Americans who die on the job typically do so at the hands of their own co-workers remains essentially unsupported (Beck & Schouten, 2000).

Another important factor to consider regarding workplace violence, despite the relatively low statistical risk of being murdered by a co-worker at work, is that the incidence of non-lethal work related violence in the form of physical assault, sexual assault, sexual harassment, telephone harassment, stalking, sabotage, theft, and verbal threat is becoming increasingly common (Fletcher et al., 2000; Miller, 1999). And, employees appear to be cognizant of this increased risk. A recent Gallup poll indicated that nearly nine out of 10 workers reported being disturbed by threats of violence in the workplace to the extent that they experienced a significant decline in work related productivity, suffered emotional distress, and even became physically sick. The same poll also revealed that two out of three employees reported feeling unsafe and vulnerable in their workplace (Labig, 1995).

Employees as Targets

Specific occupations also appear associated with an increased risk of both lethal and non-lethal work related violence. Statistics from the

NIOSH (1996) indicate that individuals in the following positions were significantly more likely to become the target of work related violence: police officer; security guard; bartender; fast food, gas station, jewelry, grocery, and liquor store cashier; taxi driver; bus driver; auto mechanic; firefighter, and *social worker* [emphasis added]. Health care workers in general (e.g., social workers, nursing assistants, pharmacists, physical therapists, psychologists, psychiatrists) also face increased risk for experiencing nonfatal, work related assaults (Beck & Schouten, 2000). Health care providers appear at greatest risk for work-related injuries due to patient violence. (Please see Chapter 7 for detailed information about the prediction, prevention, and management of patient violence.) Still other workers, in fields unrelated to the health care industry, are at significant risk for violence due to the entry of domestic abusers, stalkers, or assailants into the job site as well as disgruntled, angry clients and customers. Some concrete steps that employers can take (c.f., VandeCreek & Knapp, 2000) to help protect their employees from physical danger include:

- Schedule employees who work during evening and night hours to work in small groups, or at least in pairs (i.e., never alone)
- Install security cameras and other security devices in shops and offices, and display signs prominently that indicate their use
- Issue individual photo identification badges that employees must display prominently at all times.
- If employees experience harassment or threats from inside or outside of the workplace, encourage them to seek help via an Employee Assistance Program (EAP) and law enforcement
- If an employee is engaged in a relationship involving partner or family violence, encourage visits to an EAP and enact security protocols to prevent the entry of a known abuser into the workplace
- Assist individual employees (as well as individual store or commercial locations) in obtaining restraining orders against the entry of specific, potentially dangerous individuals into the workplace.
- Forbid employees from bringing alcoholic beverages, recreational drugs, firearms, and other weapons to the work site.
- Establish, discuss, disseminate, and clearly post a zero tolerance policy for violence in the workplace. Be sure to include verbal threats, intentional sabotage, and employee theft as well as physical abuse.

Employees as Perpetrators

Because virtually no evidence-based diagnostic protocols are available regarding the prediction of imminent violence or future violence (Runyan, Zakos, & Zwerling, 2000), many therapists who serve as industrial/organizational or EAP consultants must temper clinical decisions related to the diagnosis and prediction of violence with consummate knowledge of legal precedents and court decisions (VandeCreek & Knapp, 2000). Accordingly, a mental health provider without extensive training in forensics must be clear and direct with both employers and themselves about their own limitations in the ability to assess or predict work related violence (Beck & Schouten, 2000). For practitioners without forensic training and experience, consultation with law enforcement personnel, security experts (Beck & Schouten, 2000), legal experts, and experienced peers (VandeCreek & Knapp, 2000) becomes essential in any professional consultation.

An initial step in forensic consultation is for the mental health professional to clearly and unequivocally identify the actual client. In other words, who actually is retaining (i.e., paying for) the therapist's services? Individual employers, companies, human resource employees, EAP providers, and company medical groups all can request forensic consultations, and thus represent the mental health provider's true client. Therapists who treat a potentially violent patient through an EAP must make it clear to their patient (i.e., the company's employee) that their ultimate therapeutic responsibility lies with the patient's company, and must immediately identify any limitations in therapist-patient confidentiality.

Consultants asked to complete pre-employment assessments for applicants and fitness for duty evaluations for current employees are encouraged to avoid dual relationships by resisting the need to serve as their individual therapist in private practice or through an EAP (Beck & Schouten, 2000). In contrast, a therapist who discovers that a patient seen within the context of their own private practice has significant potential for violence has no ethical or legal obligation to that patient's employer unless that patient poses an imminent threat of work-related violence. In that instance, the therapist's ultimate responsibility remains with their individual patient, but it remains subject to all Tarasoff related statutes (also see Chapter 7).

Pre-Employment Screenings.   Forensic experts also recommend that employers engage in three distinct practices to avoid workplace violence: safe hiring, discipline, and termination (Miller, 1999). The most effective way to prevent employee incited violence or aggression is to avoid hiring violent individuals in the first place. Although it is vital for consultants to remind employers that it is not possible to predict an individual's potential for violence with 100% certainty, a number of factors can be considered in order to reduce any hiring risks (e.g., Fletcher et al., 2000).

- Because many job applicants either falsify or embellish their resumes, confirm an applicant's previous work history by contacting previous employers personally (by telephone)
- Consider a background check via security professionals (or through a typically small fee paid to the local courthouse) for records of previous arrests or other criminal activity (Beck & Schouten, 2000)
- Confirm the presence of any reported licenses, certifications, and degrees with appropriate state and local agencies or licensing boards
- Use a mental health consultant to perform an interview and gather information regarding a history of mental disorder, substance abuse, and past violent episodes, and antisocial traits
- Administer appropriate, job related psychological testing
- If warranted, screen for the presence of organic brain disease
- Honestly assess for the presence of internal, organizational dysfunction, which can lead easily to employee dissatisfaction and violence (Beck & Schouten, 2000)
- Acknowledge that various risk factors are associated statistically with an increased risk for violence, including: the male sex, an age of 20–40 (e.g., Guy et al., 1990), single marital status, the presence of diagnosable mental illness, current drug or alcohol abuse, and a low socioeconomic status
- Note that a history of previous employment problems, unresolved workers' compensation claims, and a sporadic work history also serve as risk factors (Miller, 1999)

Despite the evidence based nature of various risk factors, however, forensic consultants must advise employers not to dismiss candidates solely on the basis of one or two individual characteristics. A *pattern* of violent behavior or *numerous* risk factors for violence must be present in order to legally support a decision not to hire. In addition, the Americans with Disabilities Act (ADA, 1994) forbids employers to discriminate against a potential employee due to the presence of a mental disability or illness (e.g., manic depression; schizophrenia). However, if an employee or potential employee presents current health or safety risks (e.g., they manifest disorganized thought processes and paranoid delusions), they are subject to the same rules and standards as any other applicant or employee (Beck & Schouten, 2000). It also is vital to note that prior to any pre-employment evaluation by a mental health professional, job applicants *must* be informed that the outcome of their evaluation will bear upon the hiring decision, and the applicant must assent to the testing to be considered for employment.

Discipline and Termination of High Risk Employees. Situations also arise in which an employer may be concerned about a current employee's potential for violence, and retain a mental health consultant (or EAP member) to perform a "fitness-for-duty" evaluation. In addition to interviewing the identified employee, the consultant also may consider interviewing the worker's supervisor, co-workers, and human resource workers. Related personnel records, credit histories, medical records, and criminal records also can provide valuable information. Practitioners also should be sure to include inquires related to the employee's psychiatric history, substance use or abuse, personality characteristics, impulse control, reality testing, coping strategies, and past episodes of violence (Fletcher et al., 2000). Consultants also must be aware that employees targeted for such evaluations are likely to view them as a very real threat to their job status and even their core identity, which may serve as an additional factor in a potential escalation to violence (Miller, 1999).

   In still other situations, an employer may fear that a current employee's recent behavior (e.g., verbal threats; altered mental status) may lead to physical violence. Miller's (1999) guidelines for "safe" discipline and termination as well as Fletcher et al.'s (2000) suggestions for threat assessment now become critically important. In any disciplinary action, a careful balance should be struck between management and an individual employee. In other words, both parties should be involved in the decision making process and consider various alternatives (e.g., fines; unpaid leave; attending a specified number of therapy or EAP sessions) in order to reduce additional hostility that could lead to physical violence. The establishment of formal disciplinary review procedures (long before any incident of violence is suspected) also can reduce second-guessing by both employees and employers about appropriate protocol and procedures.

   When asked to conduct a threat assessment, consultants can consider a variety of factors in assessing the risk of violence. Indicators of concern include impulsivity, displays of weapons, a specified target of violence (e.g., a supervisor; fellow employee), a history of past violence, difficulty in accepting criticism from co-workers, holding grudges against co-workers and supervisors, blaming others for things under their own control (i.e., externalizing), limited family support, and an inability to describe thoughts and feelings surrounding previous violent incidents (i.e., limited insight; poor ego strength; Beck & Schouten, 2000). Also see Chapter 7 for additional factors related to patient (and employee) violence.

If a decision is made to terminate an employee from one's job, it should be exercised in a clear, direct, and respectful manner (Miller, 1999). For a number of interpersonal and legal reasons, the decision to fire an employee should be based upon work related behavior (i.e., failures to perform specified duties) rather than personality characteristics (i.e., having a bad attitude). If the employer believes that "the termination is hot" (i.e., conducted under hostile circumstances), the employee should be directed to leave the premises immediately—not in 24 hours or at the end of a shift. Terminated employees also should be instructed to return all employee identification badges, uniforms, keys, access codes, and other security related materials immediately. Employers also should inform terminated employees to take all personal items with them as they prepare leave, for they will not allowed to return to the building or worksite later, under any circumstances or for any reasons. Many episodes of work place violence occur after a terminated employee returns unexpectedly in a few hours or days.

To engage in humane firing practices and to avoid a potentially violent situation, information about available, company sponsored counseling and outplacement services can be provided to the terminated individual verbally and in writing. Having these types of discussions also should be conducted in a way such that the terminated employee can elect to avoid contact with supervisors or other co-workers (i.e., not feel publicly humiliated, shamed, or embarrassed.) In sum, these directives should be delivered in as respectful and humane manner as possible, but there should be no doubt by either party that the termination is absolute and final (Miller, 1999).

VIOLENCE IN SCHOOLS

Recent traumatic events such as the Columbine school shooting, and countless others, have focused increasing attention upon violence in both public and private schools. Findings from the CDC's Youth Risk

Behavior Violence Survey (1998) indicate that there were more than 170 violent, school related incidents between 1994 and 1997. The majority of these incidents involved the use of firearms and the subsequent death of students, teachers, staff members, and community members. Other alarming reports from the Youth Risk Behavior Survey (1998) suggest that nearly one in five high school students carry a weapon (e.g., gun, knife) to school on any given day, that nearly ten percent of high school students are threatened or actually injured with a weapon while on school grounds each year, and that nearly one third of all high school students have been the target of theft or vandalism of their private property (e.g., books, clothing, cars) while at school.

Of the students who reported bringing a weapon onto the school grounds, however, it remains unclear what proportion of those students carried a weapon to initiate or threaten acts of violence, or to ward off threats of violence (i.e., engage in self-protection). The CDC's 1998 report also suggests that school related violence impacts negatively upon students' education. Nearly four percent of the students surveyed reported that they had skipped school during the past year because they did not feel safe at school. Obviously, it is not possible for students to learn if they are not even attending school, or if they are too anxious or frightened to attend to class material while they are in school.

Threat Assessment

In response, many members of the public have been clamoring for mental health professionals to identify students at risk for engaging in violent behavior. The FBI recently presented a report on school related homicide, entitled "The School Shooter: A Threat Assessment Perspective" (O'Toole, 2000). The results of this report were widely publicized. Many talk shows, local news reports, and newspaper writers cited the following student characteristics, identified in the report, as significant predictors of student violence:

- The male sex
- A preoccupations with themes of violence, despair, hatred, isolation, loneliness, or nihilism, expressed in conversation or jokes
- Recurrent themes of destruction or violence (e.g., hatred, prejudice, death, mutilation, dismemberment, homicide, or suicide) in writing or artwork
- Limited ability to cope with frustration, criticism, failure, rejection, or humiliation

- A failed love relationship (i.e., experienced as a rejection)
- Symptoms of depression such as lethargy, loss of interest, feelings of hopelessness, restlessness
- Sleep and eating disorders
- An attitude of self-importance or grandiosity
- An inability to understand the feelings of others (i.e., lack of empathy)
- Demands for special treatment and consideration, consistent with perceived superiority in intelligence, creativity, and life experience
- Low self-esteem
- Uncontrollable, inappropriate, and unpredictable outbursts of anger
- An unusual fascination with violent movies, TV shows, computer games, music videos, magazines, stories, or books
- Regular searches on the internet for violent material, including evidence that material from those sites has been downloaded for review
- Preoccupation with activities related to carrying out a threat of violence (e.g., practicing with firearms; studying websites about terrorism and bombing)
- Contempt for one's parents, and possible violence in the home
- Easy access to firearms, knives, or other weapons
- Poor personal hygiene or a significant decline in one's appearance
- Drug or alcohol abuse
- Intense involvement with a gang, group, or organization that "shares a fascination with violence or extremist beliefs" (i.e., O'Toole, 2000; p. 24)

However, it is critical to note that these typical, mass media reports failed to acknowledge that although these factors are associated *statistically* with an increased risk of violence, their presence does not imply that a particular student will actually *engage* in violence. Just as many patients may exhibit warning signs for violence, yet not engage in violence (see Chapter 7), many students who display many of these aforementioned characteristics at some time in their development never engage in interpersonal violence. And, other students who display none or very few of these characteristics actually do perpetrate school related violence (c.f., Tolan, Guerra, & Kendall, 1995). Accordingly, the FBI indicated that these characteristics are not to be used as a 'profile' of a student shooter or a checklist for warning signs, but *only* as a guide to threat assessment *after* a student has actually threatened the use of violence (O'Toole, 2000).

In light of the media frenzy caused by the misrepresentation of the FBI's Shooter Report (O'Toole, 2000) in various outlets, great care must be exercised in the interpretation of any risk factors for student violence (Mulvey & Cauffman, 2001; Tolan et al., 1995). Significant concerns arise regarding the use of these findings as a literal checklist to identify certain students as high risk (e.g., identifying a student who writes creative horror stories—devoid of specific references or obvious similarities to individuals at the school—as seriously troubled or violence prone), making them the focus of staff scorn or derision. Such labeling also may violate students' civil liberties and foster a self-fulfilling prophesy in which students internalize their given label and ultimately engage in violent behavior.

Yet, many teachers are asked by their school districts to identify students who may be "having trouble" at school or home in order to target them for extra help, attention, tutoring, and meetings with the school psychologist. And, early intervention on the part of astute, concerned teachers may help prevent potentially violent (or suicidal) episodes among students. In helping teachers, school administrators, politicians, and concerned parents navigate the difficulties involved in identifying and helping at-risk students without assigning them a derisive label, mental health practitioners probably can use their clinical knowledge and skills best to help those individuals understand that student violence (as well as suicide) can never be predicted with 100% certainty.

Administrative Responses

Schoolteachers and administrators also must consider the impact of their own institutional culture upon the incidence of student violence. For example, is discipline meted out fairly among students? Is bullying tolerated, or tolerated from certain students but not others? Such inconsistencies in perceived discipline by students can suggest that aggressive behavior in a variety of forms is acceptable and engender feelings of hopelessness that encourage the utility of violent actions as a last resort.

Experts from various fields do concur that if a student threatens violence, the validity of that threat must be examined carefully, contextually (Tolan et al., 1995), and immediately (e.g., O'Toole, 2000). In response to any given threat, interviews can take place among school representatives and the student making the threat, the potential or intended victim (if specified), and the students' parents, teachers, coaches, and friends. Background information also can be gathered regarding the individual who made the threat. Similar to the criteria typically used to evaluate patient violence, care must be taken to evaluate the extent to which an individual manifests homicidal ideation, intent, or plans (identified as motive, means, and resources, from a law enforcement perspective; O'Toole, 2000). In general, the more detailed the threat or plan, the greater the risk. It also is notable that disciplinary action alone (e.g., suspension) in response to student threats may actually inflame the situation, thwart efforts at appropriate threat assessment, and cause the student to become even angrier and focused upon retaliation of additional, perceived injustices (O'Toole, 2000). Psychological or systems intervention, including family therapy and teacher consultations, may certainly provide both more immediate and long-term benefits.

An interdisciplinary team of individuals, including teachers, administrators, legal professionals, school psychologists or other mental health providers, and representatives from law enforcement appears best able to respond to actual threats of violence. Also having a specific individual assigned to the role of "Threat Assessment Coordinator" can minimize initial confusion after a threat is received because one individual is available immediately to oversee the assessment, the school's response (O'Toole, 2000), and contact with the media (if necessary). The use of law enforcement personnel to evaluate any potential threat of violence and help interview the related parties also can send an institutional message to the student making the threat, as well as to other students, that the school district will not tolerate violent behavior. Taking such threats seriously, without doing so in a rigid or frenetic manner, also gives other students the message that their safety and security is of paramount attention to the school system itself.

Efforts at Prevention

School systems also have encountered considerable press from various social groups and organizations to develop effective, violence prevention programs. Although the CDC, APA, and other prominent organizations have increased funding substantially to initiate and examine the effectiveness of various prevention programs, very few programs have modes of implementation and assessment that are amenable to rigorous scientific scrutiny. Although some well constructed pilot projects suggest that skill and content based lessons on social competence, emotional awareness, and problem solving can significantly minimize the risk of student violence (e.g., Fast Track; Conduct Problems

Prevention Research Group, 1999), results from additional, large scale, empirical studies probably will not be available for another few years.

Some current suggestions for preventing school related violence include:

- limiting unsupervised student access to school computers and the internet. Fears arise because such unlimited use may provide at risk students with detailed information about hate groups and bomb making (O'Toole, 2000). However, serious questions also must be raised in response to the censure of students' use of library and other resources (e.g., their freedom of speech).
- establishing clear, written policies regarding student violence and threats of violence, which are readily available to students, teachers, staff members, parents, and community members.
- Instituting multi-year skill-based programs that include students, teachers, parents, and community members (Bierman, 1996).

In the unfortunate instance when attempts at prevention fail and violent incidents do occur, school and community officials often follow a predetermined, strategic response to address the situation directly. One common administrative response to a critical incident is to engage in a series of Critical Incident Stress Debriefings (CISD; Mitchell, 1988). Although used by a large number of school systems, empirical support for such debriefings among students, parents, and staff members remains limited, and even controversial.

CRITICAL INCIDENT STRESS MANAGEMENT

Critical incidence stress debriefing (CISD) currently represents the most widely used intervention intended to mitigate the effects of severe trauma and stress among emergency support personnel in the world, with more than 350 "quick response" Critical Incident Stress Management (CISM) teams on call at any one time around the world (Everly & Mitchell, 1992). Although regarded with caution by many mental health professionals (e.g., Stuhlmiller & Dunning, 1999), CISD protocols have been adopted broadly by many public and private school systems, Police Benevolence Associations, various branches of the armed forces, and civil defense planners. Many high-risk industries, such as banking, mining, oil refining, commercial fishing, and chemical manufacturing, as well as other industries have adopted CISM as an essential component of their Employee Assistance Programs (EAPs). Despite this wide spread adoption of CISD in many work, school, and community related settings, however, important questions remain regarding its effectiveness (Bisson, McFarlane, & Rose, 2000; Kenardy & Carr, 2000; Paton, Violanti, & Dunning, 2000). Serious concerns even have been raised about the ability of CISM to cause unintentional harm (Conlon, Fahy, & Conroy, 1999; Stuhlmiller & Dunning, 2000).

When introduced in the early 1980's, CISM was based upon the then novel premise that crisis intervention should be multidimensional, incorporate more than one specific intervention at different points in time, and serve secondary survivors of trauma (e.g., emergency room personnel, police officers, paramedics) as well as primary survivors (Mitchell, 1983; 1988.) Another central premise of CISM is that a debriefing should occur as soon as possible after the incident occurs to decrease the intensity and duration of the typical stress response (e.g., irritability, hypervigilance, intrusive thoughts, depression, somatic symptoms, emotional numbing). CISM, as delineated by Mitchell and colleagues, features four distinct types of interventions. These include debriefings, introduced in their initial protocol (Mitchell, 1983; 1988), and the more recently introduced diffusings, demobilizations, and peer support (Everly & Mitchell, 1992; 1996).

Critical incident Debriefings require a team of CISM trained professionals, including at least one mental health provider, and an initial time commitment of two to three hours for a small group session. A diffusing requires the same CISM team with a licensed mental health professional within the context of a small group session, but with only an initial 20–40 minute time commitment. Although individuals from a variety of professions including paramedics, psychiatric nurses, police officers, fire fighters, emergency dispatchers, schoolteachers, and guidance counselors are eligible to receive training in CISM, formal protocol states that each CISM team must have at least one mental health provider (Mitchell & Everly, 1988) in order to address survivors' potentially serious problems such as suicidal ideation or a significantly impaired mental status. Peer support, also referred to as "one-on-one's," can be performed by a paraprofessional or a community based mental health professional, and requires a variable time commitment from approximately 20 minutes up to two to three days. Mobilizations, designed primarily for use after a mass casualty or community wide natural disaster, are designed to take place in a one-hour, large group session with up to 150 participants.

Anecdotal Versus Empirical Evidence

A recent Cochrane review of critical incident debriefing suggests that CISD actually may be more harmful than helpful to participants (e.g., Gist & Woodall, 2000). Forcing individuals to engage in an immediate review of a traumatic event, akin to the behavioral technique of flooding, but without individual therapeutic direction and support, may foster extended stress reactions (Conlon, Fahy, & Conroy, 1999), increased anger, high levels of blood cortisol (Stuhlmiller & Dunning, 2000) and increased alcohol consumption. Despite the Cochrane review's cautions against the use of mandatory crisis debriefings, one also may consider that most of the studies used in the Cochrane report to evaluate crisis debriefings do not provide controls for the quality of the intervention and its facilitiators.

In contrast, findings from various individual studies investigations suggest that CISM debriefings may be effective in reducing the negative, long-term effects of trauma and extreme stress (e.g., Everly, Flannery, & Mitchell, in press; Everly & Mitchell, 1997; Jenkins, 1996; Lane, 1993; Leonard & Alison, 1999; Nurmi, 1999; Robinson, 2000; Wee, Mills, & Koehler, 1999). However, the majority of these studies focus upon the reactions of emergency service workers (e.g., paramedics; police officers; firefighters; ambulance drivers; emergency room nurses) and less than one half incorporate appropriate control groups (e.g., Bisson et al., 2000; Leonard & Alison, 1999; Nurmi, 1999; Wee et al., 1999). Thus, it becomes even more difficult to evaluate the effectiveness of CISD, much less hypothesize about any specific, underlying mechanism.

Potential Population Specificity

Of all populations studied, both empirical and anecdotal reports suggest that CISD may be useful for the secondary survivors of critical incidents (i.e., emergency service workers), as initially intended (Mitchell, 1983). It also is interesting to note that when Mitchell designed the initial CISM protocols, they were designed specifically for use with emergency service providers including police officers, paramedics, emergency room personnel, dispatchers, fire fighters, and ambulance drivers. It is possible that the personality traits of individuals who often self-select into those jobs, coupled with the overall organizational culture surrounding traumatic incidents, actually may provide a situational and interpersonal context in which CISD can be more effective.

Because emergency service workers and other public servants often undertake dangerous assignments, take extreme physical and emotional risks, and endure discomfort and distress that many other people would or could not, they may be prone especially to the effects of repetitive, long-term exposure to trauma. And, despite a typically strong allegiance to one another, a number of epidemiological statistics suggest that emergency service workers are more likely to engage in ineffective coping strategies and self-destructive behavior in response to traumatic events than individuals in the general population. For example, liberal estimates suggest that while domestic violence occurs among 41% of the general population, more than 80% of police officers engage, or have engaged, in domestic abuse. Emergency service workers, as well as police officers, often are reported to have higher levels of alcoholism and completed suicide than members of the general population (c.f., Hem, Berg, & Ekeberg, 2001; Mohandie & Hatcher, 1999).

What also may help account for some of the effectiveness sometimes reported for CISD among emergency service personnel is their membership in a long-standing institutional culture that frowns upon any outward expression of grief, much less any voluntary interaction with a mental health professional. In a related discussion of "stuffing one's feelings," one police officer noted angrily, "You know, so my partner got shot and then a little kid died down the street—on my watch. What am I going to do? Am I going to sit there and cry like a big baby in my [squad] car? I don't think so. Who wants to see a cop cry? People are gonna think, 'So, who's this nut case who's allowed to carry a loaded weapon?' And you know that when we get sent to talk to [the police psychologist], it all goes right in our jacket [personnel file]. I don't need that shit! I'm not talking to anyone [a mental health professional] about anything. Never have, never will." Critical incident debriefings may allow otherwise hardened, maligned, or traumatized emergency service workers to discuss specific stress reactions among their peers (i.e., engendering social support; Jenkins, 1996), and then, if they so choose, to speak in confidence with a community based mental health provider.

Significant Controversy

Controversy also exists regarding the fiscal rather than clinical goals that underlie the extensive acceptance and even mandatory nature of CISD among various agencies and industries. Because the CISM model is recognized as a *standard of care* for the mitigation of posttraumatic stress by the United Nations, OCEA, the FBI (McNally,

1999), and many state, local, and federal agencies (Everly & Mitchell, 1997), employees in those agencies can engage in significant litigation against their employer if they are not offered CISM intervention after a job-related traumatic incident. In addition, some industrial/organizational consultants assert that immediate employer response to a traumatic event (i.e., via CISD) can make "a positive statement about the commitment of management to employee well-being" and thus reduce the cost of related legal settlements and worker compensation claims associated with traumatic stress reactions (Miller, 1999: p. 167).

Many professional organizations also function as "gate keepers" that can impact significantly upon a therapist's ability to provide services in certain business settings and to receive third party payments. Typical four-day training programs offered by organizations including the Red Cross and the International Critical Incident Stress Foundation are offered typically for a substantial fee. Formal training and certification in CISM also is important to a majority of insurance companies and Employee Assistance Programs (EAP), who will provide reimbursement for services only if a practitioner is trained and certified by one of these aforementioned agencies. And, although health care practitioners who serve on CISM teams typically provide debriefings on a pro bono basis, consistent with APA ethical guidelines that encourage volunteer service within one's local community (Linton, 1995), they may charge fees for individual therapy resulting from debriefing related referrals, usually made by the CISM team leader. Some therapists have created a marketing niche for themselves by treating traumatized fire fighters and police officers virtually exclusively.

Yet, despite the controversy surrounding the true financial benefactors of CISM and its clinical effectiveness per se, mental health professionals should at least be aware of the overall CISM protocols, recognized appropriately or inappropriately as the standard of care for many private, public, and government organizations (e.g., the FBI, Police Benevolent Associations). Even if a therapist elects not to participate in critical incident debriefings herself, familiarity with these protocols may prove useful in therapy with patients who may have participated in a debriefing themselves, in correspondence with various insurance agencies and EAPs, and in testimony as an expert witness.

Critical Incident Stress Debriefings

Mitchell and Everly (1996) suggest that a debriefing be held for individuals directly involved in the following events within a workplace or school setting: a child's death, a "line of duty death" (i.e., an emergency services worker dies on the job), a civilian dies due to the actions of an emergency services worker (e.g., an innocent bystander is killed during a high speed car chase), a mass casualty, large scale natural disasters, the suicide of a student or emergency services worker, or any school shooting. Because debriefings are so intense along a number of dimensions (e.g., time, affect), organizations are cautioned against using debriefings for other, more "minor" critical incidents. This prohibition against overuse (Mitchell & Everly, 1998) contradicts other statements in the literature that describe a virtual press for organizations to provide a mandatory debriefing following *any* traumatic event (e.g., Kenardy & Carr, 2000; Stuhlmiller & Dunning, 2000). Typically, debriefings are voluntary.

In planning a debriefing, it is vital to include everyone who experienced the event, including paramedics, emergency room personnel, teachers and supervisors, police officers, firemen (including volunteer firemen), security guards, emergency dispatchers (who typically work in physical isolation), hostage negotiators, and custodians and maintenance staff who may have cleaned up blood, debris, or worse after the event. Members of the media and government or administrative officials such as mayors, police commissioners, and school board members, unless they themselves were directly involved in the incident, are never allowed to participate in or to observe these debriefings. It is critical that the members of the debriefing are able to speak openly and honestly about what occurred, without fear of reprisals from superior officers or administrators. Of course, guaranteeing the confidentiality of a nontherapeutic group remains impossible (Stuhlmiller & Dunning, 2000).

Another critical aspect of CISD is its adherence to protocol. Some flexibility is encouraged, particularly if extreme emotional reactions occur, but the overall program is intended to be presented in its predetermined order to allow the participants to have some sense of security over the course of the intervention, and to introduce the participants slowly to the more emotionally charged aspect of intervention. The seven specific stages (Mitchell & Everly, 1996; 1998) are identified briefly in Table 4, and descriptive information for each stage will follow.

Stage 1: Introductions. The introductory phase of the debriefing is designed to promote group cohesion, establish appropriate professional limits, and highlight confidentiality. To begin the meeting, the CISM facilitator introduces himself/herself, and thanks the participants for attending the debriefing. The remainder of the CISM team introduce themselves, and the facilitator then provides an overview of the debriefing process, and outlines various ground rules.

TABLE 4. Stages in Critical Incident Stress Debriefing and Diffusings

Stage	Name	Objectives
1	Introduction	Introduce members and explain the process
2	Fact	Gather facts and dispel myths
3	Thought	Share initial thoughts
		Identify cognitive responses
4	Reaction	Identify emotional reactions
5	Symptom	Identify somatic symptoms
6	Teaching	Educate about stress reactions
		Provide stress management techniques
7	Re-Entry	Provide a transitional object (information packet)
		Offer individual discussion after the session
8	Follow-up	Promote safety and effective coping strategies
		Mobilize social support

Note: Stage 8, Follow-Up, is not identified as a formal stage in crisis debriefing by Mitchell and Everly (1996). It is included here as an additional stage by the author.

The following list identifies some of these basic guidelines for a CISM debriefing (Everly & Mitchell, 1997; Mitchell, 1983, 1988; Mitchell & Everly, 1996).

1. There is no "rank" here. No one is functioning as chief or sergeant, boss or employee. We all are equals here in this room, right now, as witnesses to this incident.
2. Everything said here in this room is confidential. Nothing leaves this room. That is one of the most important things I can tell you today. Absolutely nothing about this meeting will go in your personnel file (or "jacket" for most emergency support workers).
3. Please ask any member of the team any question at any time.
4. It is possible that some of you have no problems with this event, and you think you can handle it on your own. And, you probably are right. However, your presence here in this room will probably help other people, and we've found that people who try to handle everything by themselves often feel better even sooner if they talk things out, or even just listen.
5. You don't have to say anything if you don't want to. Your participation is voluntary, but your presence alone can help others.
6. We are here to listen, not to judge, comment, investigate, evaluate, place blame, investigate, or recommend. We just want to help you get healthy and back to work as soon as possible.
7. After this introduction, we will ask you to tell us who you are, and how you were involved in the incident. We'll give you some practical suggestions to help you get through this, and

some handouts with additional information, and numbers that you can use to reach us. We'll also be available afterward to talk individually, or one-on-one, if you want.

Stage 2: Gathering the Facts. The next phase of the debriefing is designed to foster communication among members, and participate in a basic information exchange. Participants are not asked to talk about their feelings—just about the facts. The facilitator leads the discussion and asks each participant to identify him or herself, and discuss how exactly they were involved in the incident. In other words, "What happened out there?"

Some participants have described this part of the debriefing as helpful because they often complete missing parts of a time-line, or learn about other things that happened for which they had no previous knowledge. For example, one police officer described anxiously waiting for the paramedics to arrive at the scene of a house fire. She described giving first aid to a seriously injured five year-old girl, but "not knowing enough to really help her." The little girl died on route to the hospital. The police officer felt guilty about "not doing enough, soon enough." When it came time for the paramedic in the group to talk about his involvement, he described his anger and frustration with the other drivers on the road who would not give him the right of way; "I could have gotten there 15 minutes sooner if those god damn people would have gotten out of the god damn way. With that kind of injury [smoke inhalation], 15 minutes [without oxygen] can make it a fucking lost cause." Upon hearing this piece of missing information, the police officer was able to positively reevaluate her own job performance. For other participants, however, hearing about failed rescue efforts or mistakes on the part of fellow emergency personnel can change initial feelings of competency in one's professional role to feelings of despair and derision (Stuhlmiller & Dunning, 2000).

Stage 3: Collecting Thoughts. The next phase of the debriefing is designed to serve as a transition from objective facts to an individual's cognitive and emotional response (Mitchell & Everly, 1996). The facilitator and other CISM team members ask each of the participants, "After your first adrenaline rush was over... after you came off auto pilot...what was your first thought?" Team members should be prepared for a variety of responses including silence, tearfulness, angry outbursts, attempts to blame others, gallows humor, and descriptions of emotional numbing and confusion. It is very important for team members to accept all responses at face value.

Stage 4: Eliciting Emotions.   This next stage in the debriefing process is designed to allow participants to move from the more objective arena of cognitive thought to the less objective, and presumably more stressful, arena of emotions. Each participant is asked, "What is the worst part of this for you?" Many participants describe this stage as the most difficult part of the debriefing process. Some will cry, while others will be silent. One fireman, who had witnessed the death of a young child in a fire, looked at the floor and said, "No one should have to pick a dead baby out of its crib. No one should have to do that. And I had to pick her up and bring her out to her mom. And I bring her her dead baby boy. What the fuck is that?" It can be challenging for some therapists to refrain from engaging participants in a therapeutic dialogue during the debriefing. Psychotherapy and clinical assessment can take place, but only outside of the CISM protocol, for the safety and security of all participants.

Chris.   The following vignette clarifies the need to abide by strict limits and professional parameters. A series of debriefings were scheduled for the emergency services professionals involved in the death of a police officer during a high-speed car chase (i.e., a high profile, line of duty death). One debriefing was arranged for the four paramedics who attempted to revive the officer for more than 45 minutes, who was later pronounced dead upon arrival at the hospital. Two emergency room nurses who had to deal with an unruly press corps and deliver the officer's body to the morgue were also included.

Unbeknownst to the three CISM team members and the other participants in the debriefing, this police officer's death reminded one of paramedics on the scene, Chris, of a traumatic event he experienced in his youth. A neighbor had sexually assaulted Chris when he was 12, and although he was afraid, he told his father who was a police officer. His father told him that he was proud of him for being so brave, and that he "was going to get that son-of-a-bitch if it's the last thing I do." The next afternoon, Chris's father verbally accosted the neighbor, who fled from the scene in his car. Chris's father sped after him in pursuit; Chris remembered cinders flying and his father's car fishtailing out of the driveway onto the street. Four hours later, two police officers came to Chris's home, and told his mother that his father had lost control of his car and rolled across a guardrail and into a ravine. He was killed upon impact. Chris blamed himself for his father's death, and went into the helping profession to try to "make amends" for what he did. As noted, no one in the current debriefing session, including Chris's partner, had any knowledge of this tragic, childhood event.

During the 4th stage of the debriefing when emotional reactions are elicited, Chris suddenly announced, "Guys, there's something I want to tell you … I've never told anyone this before. Not even my partner knows about this … " Fortunately, the psychologist on the CISM team interrupted him, stating "Chris, that sounds really important. But, I want you to think about this. Do you really want to share that kind of information right now, right here, with everybody like this? I'd like you to think it over for a minute." Chris paused for a few seconds and then reconsidered.

This immediate interruption of a group member who wishes to divulge a secret and test relationships within the group differs significantly from typical therapeutic responses in group therapy. However, it is vital to remember that CISM is not a form of psychotherapy. Within the boundaries established for a CISM debriefing, this type of limit setting is essential. If critical incidents cause participants to revisit previous personal issues or traumas, it also is imperative for the mental health professional on the CISM team to make an immediate assessment for danger to self or other, and to provide appropriate avenues for referral.

Stage 5: Identifying Symptoms. Each participant is asked to describe any changes they may have noticed in their body or their mind. For example, "We'd like to ask each of you to think about anything you're experiencing now, as a result of this incident … Some people describe feeling numb, having headaches, having bad dreams, trouble concentrating, being irritable, not wanting to eat, and things like that. Each person here may respond differently. These types of bodily responses are a normal response to an abnormal event. You are not crazy and you are not alone. These are just some of the different ways that our bodies attempt to deal with an abnormal amount of stress." The primary goal of this stage is to help participants to transition from their previous focus upon often-intense emotions to a somewhat more objective, ego observing state. However, critics of this stage, as well as of CISD in general (Paton et al., 2000), purport that this type of medical, pathogenic approach to trauma often elicits a self-fulfilling prophesy among participants in which they internalize the notion that any traumatic event experienced by any individual has the potential to evoke considerable anxiety, distress, and long-term effects (e.g., PTSD).

Stage 6: Psychoeducation. The goal of the sixth stage is to provide participants with specific information about critical incidence stress, what to expect in the next few days and weeks, concrete suggestions for coping (i.e., tools for stress management), the ability to engage a support system, and contact numbers for confidential help now, or in the future. In other words, psychoeducation becomes the primary goal. Some of the things shared with participants include:

1. You may feel fine now. Sometimes the effect of stress goes unnoticed for a few days, weeks, or even a few months before typical stress responses appear.
2. It is normal to experience a variety of things after being exposed to a traumatic event. These things may include physical problems such as: chills, rapid heart rate, sweating, twitches, headaches...bad memory for things related to the incident, feeling numb...insomnia, nightmares, constantly thinking about the event, being confused, and having trouble making decisions. Sometimes people's stress reactions include the ways that they behave or interact with other people including social withdrawal, increased consumption of alcohol or drugs, and avoidance of friends and family.
3. Having stress responses does not mean you are crazy or weak. By talking about the stressful event, and sharing your experience with friends and family, these stress reactions should subside sooner, and you should be able to get back to work and your normal routine sooner.
4. If you are worried about any of your symptoms, or if you feel that they are lasting too long, please see your doctor, contact anyone here on the CISM team, or call any of the numbers on the contact sheet that we gave to you right away.
5. For the next 24–48 hours, try to stay away from alcohol, caffeine, and other drugs. Your body needs a chance to rest, too. Try to eat good foods, and drink lots of water, juice, or even soft drinks. You have got to take care of yourself before you can take care of anyone else.

Detailed handouts that reiterate this information are provided to each participant. Critics note that verbal expression of one's feelings (i.e. via talking individually or in a group) is not always required for successful resolution of a traumatic incident (e.g., Pennebaker, 2000), and that forced verbal disclosure regarding the experience of traumatic events actually may promote increased levels of distress (Stuhlmiller & Dunning, 2000).

Stage 7: Re-Entry. The re-entry stage is designed to serve as a transition back to the "read world," and as a final opportunity for CISM team members to identify individuals who need immediate assistance (e.g., those who talked about wanting to die; who said they have no friends or family nearby). One summary question to ask each participant is, "Ok, now that we're about finished, how are you doing (or feeling) right now?" If participants express intense emotions (e.g., "What the fuck! This is total bullshit ... how can you just act like nothing happened?) or exhibit blunted affect and psychomotor retardation, team members are expected to engage that participant in conversation after the debriefing to further assess their mental status, and ability to remain safe.

Another vital aspect of the re-entry stage is that it provides participants a chance to talk informally with one another, and primarily with CISM team members. Some participants who were hesitant to talk in the large group may warm to the notion of speaking to a CISM team member one-on-one. For other participants, the simple act of eating or drinking with others can serve to normalize the experience, and help prevent them from feeling "crazy" or strange.

Stage 8: Follow-Up. Although not identified specifically as a formal stage in CISM debriefing (Mitchell Everly, 1996), the importance of follow-up should not be overstated. Ideally, each participant in a debriefing should be contacted in person or by telephone one or two days after the debriefing. Team members who spoke individually with someone after a debriefing should provide follow-up with that person in order to foster an increased sense of continuity and care. Otherwise, there are no formal rules for follow-up. It is not meant to approximate any form of psychotherapy or psychological assessment (unless follow-up occurs in the form of a formal referral to a mental health provider).

It also is important to note that follow-up in the context of CISM is significantly different from most mental health professionals' view of patient follow-up. Boundaries in CISM follow-up can become quite elastic, and even blurred. For example, follow-up could include driving a disoriented firefighter to the hospital to see her partner who suffered serious burns while rescuing a child, going with a paramedic to the wake of a fellow paramedic who committed suicide in the ambulance bay, having dinner and watching a ball game on the first night after a line of duty shooting if a police officer has no immediate friends or family in the area, or being present for moral support and encouragement when a policeman tells his wife that he was shot at three times without getting hurt during a robbery, but that the bullets fired from his own gun ricocheted and killed a 17 year-old boy instead. Consistent with various findings from social psychological research (Brissette et al., 2002), such in vivo support many prove quite beneficial.

Alternative Approaches

As noted, although CISM (Mitchell, 1983; 1988) may represent the most commonly used crisis intervention in the world, various experts in the field have expressed significant reservations about its use. Gist and colleagues (e.g., Gist & Lubin, 1989a,b; Gist Woodall, 2000) provide some alternative approaches to crisis intervention, which emphasize interactionist and ecological perspectives. For example, Process Debriefing (PD; Dyregrov, 1997) is another approach to large-scale crisis intervention, and is employed primarily in Western European nations. PD places its emphasis upon group process and dynamics, rather than rigid protocols (as in CISM). Interactions among group members, rather than overall cathartic reactions, are considered the restorative elements in a process debriefing. Process Debriefing also relies more upon the leadership and assessment skills of the instructor, rather than the formal structure of any rigid, standard protocol.

Recent Modifications

Critical incident stress diffusing represents one of the more recently introduced protocols in CISM by Mitchell and Everly (1996; 1998.) Diffusings were developed to provide brief group support, psychoeducation, opportunities to identify serious stress reactions, and provide additional, individual follow-up for emergency service personnel. (See Table 4 for a summary of the protocol's stages.) Critical incident stress diffusings are similar in content to critical incident debriefings, with the following clear exceptions:

- A diffusing requires only a 20–30 minute time commitment
- No formal meeting room or location is required
- Participation is strictly voluntary, and never mandatory
- The format is flexible, and does not follow a rigid, staged model

Another recently introduced component of CISM is individual peer support, often referred to by CISM team members as "one-on-one's." In practice, fellow EMS workers, rather than formally trained mental health professionals, provide individualized peer support on an as-needed basis, and after all group debriefings and diffusings. Emphasis is placed upon the notion of peer or insider support versus professional (i.e., outside, out of context) support from a mental health professional. These peer interventions are designed to foster increased perceptions of social support, provide actual (i.e., instrumental) social support, promote effective coping skills, help normalize the traumatic experience, and encourage communication between the emergency services worker and his or her family members. Peer counselors also are trained to recognize warning signs for suicidal and homicidal ideation, and in such cases to refer their assigned peer to a licensed mental health professional. Unfortunately, no empirical studies are available yet to assess the effectiveness of CISM diffusings and their related, peer support interventions, as well as the other aforementioned alternatives to formal debriefings.

Tentative Conclusions

It is difficult to come to a formal conclusion about CISM. Its widespread use as a standard of care in many institutions and businesses (c.f., Mitchell, 1983; 1988; Mitchell & Everly, 1996) often requires that mental health providers seek training in CISD in order to work in EAPs or to receive third-party payment for services. Although CISD has been identified as a generally well received intervention among participants and useful as an early screening device (Bisson et al., 2000), limited empirical evidence exists to support CISD as a buffer against the formation of PTSD or other extreme stress responses (e.g., Paton et al., 2000; Shalev et al., 2000). Findings from various empirical investigations even suggest that the use of mandatory debriefings may violate the hypocratic oath itself (e.g., do no harm), and cause significant patient distress (Stuhlmiller & Dunning, 2000).

At a minimum, however, most mental health professionals could probably agree that CISM's recent emphasis upon the inclusion of peer based, instrumental social support (via one-on-ones) promotes a salutogenic (i.e., health promoting) versus pathological approach to the experience of trauma (e.g., Paton et al., 2000), and may deliver more promising patient outcomes. Considerable research is required in order to evaluate the usefulness of these critical incident interventions; it is vital that clinicians as well as laypersons recognize that a therapeutic technique's obvious face validity in no way guarantees its internal validity.

11

Underserved Patient Populations
Children, Adolescents, Older Adults, and Minority Group Members

The experience of crisis and trauma does not limit itself to anyone based upon their age, sex, socioeconomic status, ethnicity, or race. However, the integration of that experience into one's life can be quite different depending upon various developmental and cultural factors.

Relatively little formal education in crisis intervention is available to therapists in training, and even less is available that focuses upon crisis intervention with underserved patient populations including children, adolescents, older adults, minority group members, and immigrants from other cultures. Various issues become central in treatment, including developmental issues, social supports, language or dialect, stereotypical assumptions, socioeconomic status, and religious views. Some of these critical issues will be presented here, along with available research findings. The use of case studies also will illustrate some of the typically overlooked aspects of treatment with various members of these patient populations.

CHILDREN, ADOLESCENTS, AND TRAUMA

In any setting, children must be evaluated differently from adults in response to their experience, and even definition, of trauma. The dependent nature of children upon parents and other authority figures often exacerbates various life stressors (Davidson, Inslicht, & Baum, 2000) and can pose significant barriers to treatment. The inability of many young children to verbalize their experiences and comprehend abstract concepts (e.g., the just world theory; family dynamics; external versus internal locus of control) may foster differential perceptions of trauma and the development of PTSD. What is clear is that experience of severe trauma among children (e.g., physical, sexual, and emotional abuse; natural disasters; exposure to assault or murder; accidents) often lends itself to significant delays in cognitive, biological, and interpersonal development (Davidson et al., 2000). Specific difficulties observed in children exposed to trauma include (Streeck-Fischer & van der Kolk, 2000):

- learning disabilities (i.e., difficulties differentiating between essential and non-essential information; perceptual distortions; problems with sensory integration)
- inappropriate displays of aggression against self and other (e.g., head banging; self-mutiliation)
- an increased risk of recreational drug use (Kendall-Tackett, Williams, & Finkelhor, 1993) and high-risk behavior for HIV (Streeck-Fisher & van der Kolk, 2000)
- an increased likelihood of developing cancer, heart disease, diabetes (Kendall-Tackett et al., 1993)
- changes in immune system response, including increased white blood cell counts (Ironson, Wynings, Schneiderman, Baum, Rodriguez, Greenwood, Benight, Antoni, LaPerriere, Huang, Klimas, & Fletcher, 1997)
- an increased likelihood of meeting diagnostic criteria for borderline personality disorder, dissociative disorders, eating disorders, and substance abuse in adulthood

To help prevent the development of such insidious, long-term effects, a careful review of the symptom presentation, means of assessment, and treatment of PTSD among children remains essential.

Differential Diagnostic Criteria and Symptom Presentations

Although the DSM-IV notes that children may reexperience traumatic events differently than adults (i.e., children are not required to have nightmares with content specific references to the critical incident in order to meet diagnostic criteria; APA, 1994), many symptoms of traumatic stress commonly observed among children are not included or acknowledged in any formal, DSM-IV diagnostic criteria (Ruggiero, Morris, & Scotti, 2001). Some of these symptoms include:

- social withdrawal and lack of interest in previously enjoyed toys or games
- separation difficulties (e.g., frantic attempts to remain in close proximity to caregivers; anger and rage when reunited with caregivers after a brief absence)
- regression of previously learned skills (e.g., bedwetting; use of a pacifier or other security item; lack of speech)
- magical thinking (e.g., If I am a good boy, maybe this won't happen again; I have special powers that let me see into the future.)
- inappropriate attempts to "protect" parents (e.g., I don't want to bother Mommy with stories about my bad dreams ... she seems really upset.)
- hoarding of food, toys, and other possessions
- "freezing" or emotional numbing via a catatonic like state (Streeck-Fischer & van der Kolk, 2000)
- repetitive, even compulsive, play that mimics aspects of the traumatic event
- loss of fantasy or imaginary play
- frantic attempts to maintain schedules and routines

Because these symptoms are not formally associated with a DSM diagnosis of PTSD, many experts recommend the use of empirically validated instruments for the assessment of PTSD among children (e.g., the Diagnostic Interview Schedule for Children Version IV from the National Institute of Mental Health's PTSD module; Shaffer, Fisher, Lucas, & Dulcan, 2000) as well as more "broad-spectrum" instruments (Ruggiero et al., 2001) such as the Child Behavior Checklist. Because parents often underreport the impact of traumatic events upon their children (Sternberg, Lamb, Greenbaum, Cichetti, Dawud, Cortes, Krispin, & Lorey, 1993), the assessment of PTSD remains challenging, and typically requires a comprehensive approach.

Other researchers have tried to identify factors that may predict the development of PTSD among children. Culling information from a variety of sources (e.g., LaGreca, Silverman, Vernberg, & Prinstein, 1996; LaGreca, Silverman, & Wasserstein, 1998; Vernberg, LaGreca, Silverman, & Prinstein, 1996), it appears that exposure to additional trauma after the initial incident, minority group status, high trait anxiety levels, lack of social support are uniquely predictive of PTSD up to 10 months after the initial event (LaGreca et al., 1996), and may represent risk-factors. Caution must be taken when interpreting these

results, however, because most of these studied involved children
exposed to natural disasters rather than interpersonal abuse or violence. And, children from all walks of life appear at risk.

Recent Approaches to Treatment

Many of the evidence-based treatments for PTSD among adults have
yet to be examined empirically among children (Cohen, Mannarino,
Berliner, & Deblinger, 2000). Limited empirical evidence suggests that
EMDR shows promise in symptom reduction with children (Greenwald,
2000). Although flooding represents a powerful, evidence-based technique with adults, virtually no empirical studies of flooding have been
conducted with children. This lack of empirically based investigation
into one of the more effective adult treatments for PTSD is probably in
response to the inherently anxiety producing nature of the procedure
itself. It would be reasonable to assume that such an anxiety provoking
treatment could easily overwhelm a child's already tenuous response
to a trauma, and even foster revictimization. If the use of flooding is
attempted with children, experts cite the necessity of regular attendance
at sessions and honest communication of the therapeutic process and
expectations with parents and caregivers (Ruggiero et al., 2001).
Ultimately, practitioners must determine the appropriate mode of treatment based upon clinical experience and intuition (Ruggiero et al., 2001).

Although controlled studies of family therapy are not available,
aspects of family therapy, including psychoeducation for the child's
parents, may be vital in the treatment of PTSD among children.
Numerous studies suggest that children's responses to trauma are often
mediated by parental responses to the event (McDermott & Palmer,
1999). Restrictive changes in parenting style (McFarlane, 1987),
including a lack of social activity outside of the home, and the presence of intrusive traumatic memories, particularly among mothers
(Ruggiero et al., 2001), may be responsible for this relationship. Art and
play therapy also may be useful among children who possess limited
verbal abilities, or who have regressed in their ability to articulate their
emotions and experience. A number of case studies, descriptive
research findings, and clinical anecdotes also suggest that a variety of
unconventional techniques, including the use of Big Bird from the
public television show *Sesame Street* (Davis, 1988), may be useful in
reducing the symptoms of PTSD among children.

Among these more unconventional approaches, Storm and colleagues (1994) offer a unique, integrative approach to PTSD among children. This team of therapists developed a unique approach to early

intervention and assessment via a community-wide program, which featured aspects of family therapy, art therapy, personal narratives, successful coping, gathering social support, and cognitive restructuring. The focal point of this program was the use of a specially designed workbook for students, complete with cartoon characters, suggested activities, and spaces for journaling and coloring. The workbook also served as an important transitional object, signifying the presence and support of various individuals in the community after a natural disaster left as many as one third of the children homeless. School counselors administered the program to more than 600 children exposed to a series of wildfires that left many of them initially separated from parents and caregivers, and homeless (McDermott & Palmer, 1999). The children were given the workbook, *The Bushfire and Me: A Story of What Happened to Me and My Family*, and asked to complete it with the help of their parents. Informed consent from all parties was required. Chapters in the workbook and some of its sample activities are shown in Table 5.

TABLE 5. Overview of Storm and Colleague's Workbook for Children Exposed to a Traumatic Event

Therapeutic Function	Sample Activities
Introduction: For Parents, Caregivers, and Teachers	
Provide information about stress reactions	There is no such thing as a typical reaction
Recommendations for completion	Families that use the book [together] seem to get the most benefit from the book; Keep family routines as normal as possible
Provide resources for professional help	See the appendix for resources; It is important that you have help for yourself
Chapter 1: About Me	
Personalize the experience	Draw a picture of yourself and your family
Reinforce sense of self	My hobbies and sports are:
Chapter 2: Before the Fire	
Establish percepts of normalcy	When did you first hear about the fires?
Introduce a personal narratives	If you had more time to pack, what would you have taken? Did you get caught in a traffic jam? What was that like?
Chapter 3: The Fire Came	
Debunk myths	What do you remember [about the fire]?
Provide reality testing	Were you worried someone in your family could die? Did anything bad [or good] happen to you? Where did you sleep during the fires?

TABLE 5. (*Continued*)

Therapeutic Function	Sample Activities
Identify immediate stress reactions	Did your tummy rumble? Did you want to go to the bathroom?...Did your body do anything...that surprised you?
Chapter 4: After the Fire Provide factual information	Draw a picture of your home and the places around it in your neighborhood
Allow expression of emotion	When you came home what did you see...smell...hear...touch...taste? What was the best and worst thing about coming home?
Chapter 5: People who Helped Identify supportive individuals	[Identify] who helped you [e.g., policeman, doctor, teacher, parent...]
Identify available institutional support Provide reality testing	Did you meet anyone new? Of course not...everyone is helpful...Write a list of some things that went wrong
Chapter 6: Back to School Engage effective coping strategies	As a class, make a record of plants growing back, make a class diary, notebook, or story
Instill a sense of hope and competence	Draw a picture of your friends and teachers; what bushfire stories did they have to tell? Talk about your goals for the school year
Chapter 7: Several Months Later Identify symptoms of PTSD	Did you know it can be good to talk about scary thoughts and nightmares with someone you trust? Draw a picture of one of your dreams
Review coping strategies	Because it is getting easier to think...about the fire, you may like to listen to the story of someone else, like...a firefighter or neighbor
Chapter 8: One Year Later Acknowledge anniversary effects	What might remind you of the bushfires one year later?
Promote closure and commemoration	What can you and your family do to remember and celebrate your survival of the fires?
Identify positive and negative outcomes	What advice would you give to someone if the bushfires happened in the future?

Note. Adapted from *The Bushfire and Me: A Story of What Happened to ME and my Family* (Storm et al., 1994), with permission.

Storm et al. (1994) reported that 90% of the school counselors, parents, and teachers consented to the use of the workbook. Children who completed the program were given certificates, and those who met criteria for PTSD (12%; McDermott & Palmer, 1999) were scheduled for individual or group therapy. Although no empirical evidence is available to suggest that this community-wide intervention prevented the development of PTSD symptoms, the program was deemed a success because more than 90% of the school children affected by the natural disaster, as well as their parents, were screened for early intervention and provided with appropriate treatment if necessary.

Adolescents in Crisis: Developmental Issues and Suicide

A variety of statistics indicate that out of all age groups, adolescents make the highest number of suicide attempts (Jamison, 1999). However, such statistics also show that adolescents are more likely to attempt rather than actually complete a suicide attempt. Their primary methods of suicide often include less lethal approaches (i.e., compared to firearms and falls) such as overdosing, cutting, and hanging. In other words, some teens who commit suicide can be resuscitated via a visit to the local emergency room. Because this type of information has become available for public consumption, many laypersons often misinterpret this information to mean that young adults only threaten to commit suicide in order to gain attention. Their attempts are often considered ineffective and "just for show." Caregivers may even be told to ignore their teen or "tell them to shape up." Unfortunately, this type of public nonchalance (or "tough love") regarding young adults' mental health is also the kind that can lead to a teenager's untimely death.

Although a large number of teenagers do recover from suicide attempts, a large number of teenagers die from their attempts. It also is interesting to note that debriefings with teenagers who were resuscitated after serious suicide attempts often reveal that these teens did not actually intend to kill themselves, but only become sick enough to require medical (and psychological) attention. However, a number of misconceptions and situational factors often turned their "less dangerous," calculated attempt into very serious, deadly, often impulsive attempts. For example, some teens noted that they clearly underestimated the number of pills they could take and still remain conscious for a certain period of time. Other young adults described things "getting out of hand" after consuming even a small amount of alcohol or other recreational drugs (e.g., Jamison, 1999). The resulting changes in perception, difficulties in controlling impulses, and decreased

sensitivity to pain may account for their sudden change to more lethal
suicide attempts. Still other teens describe a terrible situation in which
they feel that they have to "up the ante" just to get their parents' attention (e.g., "If you don't let me go out I'm going to cut my throat right
here, right now!), and slice deeper or fall farther than they had initially
intended. In that moment, these teens report that they would rather
risk death than lose face by backing down from a power struggle or
confrontation (e.g., Sells, 1998). In sum, *any* suicide threat or attempt
made by a teen must be taken seriously.

   Still other teens describe a day-to-day existence filled only with
"mental pain and torture," and attempt suicide in order to escape from
the devastating symptoms of an often undiagnosed, untreated mental
illness. The parents of adolescents who make suicide attempts often
respond, "I really just thought he was a moody kid, like virtually all
teenagers get. I just thought he would grow out of it, and that it made
him feel better by hanging out with his friends … she said that doing
family things together was like baby stuff." Just as many members of
the public maintain unfavorable stereotypes regarding elderly adults,
many adults often maintain similar, negative stereotypes about
teenagers, who normally appear "brooding, selfish, arrogant, awkward,
embarrassed, and depressed." The gangs and close knit peer groups
that many adolescents use as a substitute family typically do not provide the intended supportive relationships and unconditional positive
regard. Thus, although confidentiality is often a significant issue for
adolescents in treatment, every attempt should be made to include parents and caregivers in treatment (e.g., individual and family therapy).
Educating parents about limit setting, appropriate discipline, and
recovering love and respect in the parent-child relationship also can be
invaluable, and impact positively upon the entire family system (Sells,
1998).

   When working with a suicidal teen, it becomes especially
important to address developmental issues, including dependency
upon others (i.e., family members or guardians) and a typical inability
to acknowledge the permanence of their actions. Sometimes a serious
suicide attempt can be thwarted with the discussion that results from
the simple question, "So, where do you think you will go after you die?
What do you think it will be like?" Many adolescents fantasize about
suicide as a way to "get back at someone," make someone suffer or feel
guilty about how they treated them, or become reunited with a lost
friend or loved one. (Also note that a teen whose only goal is to find
relief from overwhelming psychic pain via untreated mental illness
would be treated somewhat differently.)

When asked to explore their thoughts regarding the final outcome of their suicide, some teens may acknowledge that they "really hadn't thought much about what it would be like" for them after the funeral, or about what would happen to them a few years later, after many people (i.e., especially the ones they wanted to anger or imbue with guilt) have forgotten about them and are even enjoying their day-to-day lives. Some adolescents with strong religious beliefs may examine fears that they will go to hell or somehow be punished for killing themselves. Although this approach initially may appear cruel, it can often allow teens to acknowledge the consequences of their actions. And, as one 17 year-old patient stated, "You know, this is kind of cool. I realize that I really want to piss [my friends] off, and now I can figure out a way to do it, and even be around to see it. I don't have to die to piss anyone off, and I can probably even do it better while I'm alive. Fuck them!" (Also note that the therapist would encourage and condone only assertive, and not aggressive, responses.) Thus, real problem solving and an analysis of more deep-seated problems, in which the patient now views herself as an active and effective change agent, can begin.

ELDERLY ADULTS IN CRISIS

As noted previously in Chapter 6, older adults present a significantly higher risk of completed suicide than any other age group. Older adults who attempt suicide often select highly lethal approaches, including firearms and jumping from great heights. When someone shoots themselves in the head or jumps from a five-story balcony, there is little that anyone can do to circumvent the process, or help the person recover afterwards. Thus, suicide risk among older adult patients cannot be underestimated, and must be taken very seriously. Risk factors for this population, which always must be viewed with caution because individuals who fit none of these categories often commit suicide, include being male, single, widowed, or divorced, having one or more chronic health problems (e.g., clinical depression), having limited financial resources, living alone, and having a significant drug or alcohol problem (Hendin, 1995; Jamison, 1999).

Depression is not a Sign of "Normal" Aging

To complicate the clinical picture, older adults in this current cohort were raised in an era in which individuals did not label mood disturbances as depression per se. Instead, people were instructed to "pull themselves up by their bootstraps" and not "cry over split milk." Generational differences also include a significant degree of embarrassment and shame in the need to seek help from someone, much less a psychologist, psychiatrist, or other mental health professional. Many older adults assume incorrectly that the only people who seek help from therapists are seriously and chronically mentally ill (i.e., psychotic, schizophrenic, "just plain crazy").

Sometimes changes in the marketing of services can help older adults avoid feelings of shame, and actively seek treatment. For example, one 78 year-old man would not seek treatment for his major depression until he was offered "counseling...similar to what you would do with your pastor or a trusted friend" instead of "psychotherapy," which he identified as "psycho-babble crap...for people who are dumber than a sack of hammers and just plain nut cases." Because many older adults from this current cohort report that religion plays a very important part in their lives, activating an older adult's church related support system can be helpful. Older adults also are more likely to seek treatment if their pastor supports their decision, and even accompanies them to their first appointment.

It also is critical to note that the clinical presentation of depression itself often varies widely between younger and older adults. Many older adults do not express sentiments that they are sad, depressed, or tearful. Instead, they are more likely to report feeling bored or irritable, and discuss a variety of somatic complaints such as headache, backache, joint pain, dizziness, and stomach upset. It also can be difficult to determine if an older adult is significantly depressed because some of the typical indicators (e.g., an inability to perform work-related tasks; impaired social relationships) are not as valid among elderly adults who are retired or who live alone, unable to drive or ambulate independently.

Worse still, many family members and friends of many depressed elders often assume that becoming quiet, depressed, irritable, and socially withdrawn is simply a "normal" function of aging (Hillman, 2000). Many health care professionals themselves are often unaware of the creative and low cost senior care programs offered in their local community. Psychoeducation thus may become one of the more effective ways for mental health professionals to combat the increase in depression, suicide, and other crises among older adults.

Borderline Personality Disorder: Differential Symptom Presentation

Another aspect of crisis intervention involves the long-term sequelae of trauma, including the possible development of (BPD). When asked to think about a patient suffering from BPD, many clinicians' initial thoughts turn to young men and women who engage in dramatic, impulsive behaviors such as reckless driving, alcoholic or drug related binges, one night stands with various sexual partners (typically involving unprotected sex), gambling to excess, and self-mutilation. Very rarely do clinicians identify an elderly patient as suffering from BPD. And, epidemiological studies do suggest that the base rate of BPD among elderly adults is significantly lower than that observed among young and middle-aged adults (Zweig & Hillman, 1999).

One possible explanation for this dramatic decrease in the prevalence of BPD in later life is that individuals with this disorder "burn themselves out," and engage in life-threatening behaviors that literally prevent most of them from reaching old age. However, this notion that individuals with BPD simply "run out of steam," is not supported by other studies in which a number of older adults diagnosed *clinically* with BPD did not receive an official diagnosis when evaluated according to the strict diagnostic protocols of the DIB-R and the DSM-IIIR (Rosowsky & Gurian, 1991; also see Zweig & Hillman, 1999). In response, Sadavoy (1996) suggests that although some manifestations of psychopathology may change, its core remains.

For example, an older adult who lives alone on a small, fixed income, unable to ambulate independently, and completely dependent upon family members for support would not even have the opportunity to engage in reckless driving, alcoholic binges, or one night stands. Other clinicians (e.g., Zweig & Hillman, 1999) assert that individuals suffering from BPD may show a marked decrease in symptoms during mid-life in response to defined roles and structure as employees and parents, only to experience a resurgence of symptoms when they lose the stabilizing influence of work (due to retirement) and face additional stressors of aging such as increased likelihood of chronic illness, social stigma, and overall physical decline. The loss of identifiable social roles and relationships, often endemic in later life, also are likely to pique existing fears of abandonment.

Thus, it may be appropriate to identify more flexible diagnostic criteria for the presence of BPD in later life, that incorporate the influence of potential, significant declines in physical health and environmental resources. Definitions of self-injurious or damaging behavior could be expanded to include missing important doctors' appointments, smoking or drinking against doctors' orders, impulsively storming out of family gatherings when the patient is dependent upon family members for help, spending $150 dollars on non-essential items when the patient's fixed income leaves only $10 for food during the rest of the month, taking too many prescription drugs, and refusing to eat (i.e., anorexia). Identity disturbances may be expanded to include issues that revolve around changes in one's physical appearance rather than a more subjective sense of "Who am I?" Patterns of intense, unstable relationships may be extended to consider relationships with formal and informal caregivers. (Some elderly adults may not have access to a large number of social contacts due to health constraints or other physical limitations.) For example, an elderly patient may have significant difficulty in establishing and maintaining a relationship with one particular caregiver. Many elderly adults diagnosed clinically with BPD have been reported to "fire" their home health care aids (for ambiguous reasons) faster than related social service agencies can find replacements.

Affective instability and chronic feelings of emptiness also may present themselves in different focal symptoms among elderly adults. For example, many older adults diagnosed with BPD manifest a number of somatic symptoms and complaints that have no identifiable medical origin. Just as many older adults with clinical depression identify with the presence of chronic headaches, backaches, and other somatic symptoms instead of more emotive statements such as "I feel sad, hopeless, or worthless" (e.g., Hillman, 2000) it stands to reason that older adults with BPD will communicate psychological distress primarily through the presence of unpleasant, bodily sensations.

Some elderly patients diagnosed with BPD also appear to manifest psychosomatic symptoms that mimic the experience of early trauma, perhaps linked with the common PTSD symptom of reexperiencing the traumatic event. For example, one homebound 73 year-old woman, Ester, required almost daily visits to the Emergency Room for management of severe asthma attacks. (She came to depend upon her interaction with the ambulance crew and hospital workers as her primary form of socialization, which served as significant secondary gain in response to her poor compliance with prescribed, home based treatments.) In therapy, Ester described how her mother would choke her virtually into unconsciousness whenever she cried out of fear or loneliness. When asked when her asthma attacks first began, Ester noted that they started a few months after her mother died. It is as though Ester was able to minimize her psychic separation from her mother by (unconsciously) reexperiencing these traumatic episodes of choking in the form of very real, serious asthma attacks.

As a caution, clinicians must take care to make appropriate, differential diagnoses between BPD and clinical depression among older adults. Although it is possible and even likely that older adults may suffer from both disorders, the emergence of BPD in late life is unlikely, whereas the emergence of depression in late life is more common. It also is vital to gather enough social history to establish that a elderly patient would have met DSM criteria for BPD in their early adulthood. As a final caution, it is important for therapists to note that older adults suffering from BPD are less likely to engage in self-mutilating behavior than their younger cohorts with the disorder, these elderly adults are significantly more likely to make a lethal (i.e., completed) suicide attempt.

Because a large proportion of nursing home residents appear to suffer from a personality disorder, which may account for their placement in an institution if they were unable to develop supportive relationships with spouses, family members, or children, psychologists working in long-term care can probably expect to work with at least one elderly patient with BPD in treatment (Hillman, 2000). Many elderly patients with personality disorders are brought to the attention of staff psychologists or outside therapy consultants due to their apparently focal role in institutional disruption. Due to these patients' difficulties in viewing individuals as integrated wholes, it is not uncommon for elderly individuals with BPD to generate friction among staff members by professing their extreme and often rapidly vacillating views (e.g., You know, Sue let me eat my dinner early. I guess you just don't stack up; How am I supposed to work with you? I only want to work with Allison!; "Right now, you are my most favorite nurse. I can't imagine anyone who could be better at anything than you).

Due to their sensitivity to interpersonal dynamics (borne out of a need for prediction in the service of self-protection), coupled with a limited ability to focus upon the needs and feelings of others, elderly patients with BPD also often demand special treatment or favors (e.g., "I am going to sit here in this room and rot unless you let me get another roommate [for the third time this month] ... what a pain in the ass ... and you know I can make life difficult for everyone around here if you don't let me do it."). And, out of desperation, many staff members submit to these special requests in a desperate attempt to avoid continued conflict. Unfortunately, this type of assent only serves as reinforcement for this type of inappropriate behavior.

To respond effectively to the needs of an elderly patient with BPD within the context of an institutional setting or nursing home, the following guidelines may be useful:

- Therapists can expect to provide as much support and guidance to staff members as to their own patients.
- Patient confidentiality and the extent to which treatment information will be shared among health care professionals and other staff members *must* be discussed very specifically with patients at the initiation of any treatment or consultation.

- Therapists can guide staff members—including food service workers, janitors, transportation workers, and security personnel as well as nurses, physicians, and occupational therapists—in the development of a concrete, written, comprehensive treatment plan to be followed by every member of the treatment team—without exception.
- If a patient engages in inappropriate behavior (e.g., throwing plates; kicking a staff member), specific institutional responses must be identified ahead of time so that important decisions are not made arbitrarily, in anger or haste.
- Preparing staff members for the impact of patient idealization and devaluation can be helpful. Knowing that a patient's perceptions are derived from difficulties with insecurity and a low tolerance for (both positive and negative) affect can help make it easier for staff members to work *with* patients rather than react to them.
- Consistency in staffing can provide patients suffering from BPD with some sense of stability in response to painful, internally vacillating states.
- Concrete representations (i.e., literal reminders or likenesses) of family members, previous club or work affiliations, hobbies and outside interests, and even staff members, in the form of prominently displayed pictures and prized possessions also can help assuage a patient's lack of internalized objects, and feelings of image disturbance and emptiness.
- Helping patients focus upon current strengths as well as the generation of new skills and abilities can help minimize the narcissistic injury associated with unexpected bodily changes.
- Assertiveness training can empower patients suffering from BPD to get their needs met while maintaining appropriate interpersonal relationships. Although unfortunate, it is easy to recognize that the quality of interpersonal relationships between patients and caregivers can be essential for the delivery of quality patient care in institutional settings.

In sum, the best approach to treatment with an elderly patient with BPD in long-term care is to provide both the patient and staff with some degree of structure, consistency, and skill.

HIV Infection in Later Life

The vast majority of laypersons, and even many health care professionals (Hillman, 1998), regard AIDS as a problem of youth. However, more than 10 percent of all reported AIDS cases are among adults over the age of 50, with one quarter of those cases among adults over the age of 65. In other words, more elderly adults have died of AIDS than soldiers have died in the Vietnam War (Hillman & Stricker, 1998). Consider the following:

- Studies show that the majority of men and women over the age of 50 view condoms only as an unnecessary form of contraception (Stall & Catania, 1994). Many older adults also have misconceptions that it is OK to reuse condoms (to save money), to use oil based lubricants (e.g., Vaseline), to use sheepskin condoms, and to store condoms in the freezer to increase shelf life.
- More than one third of all seriously ill AIDS patients are cared for by older parents and grandparents. Many elderly caregivers do not understand universal precautions, and contract AIDS by coming into contact with infected bodily fluids while adjusting catheters or changing the dressings on open wounds (Hillman, 2000; Levine-Perkell, 1996).
- Cases exist in which older adults have contracted HIV by sharing needles for prescribed insulin injections (Hillman, 2000) as well as for illicit, IV drug use (e.g., Levy, 1998).
- The early symptoms of HIV infection in older adults often appear as confusion and memory loss, and are misdiagnosed by health care providers as Alzheimer's disease, dementia, depression, or "signs of normal aging" (Hillman, 2000; Hillman & Stricker, 1998). By the time the older adult develops AIDS, it often is too late to begin effective treatment.
- Older adults who become infected with HIV develop AIDS faster and die sooner than younger adults. Protease inhibitors and other AIDS medications do not work as well with older adults due to their increased incidence of severe side effects.

Compared to younger adults, adults over the age of 50 also appear to maintain less accurate knowledge of HIV and its transmission (Mack & Bland, 1999; Ory & Mack, 1998), and to underestimate their risk of infection (Rose, 1996). Consistent with these misperceptions of risk, older adults who engage in high-risk behavior are six times less likely to take necessary precautions (e.g., use condoms) against HIV infection, and four times less likely to engage in voluntary testing than younger adults (Stall & Catania, 1994). Due to ageist attitudes and differential symptom presentations, AIDS also is less likely to be diagnosed among older adults (Hillman, 1998), leading to increased mortality and an overall decrease in quality of life (Hillman, 2000).

Issues regarding older adults and HIV also tend to be different from those among younger cohorts, and from other high-risk groups in general (e.g., IV drug users). For example, ageist attitudes that older adults do not engage in high risk behaviors, such as heterosexual activity, homosexual activity, and IV drug use, contribute to incorrect assumptions that elderly people themselves are not susceptible to AIDS (Ory, Zablotsky, & Crystal, 1998). As a result, rates of heterosexual transmission actually have been increasing among older and middle-aged adults rather than decreasing, as is the case with most younger age groups (CDC, 1998).

Once infected with HIV, older adults typically display different symptoms than younger adults. For example, older adults appear to display more neurological and cognitive deficits in the early stages of infection than younger adults (National Institute on Aging, 1988). These symptoms associated with HIV Associated Dementia Complex often mimic those of Alzheimer's Disease (Hillman & Stricker, 1998), which can lead to difficulties in making a timely and accurate diagnosis. Even if a diagnosis is made, it may be kept "secret" due to fear and embarrassment on the part of spouses and family members who do not want to reveal their relative's HIV status, even on a death certificate (Hillman, 2000). Without primary prevention, including the development of an accurate knowledge base among mental health professionals, the increasing rate of HIV infection among older adult men and women can only be expected to increase.

MINORITY GROUP MEMBERS

Attention to cross- and multi-cultural issues in crisis intervention is essential. Although the overall therapeutic process among patients and therapists from dissimilar backgrounds remains significantly more similar than different, some general considerations and knowledge base can help foster the therapeutic relationship, and provide greater entrée to clients' support networks and services. In response to a need for brevity, the following discussion of these issues will certainly appear limited. Despite these inherent limitations, however, several vital, overarching concepts and recommendations can be advanced.

General Recommendations and Considerations

To foster rapport and mutual understanding, some general suggestions can be offered in work with members of different a culture, ethnicity, or religious background.

1. Probably the first, and most essential, consideration for therapists is to never assume anything about a patient, based upon his or her

background. For example, a patient may possess Asian features, but reveal that she was adopted and raised in Europe; making assumptions regarding traditional Asian family practices could prove disastrous. Some therapists may be unaware that cultural norms often vary widely among Latinos, whose origins may be Puerto Rican, Dominican, Cuban, Haitian, Columbian, Spanish, or Mexican, among others. In other words, having a general understanding of certain cultural and religious groups can begin to provide a knowledge base for therapists, but only when this information is made explicit and confirmed, denied, or modified through direct communication with a patient.

2. To counter the impact of value-laden assumptions, therapists can model appropriate behavior for their patients by carefully and respectfully asking questions. However, therapists also must be cautioned about becoming so enamored with learning about their patient's cultural background that they lose track of the central issue in treatment.

3. If there is dissimilarity among patient and therapist, particularly if the therapist is presumed to be from the majority culture, meeting patients in their neighborhood, their church, or their community center (i.e., on their own turf) can immediately establish a sense of respect for that patient's own, unique situation and needs. Interacting with a patient in their own environment also indicates that the therapist is willing to "take a one down position" and view the patient as the expert in their own treatment (Sells, 1998, 2001).

4. To encourage communication regarding possible differences, therapists also can make statements such as, "If I ever do or say anything to disrespect you, or any aspect of your culture [or religion], which I would only do by accident, please tell me and set me straight. I don't ever want to say anything that is disrespectful. You are the expert here. Can I count on you to let me know, right away, if I say something that doesn't sound right, or is hurtful or disrespectful in any way? That is very important to me" (c.f., Sells, 1998).

5. If patient-therapist differences are apparent, it is vital that therapists acknowledge them, and work within the patient's cultural or familial system. For example, in crisis intervention with a Korean family, who ascribes to traditional values, the therapist would acknowledge the family hierarchy, and always address the father first, even if he were not the identified patient. Labeling symptoms as "mental illness" would be avoided, at least initially, and the therapist would take on the role of "expert," as indicated by cultural traditions.

6. It is vital to make all parties aware of the therapist's legal and ethical responsibilities (e.g., mandatory reporting of imminent, homicidal behavior toward a specific individual), while emphasizing the nature of patient-therapist confidentiality. For example, if a patient

is an illegal alien, therapists can review confidentiality issues to thwart fears that interaction with a therapist could result in arrest or deportation.

7. If a language barrier is present, therapists should carefully evaluate the use of a translator. As indicated in the APA (1992) ethical guidelines, therapists are required to seek the use of a translator when the need is obvious and present. However, locating and employing a translator can be difficult, and the costs may be prohibitive. A creative approach is often required. In one institutional setting, for example, due to a lack of available translators, a member of the food preparation staff was recruited to serve as a translator, with excellent results. Yet, additional problems arise regarding confidentiality and the general inability to determine if any translator is able to interpret the patient's statements accurately. If determined to be in the patient's best interest, therapists also may consider a referral to a native speaking therapist.

8. Therapists can still present their own, unique opinions in response to their patient's background, without being disrespectful. For example, a therapist might simply say, "You know, I myself am not familiar with arranged marriages. Most teenagers in the US would not even consider having one. But, you are upset and concerned that your son will not consider one. I just want you to know that, in accord with your beliefs, I am willing to work with you on that issue ... I might have to ask you some questions from time to time, and have you clarify some things for me, but I want you to know that I respect your beliefs, and want to work with you in a way that is respectful to you and to them." It also is important to note that, in this case (as would be in any other), the therapist did not make any promises about changing the behavior of others or feign adherence to the patient's belief system, but rather extended a willingness to explore, understand, respect, and empathize.

9. Recent evidence also suggests that many psychotropic medications are metabolized differently among members of various ethnic groups and racial backgrounds (see Lin, Poland, & Nakasaki, 1993). For example, African-American and Asian patients have been found to metabolize antidepressant and antipsychotic medication at a significantly lower rate than members of other ethnic groups. Due to this difference in chemical processing, many patients of African-American heritage may inadvertently be receiving excessive doses of medication, and experience a higher degree of side effects. Therapists often can help their patients interface more effectively with their psychiatrists (as well as other medical health providers) and open additional areas of inquiry.

Cross-Cultural Factors

Although these findings must be regarded only as potential starting points in any formal assessment of a patient's belief system, some patterns have been reported among various ethnic and religious groups regarding the stigma often associated with mental illness and suicide. In traditional Asian culture (again, note that vast differences in cultural beliefs and customs exist among different Asian subgroups including Koreans, Chinese, Japanese, and Philippines), significantly great emphasis is placed upon the family (particularly the father) or group, rather than the individual. Because familial ties are so important, any type of problem observed or presented publicly among one family member is expected to reflect negatively, and virtually permanently, upon all family members.

Mental illness is considered extremely shameful, and many Asian families will deny its presence or refuse to seek professional help out of fear. Many Asian immigrants describe somatic symptoms and "problems with eating" in order to convey a sense of personal distress, without being ashamed to admit emotional distress. (In the US, many elderly adults were raised to believe that people facing hardships simply "pull themselves up by their bootstraps," and present with similar, primarily somatic depressive symptoms.) And, in some Asian subcultures, such as the traditional Japanese middle and upper class, suicide is often seen as the only way to escape from a problem (e.g., not passing qualifying examinations to attend a prestigious school), or to remove shame from one's family. Hsu and others (e.g., Tseng & Hsu, 1991) have written extensively about these types of issues, and offer a wealth of initial guidelines and recommendations.

In traditional Indian culture, individuals often engage in some form of familial, arranged marriage, take notice of differences in cultural (i.e., caste) systems, and embrace spirituality as a resource. Within the context of an arranged married, even the more modern variety in which the potential husband and wife are able to politely turn down or "choose from" a number of acceptable, parentally identified mates, Indian men and women often speak about marrying into an entire family rather than marrying just one individual. Representatives from both families often make formal appointments to visit each other's homes and businesses (typically before the potential bride and groom have even been introduced), to discuss everything from cooking to education to bank accounts. The presence of alcohol abuse or mental illness, even among distant cousins or in-laws, is considered reason enough to withdraw from any marriage contract.

Traditional Indian culture also suggests that it is improper for any-one to discuss sexuality or sexual relations, even among mothers and daughters, and fathers and sons. Subsequently, some experts suggest that within the next two decades, India will overtake Africa as the number one country in the world with the greatest number of AIDS cases (Roth, Krishnan, & Bunch, 2001). Therapists must consider very carefully the high stakes often perceived among Indian patients who seek help and support from, or are assigned or court ordered to see, a mental health professional.

In many Latino cultures, a patriarchal family structure, strong beliefs in Catholic doctrine, and the presence of machismo permeate virtually all interpersonal relationships (Kazarian & Evans, 2001). The notion of machismo suggests that Latino men are driven by immense, and often insatiable, sexual urges. It is expected that men have multi-ple sexual partners in order to satisfy their needs, and that the use of a condom is unacceptable because it both violates traditional, Catholic doctrine and robs a man of his sexual pleasure. Women are not expected to receive much sexual pleasure. (The rate of new AIDS cases is rising rapidly among Latino populations.) Some members of tradi-tional Latino culture also espouse that if a man hits or beats his wife or girlfriend, it represents a show of affection and romantic attraction (c.f., McFarlane, Wiist, & Watson, 1998). Above all else, as noted pre-viously, therapists must be sure to investigate their patients' cultural beliefs rather than rely upon stereotypical assumptions.

In contrast with traditional Indian and Latino culture, traditional African-American culture typically follows a matriarchal family struc-ture. Women's roles are often clear-cut and defined as mother, sister, aunt, spiritual leader, keeper of traditions, disciplinarian, teacher, and social coordinator. Grandmothers often have a special place in the fam-ily, and exert significant influence regarding the day-to-day function-ing of the family. Spirituality is often important, and can serve as a valuable anchor in times of crisis or stress. Many therapists are trained in professional programs that fail to offer any coursework in spiritual-ity, and often assume that patients who are deeply religious would ben-efit more from pastoral counseling. In contrast, the use of an already established support system (i.e., the church) can be utilized in any therapeutic crisis, regardless of a therapist's particular orientation.

Individuals from marginalized groups also may be hesitant to engage in, or even seek treatment. One Russian immigrant noted, "Yeah. I'm supposed to tell my therapist everything [laughed]. I just came from a communist country where you could get put in jail for just saying the wrong thing. I still have to tell myself that I can say out loud, in the open, what I think in my head ... I am still used to automatically keeping those thoughts in my head, where they can't hurt me [laughed again.]" One African-American woman made somewhat similar comments when she stated, "It's hard to trust people in the establishment. I know they are doctors, and that they are supposed to help. But, you know, I remember Tuskegee, and I don't know how far I want to go with [toward trusting] these people." Addressing such caution and distrust within the context of the therapeutic relationship is not always easy for clinicians, but requisite.

Phyllis: Deconstructing a Suicide Attempt. Consider the case of Phyllis, a 67 year-old African-American woman who was admitted to a day treatment program after a serious suicide attempt. Phyllis was a feisty woman who outlived three husbands (and currently had a boyfriend), raised eight children, had a close knit extended family, and more than 12 "grands" (grandchildren). Phyllis served as the matriarch of her family, and was active in church, politics, and the local community. She also had been one of the only African-American employees (much less an African-American woman) to reach a certain pay scale in the government bureau where she worked before retirement. She described facing considerable discrimination at work, in which "I had to prove myself with my test scores ... they had no choice but to promote me then ... I never let them see what was going on inside me, either ... they would never know how much they upset me." Two months before her admission to the day program, Phyllis had fallen from her fourth story bedroom window, and required surgery and extensive rehabilitation to repair a broken knee, elbow, collarbone, and pelvis.

After her admission to the day hospital program, it took more than three sessions with her individual therapist for Phyllis to actually recount the details of her suicide attempt. (Her therapist wanted both of them to understand the factors that led up to her suicide and also provide enough cognitive dissonance to make future attempts significantly less palatable.) Phyllis initially changed the subject, and commented, "that [my suicide attempt] was just so silly ... I don't need to talk about it ... let's just leave that crazy thing in the past." To avoid discussing her suicide attempt, she also made jokes and attempted to focus upon the difficulties of other patients. With gentle prodding and an explanation for the need to review the tragic event, however, Phyllis consented.

Phyllis described the two months before her suicide attempt as "absolutely terrible and frightful." She experienced a stroke, and temporarily lost control over the left side of her body. She could not easily venture out of her home, and was embarrassed to use her walker and cane. Her speech was slurred, and she had trouble getting people to understand what she was saying. She described lying for hours in her bedroom, looking out the window, thinking "what a waste I am ... just sitting here doing nothing." Phyllis also was upset that her son and daughter-in-law took time off from work to help take care of her; "they have their own lives and children, they didn't need to make such a fuss over me." She also refused to let her boyfriend help her with daily needs such as dressing, bathing, and toileting because she didn't want him "to see me like that ... I've always been a stone cold leader, and I've always been the one to take care of other people."

During her next session, Phyllis quietly described "the last straw," when she decided to go out the window. Phyllis spoke so softly that her therapist often had to ask her gently to repeat what she had said. In sum, Phyllis described a bitter divorce between one of her sons and daughter-in-law. She said that her daughter-in-law had "turned the other way," and announced that she was a lesbian. Interestingly, Phyllis was not that upset about her ex-daughter-in-laws sexual orientation. Rather, Phyllis described being devastated by the news because she was *the last in the family to know.* She felt that she wasn't needed anymore, and that she was no longer a valued part of the family.

Phyllis spoke about her suicide attempt in a quiet voice, tinged alternatively with elements of sadness and wry humor. Phyllis said that when she knew she was alone at home, she pushed the screen out of her fourth floor bedroom window. She said, "You know, I was too fat to get out the window! I just couldn't get it all out there at one time ... So I was hanging out of the window, with my caboose sticking right out. And I got stuck. I couldn't go in or out, and I started thinking, 'I don't want to go! I really don't' but I couldn't get back in my room. I don't know how long I hung there, with my arms and hands pressed against the sill ... it might have been 15 minutes. I'm kind of surprised no one starting honking their horn or something seeing my butt up there in the air ... Then I could hear the window pulling out of the wall."

Phyllis continued her story. "The next thing I know, I'm lying on the ground, in the bushes behind my sidewalk. I must have fell on top of my neighbor's van, and rolled off it into the bushes. That's the only way the doctors figured out I could have survived, plus with the damage to the van and all. I couldn't get up." When asked how she received help, she said softly, "Well, I lay there for eight hours ... I could hear people walking by on the sidewalk and the street." When asked why she did not call out for help, Phyllis responded in a husky voice, "I was too embarrassed and ashamed." Phyllis said that her boyfriend found her when he had come over to visit after work. He initially thought Phyllis was joking around. She said, "Yeah, James kept asking me why I was playing around in the bushes." Phyllis was then taken to the hospital for surgery.

Phyllis related that she "had hurt [her] family more than [she] had hurt [herself.]" She looked at their faces one day and said, "Oh, my god! You look more tired and upset than I do!" In the day hospital program, Phyllis began to talk about some of her issues, and soon became one of the most liked patients in the program among both patients and staff. (It was easy for staff to become lulled into thinking that Phyllis was no longer depressed because she was so socially active and cheerful.) Phyllis always had time to listen to a fellow patient's concerns. She began to walk about much more easily, and resumed many of her church and community activities. In therapy, Phyllis developed concrete plans and goals for her immediate future. Then, the bad news hit.

During her last appointment with her orthopedic surgeon, he noticed that Phyllis was limping. She admitted reluctantly that she was in constant pain, but that she did not want to bother anyone about it. Further tests revealed that Phyllis would need needed hip replacement surgery. That would mean Phyllis would find herself back in bed, unable to ambulate independently for weeks at a time. In other words, this procedure would send Phyllis right back into the same situation she was in before her previous suicide attempt. Although Phyllis became despondent, she refused to discuss the impending surgery at the day hospital program stating, "Everything will be OK."

Again, Phyllis's therapist insisted that they talk about the upcoming surgery, and make specific plans ahead of time to help Phyllis make it through the ordeal. Fortunately, Phyllis was able to expand upon her plans for the future. She had always wanted to earn a college degree, and with the help of the team social worker, made arrangements through the local community college to complete two televised, independent study courses while she was recuperating. Phyllis also agreed to a family meeting, and with her therapist's support she was able to articulate her needs and concerns to her family members. She also made requests for specific, instrumental needs, but on her own terms. For example, if someone were coming over to help for the day, Phyllis would ask her specifically to perform two or three chores, and to discuss how they could help with her bathroom needs while affording the maximum privacy possible.

Phyllis's family members were pleased to be included in her recovery plans, and were able to tell her that they felt much better when she could talk to them about her needs and wants. Spontaneously, family members asked Phyllis if they could all share a weekly meal at her home (they would bring and make the food) so that Phyllis could continue to "keep her place" in the family. Her minister also agreed to visit her twice a week to discuss scripture and "what was going on at church." Phyllis also agreed to get a home health aid for the first two weeks after her surgery, and arranged for weekly therapy sessions over the telephone.

Overall, Phyllis's therapist felt considerable anxiety regarding her patient's hip surgery. She had to take Phyllis at her word that she would not hurt herself, but her previous history of a typically lethal suicide attempt gave her the impetus to make a series of thorough, concrete plans with a wide variety of support systems. From a dynamic perspective, Phyllis and her therapist also worked through some issues in which Phyllis perceived her therapist as an oppressor, who forced her to discuss issues that she did not want to. A few challenging sessions (for the therapist!) were spent talking about cultural differences among the two women, and about difficulties in establishing trust and rapport. Eventually, Phyllis said that she was OK with her therapist "pushing" her so much. She was able to see past the cultural difference, and parallel process of oppression, to the insight that she was entitled to ask for help from others, just as she prided herself on doing for others.

12

The Future of Crisis Intervention

With the tragic events of Columbine and September 11th fresh in the minds of Americans, as well as individuals around the world, psychology as a profession should embark upon a mission to educate individuals about crisis and trauma, to engage in treatment models that employ a variety of professionals in a variety of settings, and to develop effective, evidence-based approaches to prevent the occurrence of such future disasters.

WRAP-AROUND SERVICES

An emerging trend in crisis intervention and trauma counseling is the use of wrap-around or therapy support services (TSS). Therapists in these program may be asked to perform a variety of activities related to crisis management, including assessment, intervention, and follow-up. Therapists typically make visits to a patient's home, and assess for dangerousness to self and others, look for any drug reactions, offer counseling, encourage effective coping strategies, coordinate social supports, and even provide assistance with instrumental needs such as transportation to a doctor's appointment or pharmacy. Patient populations range from children to older adults, from individuals to entire families in crisis. Individuals in need of services also come from a wide range of incomes, educational backgrounds, religious affiliations, and cultural and ethnic groups.

Costs and Benefits

Many states have made these in-home or wrap-around services a guaranteed benefit for residents with certain disabilities or psychiatric diagnoses (e.g., autism; mental retardation; schizophrenia). In response, employment opportunities have soared for individuals with masters and bachelor level degrees. Other social service agencies provide, and HMOs often pay for, wrap-around services because they can provide a realistic assessment of a patient's home and social setting as well as offer a generally seamless continuum of care. (One TSS provider explained, "Seeing patients in their home instead of an office is like going from black and white TV to color with surround sound.") Agencies and HMOs also may endorse the use of these services because the total cost of TSS and wrap around services is significantly less than that for traditional psychotherapy with a licensed mental health provider (e.g., psychologist or social worker), inpatient treatment, and institutionalization.

Although there is limited empirical evidence regarding the usefulness of the wrap around services, significant benefits for patients may be associated with their implementation. TSS and wrap-around providers can provide critical testimony in court decisions regarding involuntary hospitalization, nursing home, and foster care placements. Because much of an individual's behavior is situation specific (Jones & Nisbett, 1972), many patients present very differently at home than in their therapist's office. In home providers literally can check on the contents of a patient's kitchen (i.e., is there enough food in the refrigerator; is it healthy food; is it spoiled), observe how clean, dirty, or crowded their patient's home is (e.g., do they share a one bedroom apartment with eight other people), observe how relatives and neighbors treat their patients, note the number, type, and health status of pets in the home, and more realistically assess the patient's environmental and social stressors (e.g., are the parents emotionally abusive, is there a heavy presence of drug dealers and crime in the neighborhood). In home service workers also may be able to have conjoint sessions or meetings with their patients' friends, who may influence their behavior as much, or even more, then their own family members.

Despite these potential benefits to patients regarding the use of home services, many of the individuals hired to provide those services receive limited training and supervisory or administrative support. In home providers may not have the diagnostic skills or experience to identify someone who is chronically mentally ill. Patients also may feel that they have limited privacy in their own homes, and resent the presence of any mental health provider. For TSS providers, the work is often exciting and challenging, but potentially dangerous and relatively low paying. Thus, the turnover rate among staff tends to be high. Additional issues in home care treatment can include poorly delineated environmental and personal boundaries, an initial lack of structure, unfamiliar or unsafe environments, multicultural issues (e.g., among Chinese immigrants, a hunger strike can represent a suicidal gesture or familial attack), powerful group and family dynamics, potential exposure to infectious diseases (e.g., drug resistant tuberculosis), a lack of daily interaction with (professional) peers, and intense countertransference. Certainly, rigorous empirical investigations of home based treatments is needed.

Suggestions for Delivery

Some basic guidelines can be offered to help minimize the impact of some of these potentially problematic issues.

- Get a thorough pre-briefing before arriving on scene.
- Know where to park. Ask colleagues for suggestions or advice, and if possible, leave early enough for an appointment to check out the area.
- Always carry a cell phone and beeper.
- Dress to "fit in," not to impress. Become familiar with the current stock language regarding music, entertainment, and drug use. Also become familiar with local gangs' colors, and avoid wearing them in their area.
- Go in pairs if possible.
- Make sure you have an easy exit.
- Do not appear bashful, intimidated, or subtle. It is helpful to be honest and straightforward. Consider both your tone of voice and body language.
- Structure the setting as much as you can. In other words, know how much noise and activity you can handle. It is not uncommon for babies to be screaming, people to be yelling, and music to be blaring upon arrival at a home. It is appropriate to set limits on the volume of the TV and the numbers of people who may walk in and out of the room during a session.
- Invoke the rights of the patient. For example, if a patient's parent is swearing at him and calling him names, the TSS worker might state, "Swearing at J. is not helpful. Let's see if we can find another way for you to get you point across to him."

- Invoke your own rights as a professional. For example, a TSS worker may say, "I cannot help you if I cannot hear you over this yelling and screaming. You must keep your voices down so that we can work on this together" or "I want to assist you, but I cannot accept being called names...I will leave if you continue to use foul language."
- At the first sign of trouble, leave the premises. *This is probably the most important edict for in home providers.* Call for help or assistance from your car or the street. Remember that you cannot help someone else if you are in danger yourself.

Initial Experiences

One wrap-around service provider, Barbara, recounted one of her early home visits, in which she was asked to help manage a domestic dispute. Barbara described going alone to an apartment building in a run down section of town. She parked her car on the street, where a co-worker had advised her it was safe. When Barbara found the apartment she knocked on the door, and heard adults shouting and a baby crying. No one answered, and she tried the door. It was unlocked. Barbara pushed the door open, and could see two women in the kitchen (one of whom was presumably the baby's mother), fighting about money towed o each other for drugs. Barbara walked into the living room and announced who she was and that she was there to help. The woman holding the baby turned to Barbara and said, "Yeah, right. And who the fuck you are you anyway? And what the hell are you doing coming into my goddamn house? No one asked you here. Get the fuck out." During the shouting, the second woman grabbed the baby from the first woman, threatening her, "Ok, bitch. I'm going to drop the baby if you don't settle this up with me right now. You owe me big and I am not going to take some bullshit excuse for an answer." The second woman held the baby by the shoulders and had her sitting unsteadily on the edge of the kitchen counter.

Barbara immediately asked the two women in a low, calm voice to please put the baby down so that they could talk. In response, the woman holding the baby grabbed a pot [fortunately an empty one] off of the stove and threw it Barbara. While distracted by the sound, the first woman reached over and smacked the other hard on the face. In retaliation, the second woman grabbed at the first woman's hair. In the scuffle, the second woman let go of the baby, and it fell from the counter to the floor. Barbara didn't see the baby land on the floor (her view was blocked), but she said that all she could think about was getting to the baby to see if it were hurt. At this point, the second woman grabbed a knife from an open drawer, and began slashing at the air in front of the first woman.

Barbara tried to decide what to do. Both women were now ignoring the screams of the baby, but Barbara was afraid that she would be hurt if she tried to get between the two women and get the baby out of the kitchen. Barbara ran back to the living room, crouched by the front door, and called the police in a hoarse whisper. Within five minutes, the police arrived with their weapons drawn, and safeties off. Barbara said that she had no idea that the police would rush into the apartment with their weapons drawn, and gain control of the situation by barking orders and forcing people to the ground. Barbara was absolutely terrified as she was ordered to show her hands in the air, and get on the floor with everyone else. Ultimately, the infant was delivered, uninjured, into protective custody. Barbara later found out that neither women was the baby's mother; the first woman was babysitting for her boyfriend's sister.

Looking back on the incident, Barbara notes, "I don't think I realized at the time how dangerous the situation was. [Domestic violence calls are among the most potentially violent and unpredictable for police officers.] No one knew I was there until I called for the police. If I got hurt, I couldn't have helped that baby anyway...I tell everyone who works in this field to get help managing your stress, and to make sure that you leave the apartment, house, or whatever, if you think something is about to go wrong. It can be very difficult to do in that moment, but remember that you can always go back and address things later. It also is critical to help managing your stress." Barbara added with a sheepish smile that she gained 20 pounds during her first year as a wrap-around provider. But, she also noted that in her three subsequent years on the job, she lost the weight, "got a handle on my stress issues," has made a significant difference in a few people's lives, and has never had a boring day.

ALTERNATIVE AND COMPLEMENTARY MEDICINE

Another approach to crisis intervention, particularly in conjunction with stress management, is the use of alternative and behavioral medicine. Often employed as an adjunct with traditional psychotherapy or crisis intervention, and thus referred to as complimentary alternative medicine (CAM), members of the general public have been showing active support for these alternative approaches. The largest numbers of consumers of CAM include men and women over the age of 65, and between the ages of 25 and 49. The reasons cited most frequently for treatment include back and neck problems, typically associated with trauma and stress, anxiety, and headache. Most consumers are college educated and from a higher socioeconomic status (Eisenberg, Davis, Ettner, Appel, Wilkey, Van Rompay, & Kessler, 1998).

Many insurance companies now offer third party payment for a variety of CAM services, including mind-body medicine (e.g., biofeedback, mindful meditation, guided imagery—which are already practiced by many mental health providers) and manipulative and body based systems (e.g., massage therapy, osteopathy, acupuncture). However, many insurance companies who now support CAM treatment have not done so specifically in response to treatment efficacy, but because offering CAM benefits allows them to attract increasing numbers of more young, generally healthy policy holders (Pelletier, 2000). In other words, most CAM consumers have lower overall health care costs than other segments of the population, and typically have the means to pay for their premiums on time and in full.

Despite the purely monetary gains associated with CAM in the insurance industry, recent findings from NIH study centers (Couzin, 1998) and Cochrane reviews (Ezzo, Berman, Vickers, & Linde, 1998) suggest that certain CAM modalities represent effective, evidence based treatment for various ailments under certain conditions for certain patients. (In a radical departure from previous funding initiatives, the NIH recently instituted a series of exploratory pilot projects that allowed researchers to conduct controlled studies of various CAM approaches, and upgraded their Office of Alternative Medicine to a National Center for Complementary and Alternative Medicine in 1998; Pelletier, 2000.) Some of these more striking, empirically based findings include consistent support for the use of mind-body medicine, including meditation, biofeedback, self-hypnosis, and prayer for treatment of high blood pressure, coronary heart disease, chronic pain, and arthritis (Pelletier, 2000), and for immuno-enhancement, particularly after a traumatic or stressful event. Both medical and mental health practitioners may be interested in the outcome of these studies because experts suggest that by the year 2020, the top ten most frequent causes for global infirmity will include traffic accidents, war, severe depression, and AIDS (Pelletier, 2000), all intimately associated with crisis intervention and trauma counseling.

Self-Directed Techniques

Three mind-body techniques that have begun to receive attention as adjuncts in crisis intervention and trauma counseling include meditation, biofeedback, and self-hypnosis. One way to define these constructs is that they represent "a self-directed practice that quiets the mind and relaxes the body" (Pelletier, 2000: p. 64).

Two forms of meditation that have received a significant degree of empirical study include mindfulness meditation (Kabat-Zinn, Lipworth, Burney, 1985), in which an individual is encouraged to focus upon one's thoughts and bodily sensations without judging or evaluating them, and transcendental meditation in which an individual is encouraged to silently repeat a mantra while acknowledging and then dismissing any intrusive thoughts. Biofeedback, practiced typically by psychologists for more than 30 years, allows individuals to alter bodily functions (e.g., heart rate, blood pressure, respiration) via the presence of a literal feedback loop that indicates their level of progress. Self-hypnosis and guided imagery also may involve training or coaching by a therapist, but the locus of change and control remains with the patient.

A variety of rigorous, empirical studies suggest that self-directed mind-body therapies such as meditation, biofeedback, self-hypnosis, and mental imagery can be used to (c.f., Pelletier, 2000):

- lower blood pressure
- reduce perceptions of pain, anxiety, and depression
- decrease emotional reactivity to stressful life events
- increase the production of immune cells (i.e., lymphocytes)
- decrease levels of cortisol (a hormone typically released under stress in the bloodstream.
- improve blood sugar stability in diabetics
- increase tolerance to chemotherapy
- reduce sleep irregularities
- improve blood circulation to the extremities
- decrease the frequency of asthma attacks

Because such self-directed mind-body techniques appear so effective in producing positive, systemic changes, their use as adjuncts in crisis intervention and trauma counseling already is relatively common. Another additional benefit of these self-directed techniques is that the patient, not the practitioner, controls or directs the process. For individuals subjected to traumatic events, the use of such self-directed techniques can only serve to increase a survivor's sense of personal power, control, and effectiveness.

Spirituality

Spirituality continues to be one of the most overlooked patient resources in both psychotherapy and crisis intervention per se. Few graduate programs in psychology offer coursework in spirituality, and many practitioners (and laypersons) believe that someone who his quite religious is best served by seeking specifically pastoral-related counseling or care. As noted previously, however, spirituality in virtually any form (e.g., membership in a congregation; joining a prayer group; possessing a sense of greater purpose or hope) can foster increased social support and stress relief for individuals in crisis. An increasing number of controversial, but well-controlled scientific studies also support the role of prayer and spirituality in physical and psychological healing (Chamberlain & Hall, 2000; Pelletier, 2000; Schlitz & Braud, 1997).

One of the more commonly cited, early studies regarding the impact of prayer (i.e., "prayer at a distance" versus forms of person-to-person faith healing or the laying on of hands) is that of Byrd (1988), a cardiologist at the University of California School of Medicine in San Francisco. He found that half of the 383 newly admitted patients to the Coronary Care Unit, who were randomly selected to be prayed for by individuals unknown to them, fared significantly better on various measures of care including a decreased need for antibiotics and a lower likelihood of developing pulmonary edema. Patients who were prayed for also required less frequent CPR, were less likely to be put on a ventilator, and had shorter stays in the hospital. It also is interesting to note that in this double-blind study, neither patients nor doctors knew that any patients on the unit were being "prayed for." Significant criticism also has been raised that patients in this study who may have held beliefs that religion or prayer was negative or somehow immoral had their beliefs violated in a breach of ethical protocol.

Additional researchers (Harris, Gowda, Kolb, Strychacz, Vacek, Jones, Forker, O'keefe, & McCallister, 1999; Sicher, Targ, Moore, & Smith, 1998) have attempted to replicate Byrd's (1988) findings with some degree of success. In these studies, however, patients who comprised the subject pool of randomly selected, possible prayer recipients were first screened to determine their religious beliefs and feelings about prayer in general.) Many of these studies also engaged additional controls regarding the type of prayer used as an intervention (e.g., general well-wishes versus religion specific) and the "experience" of the individuals employed to provide prayer.

Notably, Harris et al.'s (1999) study, published in the *Archives of Internal Medicine*, of more than 990 newly admitted patients to a coronary care unit, assigned randomly to receive prayer or not, revealed that patients who were prayed for had similar lengths of hospital stays, but were significantly less likely to require major surgery and require intra-aortic balloon pumps. Prayed for patients also had a significantly better course scores (i.e., independently evaluated chart reviews that identify treatment outcomes) than those who did not receive prayer. AIDS patients in Sicher et al.'s study (1998) who were randomly assigned to receive prayers unknowingly from a variety of spiritual healers (i.e., Catholic priests, Protestant ministers, Jewish rabbis, Native American healers, Buddhist monks, and graduates of secular meditative programs) required significantly fewer inpatient hospitalizations, fewer total days of hospitalization, and fewer additional diagnoses of AIDS-related diseases. Statistical analyses also revealed that the religious or secular background of the individuals providing prayer was unrelated to the positive effect of that prayer.

Thus, practitioners are probably safe to assume that spirituality and prayer, unrelated to any specific religious belief or dogma, represent a possible source of healing above and beyond any related aspects of social support. Even if the impact of prayer alone upon psychological health and immune function is found to be spurious in later studies, its current use appears to provide patients with no type of detrimental or ill effects. Thus, the potential benefits of spirituality (and prayer) in conjunction with crisis intervention and trauma counseling cannot easily be discounted.

Physical Manipulation and Touch

Developmental psychologists have long appreciated the value of touch in the infant-caregiver relationship, and numerous studies suggest that infant massage can help premature infants, who often are not able to receive consistent contact with their primary caregiver due to the presence of feeding tubes and monitors, gain weight faster and stabilize their core body temperature sooner than those infants not provided with therapeutic massage (Field, 1998). Within the context of family therapy in response to serious child behavioral problems, some practitioners (e.g., Sells, 1998) even "prescribe" daily hugs between sets of parents and children in crisis. However, the therapeutic use of touch and bodily manipulation (e.g., acupuncture, massage therapy) among adults has only begun to receive rigorous scientific attention.

Various empirical studies, including those sponsored by the NIH, suggest that the ancient Chinese use of acupuncture may help alleviate depression (Ernst, Rand, & Stevinson, 1998), reduce relapse in treatment of narcotic drug abuse (Lipton, Brewington, & Smith, 1994), as well as reduce the severity of chronic neck (Coan, Wong, & Coan, 1982), lower back (Laitinen, 1976), tension headache, and menstral pain (Helms, 1987), increase immune system functioning, and minimize the nausea often associated with chemotherapy, morning sickness (De Aloysio & Penacchioni, 1982), and recovery from general anesthesia (Ho, Jawan, Fung, Cheung, & Lee, 1990). Interestingly, many of these positive effects related to depression and pain perception were found only when the use of acupuncture was coupled with a supportive, therapeutic relationship (Pelletier, 2000).

Massage therapy, which actually has a long history within the context of the healing arts (Field, 1998), has been explored recently as an adjunct to crisis intervention and trauma counseling. Empirical data suggest that the use of massage therapy as a stress reduction or crisis intervention can reduce perceptions of anxiety and depression (Ernst et al., 1998), lower the rate of respiration, increase "natural killer cell" activity in the immune system (Zeitlin, Keller, Shiflett, Schleifer, & Bartlett, 2000), decrease salivary cortisol levels, and even mitigate symptoms associated with PTSD (Field, Seligman, Scafidi, Schanberg, 1996). Thus, although mental health practitioners typically abstain from physical contact with patients in order to better facilitate the verbalization and articulation of the patient's thoughts, feelings, and actions (as well as to avoid inappropriate therapist-patient interactions such as romantic relationships and reenactments of control or abuse), the adjunctive use of massage therapy to traditional psychotherapy may allow some patients to experience enough decrease in unpleasant somatic symptoms to better tolerate the evidence-based interventions often used to treat PTSD (e.g., flooding; exposure therapy).

Integration with Crisis Intervention and Counseling

Although mental health practitioners themselves cannot or should not administer various CAM approaches within the context of a therapeutic relationship (e.g., massage therapy; accupunture), it behooves us as professionals to become familiar with recent empirical findings in order to better counsel our patients about their treatment options, and to help them understand the benefits and limitations of the various forms of CAM. The recent trend in which many insurance companies and medical centers now accept many aspects of CAM (e.g., Pelletier, 2000) certainly reinforces the valuable work that many mental health providers have been providing for decades in the areas of biofeedback, guided imagery, and self-hypnosis. In response, some clinicians have opted to make alternative medicine a hallmark feature of their practice by establishing group practices that include alternative medicine providers (e.g., licensed massage therapists; acupuncturists) as members. In sum, it is likely that CAM, in a variety of forms, has the potential to positively influence the outcome of psychotherapy, and assuage some of the potentially negative impact of personal crisis and trauma.

CALL FOR A RENEWED FOCUS ON EDUCATION AND PREVENTION

Although a number of advanced have been made in the treatment of PTSD and other stress related disorders, experts in the field indicate that increased attention to basic education in crisis intervention and trauma counseling remains crucial for mental health providers. As noted by the APA task force on Education and Training in Behavioral Emergencies (2000), the lack of formal coursework and training available to mental health professionals must be addressed. And, just as the field of Positive Psychology attempts to focus upon positive and protective aspects of personality (c.f., Seligman & Csikszentmihalyi, 2000), the field of crisis intervention and trauma counseling may benefit from such an emphasis on prevention, and the strengthening of restorative human factors even before an individual is exposed to a traumatic event or in crisis.

References

Abeles, N., Cooley, S., Deitch, I. M., Harper, M. S., Hinrichsen, G., Lopez, M. A., & Molinari, V. A. (1998). What practitioners should know about working with older adults. *Professional Psychology: Research and Practice, 29*, 413–427.

Adler, G. (1993). The psychotherapy of core borderline psychopathology. *American Journal of Psychotherapy, 47*, 194–205.

Albrecht, S. (1996). *Crisis management for corporate defense.* New York: Amacom.

American Psychological Association. (1992). Ethical principles of Psychologists and code of conduct. *American Psychologist, 47*, 1597–1611.

American Psychological Association. (1993). *Violence and youth: Psychology's response.* Washington, DC: Public Interest Directorate, American Psychological Association.

American Psychological Association. (1994, November 11). *APA panel addresses controversy over adult memories of childhood sexual abuse* ([Press release]. Washington, DC: Author).

American Psychological Association. (1994). *Diagnostic and statistical manual of mental disorders.* 4th ed. Washington, DC: American Psychiatric Association.

American Psychological Association. (2000). *Report on education and training in behavioral emergencies.* Washington, DC: Section on Clinical Emergencies and Crises (Section VII, Division 12), American Psychological Association.

Americans with Disabilities Act of 1990, 42 U.S.C. Section 12101, et seq.

Applebaum, P. (1985). Tarasoff and the clinician: Problems in fulfilling the duty to protect. *American Journal of Psychiatry, 142*, 425–429.

Appelbaum, S. A. (1975). Parkinson's law in psychotherapy. *International Journal of Psychoanalytic Psychotherapy, 4*, 426–436.

Avery-Leaf, S., Cascardi, M., O'Leary, K. D., & Cano, A. (1997). Efficacy of a dating violence prevention program on attitudes justifying aggression. *Journal of Adolescent Health, 21*, 11–17.

Baird, B. N. (1999). *The internship, practicum, and field placement handbook: A guide for the helping professions.* Upper Saddle River, New Jersey: Prentice Hall.

Baldwin, B. A. (1979). Training in crisis intervention for students in the mental health profession. *Professional Psychology: Research and Practice, 10*, 161–167.

Ballenger, J. C., Davidson, J. R. T., Lecrubier, Y., Nutt, D. J., Foa, E. B., Kessler, R. C., & McFarlane, A. C. (2000). Consensus statement on posttraumatic stress disorder from the international consensus group on depression and anxiety. *Journal of Clinical Psychiatry, 61*, 60–66.

Bandura, A., Ross, D., & Ross, S. A. (1961). Transmission of aggression through imitation of aggressive models. *Journal of Abnormal and Social Psychology, 63*, 575–582.

Beauford, J. E., McNeil, D. E., & Binder, R. L. (1997). Utility of the initial therapeutic alliance in evaluating psychiatric patients' risk of violence. *The Journal of American Psychiatry, 154*, 1272–1276.

Beck, J. C. (1982). When the patient threatens violence: An empirical study of clinical practice after Tarasoff. *Bulletin of the American Academy of Psychiatry and the Law, 10*, 189–201.

Beck, J. C., & Schouten, R. (2000). Workplace violence and psychiatric practice. *Bulletin of the Menninger Clinic, 64*, 36–50.

Beck, R. W., Morris, J. B., & Beck, A. T. (1974). Cross-validation of a suicide intent scale. *Psychological Reports, 34*, 445–446.

Beitchman, J. H., Zucker, K. J., Hood, J. E., daCosta, G. A., Ackman, D., & Cassavia, E. (1992). A review of the long-term effects of child sexual abuse. *Child Abuse and Neglect, 16*, 101–118.

Ben-Amos, D. (1994). Bettelheim among the folklorists. *Psychoanalytic Review, 81*, 509–535.

Bernstein, E. M., & Putnam, F. W. (1986). Development, reliability, and validity of a dissociation scale. *Journal of Nervous and Mental Disease, 174*, 727–735.

Bero, L., & Rennie, D. (1995). The Cochrane Collaboration: Preparing, maintaining, and disseminating systematic reviews of the effects of health care. *Journal of the American Medical Association, 274*, 1935–1938.

Berry, D. B. (1996). *The domestic violence sourcebook*. Los Angeles, CA: Lowell House.

Bierman, K. L. (1996). Integrating social-skills training interventions with parent training and family-focused support to prevent conduct disorder in high-risk populations: The Fast Track multisite demonstration project. In C. F. Ferris, & T. Grisso (Eds.), *Understanding aggressive behavior in children*. New York: New York Academy of Sciences.

Binder, R. L., & McNeil, D. E. (1996). Application of the Tarasoff ruling and its effect on the victim and the therapeutic relationship. *Psychiatric Services, 47*, 1212–1215.

Bisson, J. I., McFarlane, A. C., & Rose, S. (2000). Psychological debriefing. In E. B. Foa, T. M. Keane, & M. J. Friedman (Eds.), *Effective treatment for PTSD: Practice guidelines from the International Society for Traumatic Stress Studies* (pp. 317–326). New York: Guilford.

Black, S. T. (1993). Comparing genuine and simulated suicide notes: A new perspective. *Journal of Consulting and Clinical Psychology, 61*, 699–702.

Blanchard, E. B., & Hickling, E. J. (1997). *After the crash: Psychological assessment and treatment of survivors of motor vehicle accidents*. Washington, DC: American Psychological Association.

Bogal-Allbritten, R. B., & Allbritten, W. L. (1985). The hidden victims: Courtship violence among college students. *Journal of College Student Personnel, 26*, 201–204.

Bongar, B., & Harmatz, M. (1991). Clinical psychology graduate education in the study of suicide: Availability, resources, and importance. *Suicide and Life-Threatening Behavior, 21*, 231–244.

Bowman, E. S., & Coons, P. M. (2000). The differential diagnosis of epilepsy, pseudoseizures, dissociative identity disorder, and dissociative disorder not otherwise specified. *Bulletin of the Menninger Clinic, 64*, 164–180.

Bremner, J. D. (1999). Does stress damage the brain? *Biological Psychiatry, 45*, 797–805.

Bremner, J. D., Narayan, M., Staib, L. H., Southwick, S. M., McGlashan, T., & Charney, D. S. (1999). Neural correlates of memories of childhood sexual abuse in women with and without posttraumatic stress disorder. *American Journal of Psychiatry, 156,* 1787–1795.

Brissette, I., Scheier, M. F., & Carver, C. S. (2002). The role of optimism in social network development, coping, and psychological adjustment during a life transition. *Journal of Personality and Social Psychology, 82,* 102–111.

Brock, T. C., Green, M. C., & Reich, D. A. (1998). New evidence of flaws in the Consumer Reports study of psychotherapy. *American Psychologist, 53,* 62–63.

Brown, G. K., Beck, A. T., Steer, R. A., & Grisham, J. R. (2000). Risk factors for suicide in psychiatric outpatients: A 20-year prospective study. *Journal of Counseling and Clinical Psychology, 68,* 371–377.

Buckley, T. C., Blanchard, E. B., & Neill, W. T. (2000). Information processing and PTSD: A review of the empirical literature. *Clinical Psychology Review, 20,* 1041–1065.

Byrd, R. C. (1988). Positive therapeutic effects of intercessory prayer in a coronary care unit population. *Southern Medical Journal, 81,* 826–829.

Cantagallo, A., Grassi, L., & Della Sala, S. (1999). Dissociative disorder after traumatic brain injury. *Brain Injury, 13,* 219–228.

Carlson, E. B., & Putnam, F. W. (1993). An update on the Dissociative Experiences Scale. *Dissociation, 6,* 16–27.

Centers for Disease Control and Prevention. (1998). AIDS among persons aged >50 years: United States. *Morbidity and Mortality Weekly Review, 47,* 21–27.

Centers for Disease Control and Prevention. (1998). Youth risk behavior surveillance-United States, 1997. *Morbidity and Mortality Weekly Review, 47,* 1–89.

Chamberlain, T. J., & Hall, C. A. (2000). *Realized religion: Research on the relationship between religion and health.* Philadelphia, PA: Tempelton Foundation Press.

Chemtob, C. M., Bauer, G. B., Hamada, R. S., & Pelowski, S. R. (1989). Patient suicide: Occupational hazard for psychologists and psychiatrists. *Professional Psychology: Research and Practice, 20,* 294–300.

Chemtob, C. M., Tolin, D. F., van der Kolk, B. A., & Pitman, R. K. (2000). Eye movement desensitization and reprocessing. In E. B. Foa, T. M. Keane, & M. J. Friedman (Eds.), *Effective treatment for PTSD: Practice guidelines from the International Society for Traumatic Stress Studies* (pp. 333–335). New York: Guilford.

Choi, N. G., & Mayer, J. (2000). Elder abuse, neglect, and exploitation: Risk factors and prevention strategies. *Journal of Gerontological Social Work, 33,* 5–25.

Coan, R., Wong, F., & Coan, P. L. (1982). The acupuncture treatment of neck pain: A randomized controlled study. *American Journal of Chinese Medicine, 9,* 326–332.

Cochrane B., Kate, A., Lofchy, J. S., & Sakinofsky, I. (2000). Clinical rating scales in suicide risk assessment. *General Hospital Psychiatry, 22,* 445–451.

Cohen, J. A., Mannarino, A. P., Berliner, L., & Deblinger, E. (2000). Trauma-focused cognitive behavioral therapy for children and adolescents: An empirical update. *Journal of Interpersonal Violence, 15,* 1202–1223.

Conduct Problems Prevention Research Group. (1999). The initial impact of the fast track prevention trial for conduct problems: II. Classroom effects. *Journal of Consulting and Clinical Psychology, 67,* 648–657.

Conlon, L., Fahy, T. J., & Conroy, R. (1999). PTSD in ambulant RTA victims: A randomized controlled trial of debriefing. *Journal of Psychosomatic Research, 46,* 37–44.

Couzin, J. (1998). Beefed-up NIH center probes unconventional therapies. *Science, 282,* 2175.

Croft, R. J., Klugman, A., Baldeweg, T., & Gruzelier, J. H. (2001). Electrophysiological evidence of serotonergic impairment in long-term MDMA ("ecstasy") users. *American Journal of Psychiatry, 158,* 1687–1692.

Damasio, A. R. (1994). *Descartes' error.* New York: Avon.

Darley, J. M., & Batson, C. D. (1973). "From Jerusalem to Jericho": A study of situational and dispositional variables in helping behavior. *Journal of Personality and Social Psychology, 27,* 100–108.

Davanloo, H. (Ed.). (1980). *Short-term dynamic psychotherapy.* New York: Jason Aronson.

Davidson, L. M., Inslicht, S. S., & Baum, A. (2000). Traumatic stress and posttraumatic stress disorder among children and adolescents. In A. J. Sameroff, M. Lewis, & S. M. Miller (Eds.), *Handbook of developmental psychopathology (2nd ed.)* (pp. 723–737). New York: Kluwer Academic/Plenum Publishers.

Davidson, M. W., & Range, L. M. (1999). Are teachers of children and young adolescents responsive to suicide prevention training modules? *Death Studies, 23,* 61–71.

Davidson, M. W., & Range, L. M. (2000). Age appropriate no-suicide agreements: Professionals' ratings of appropriateness and effectiveness. *Education & Treatment of Children, 23,* 143–148.

Davies, J. M., & Frawley, M. G. (1994). *Treating the adult survivor of childhood sexual abuse: A psychoanalytic perspective.* New York: Basic Books.

Davis, E. P. (1988). Big Bird teaches fire and hurricane safety. In M. Lystad (Ed.), *Mental health response to mass emergencies: Theory and practice* (pp. 311–320). New York: Bruner/Mazel.

De Aloysio, D., & Penacchioni, P. (1992). Morning sickness control in early pregnancy by Neiguan point acupressure. *Obstetrics & Gynecology, 80,* 852–854.

Deutsch, F. M., & Lamberti, D. M. (1986). Does social approval increase helping? *Personality and Social Psychology Bulletin, 12,* 149–158.

Diener, E. (2002). *Subjective well-being: The science of personal feelings of happiness, life satisfaction, positive emotions, and fulfillment.* Presented at the APA's Division 2 Teaching of Psychology Conference, St. Petersburg, FL.

Diener, E., & Seligman, M. E. (2002). The happiest people. *Psychological Science, 13,* 81–84.

Diener, E., Suh, E. M., Lucas, R. E., & Smith, H. L. (1999). Subjective well-being: Three decades of progress. *Psychological Bulletin, 125,* 276–302.

Dineen, T. (2000). *Manufacturing Victims: What the psychology industry is doing to people.* New York: Robert Davies.

Drabman, R. S., & Thomas, M. H. (1974). Does media violence increase children's tolerance of real-life aggression? *Developmental Psychology, 10,* 418–421.

Dutton, D. G., & Painter, S. (1993). The battered woman syndrome: Effects of severity and intermittency of abuse. *American Journal of Orthopsychiatry, 63,* 614–622.

Dyer, C. B., Pavlik, V. N., Murphy, K. P., & Hyman, D. J. (2000). The high prevalence of depression and dementia in elder abuse or neglect. *Journal of the American Geriatrics Society, 48,* 205–208.

Dyregrov, A. (1997). The process in psychological debriefings. *Journal of Traumatic Stress, 10,* 589–605.

Ebert, B. W. (1987). Guide to conducting a psychological autopsy. *Professional Psychology: Research and Practice, 18,* 52–56.

Eisenberg, D. M., Davis, R. B., Ettner, S. L., Appel, S., Wilkey, S., Van Rompay, M., Kessler, R. C. (1998). Trends in alternative medicine use in the United States. *Journal of the American Medical Association, 280,* 1569–1575.

Ernst, E., Rand, J. I., & Stevinson, C. (1998). Complementary therapies for depression: An overview. *Archives of General Psychiatry, 55,* 1026–1032.

Everly, G. S., & Boyle, S. H. (1999). Critical Incident Stress Debriefing (CISD): A meta-analysis. *International Journal of Emergency Mental Health, 1,* 165–168.

Everly, G. S., Flannery, R., & Mitchell, J. (2000). CISM: A review of the literature. *Aggression and Violent Behavior: A Review Journal, 5*, 23–40.

Everly, G. S., & Mitchell, J. T. (1992). *The critical incident stress debriefing process (CISD) and the prevention of occupational post-traumatic stress.* Paper presented at the Second American Psychological Association and NIOSH Conference on Occupational Stress, Washington, DC.

Everly, G. S., & Mitchell, J. T. (1997). *Critical incident stress management (CISM): A new era and standard of care in crisis intervention.* Ellicott City, MD: Chevron Publishing Corp.

Eyman, J. R., & Eyman, S. K. (1991). Personality assessment in suicide prediction. *Suicide & Life-Threatening Behavior, 21*, 37.

Ezzo, J., Berman, B. M., Vickers, A. J., & Linde, K. (1998). Complementary medicine and the Cochcrane Collaboration. *Journal of the American Medical Association, 280*, 1628–1630.

Feldman-Summers, S. (1996). Litigation pitfalls for the psychotherapist whose client "first remembers" childhood sexual abuse during therapy. *Women and Therapy, 19*, 109–122.

Feldman-Summers, S., & Linder, K. (1976). Perceptions of victims and defendants in criminal assault cases. *Criminal Justice and Behavior, 3*, 135–150.

Field, T. M. (1998). Massage therapy effects. *American Psychologist, 53*, 1270–1281.

Field, T., Seligman, S., Scafidi, F., & Schanberg, S. (1996). Alleviating posttraumatic stress in children following Hurricane Andrew. *Journal of Applied Developmental Psychology, 17*, 37–50.

Figley, C. R. (Ed.). (1995). *Compassion fatigue: Coping with secondary traumatic stress disorder in those who treat the traumatized.* Philadelphia, PA: Brunner/Mazel.

Fine, C. G. (1999). The tactical-integration model for the treatment of dissociative identity disorder and allied dissociative disorders. *American Journal of Psychotherapy, 53*, 361–376.

Fletcher, T. A., Brakel, S. J., & Cavanaugh, J. L. (2000). Violence in the workplace: New perspectives in forensic mental health services in the USA. *British Journal of Psychiatry, 176*, 339–344.

Foa, E. B., Hearst-Ikeda, D., & Perry, K. J. (1995). Evaluation of a brief cognitive-behavioral program for the prevention of chronic PTSD in recent assault victims. *Journal of Consulting and Clinical Psychology, 63*, 948–955.

Foa, E. B., Keane, T. M. & Friedman, M. J. (Eds.) (2000). *Effective treatment for PTSD: Practice guidelines from the International Society for Traumatic Stress Studies.* New York: Gilford.

Foa, E. B., Rothbaum, B. O., Riggs, D., & Murdock, T. (1991). Treatment of PTSD in rape victims: A comparison between cognitive-behavioral procedures and counseling. *Journal of Consulting and Clinical Psychology, 59*, 715–723.

Foley, L. A., & Pigott, M. A. (2000). Belief in a just world and jury decision in a civil rape trial. *Journal of Applied Social Psychology, 30*, 935–951.

Franklin, A. J., Carter, R. T., & Grace, C. (1993). An integrative approach to psychotherapy with Black/African Americans: The relevance of race and culture. In G. Stricker & J. R. Gold (Eds.), *Comprehensive Handbook of Psychotherapy Integration* (pp. 465–479). New York: Plenum Press.

Fredrickson, B. L. (2001). The role of positive emotions in positive psychology: The broaden-and-build theory of positive emotion. *American Psychologist, 56*, 218–226.

Freedman, J. L., & Fraser, S. C. (1966). Compliance without pressure: the foot-in-the-door technique. *Journal of Personality and Social Psychology, 4*, 195–202.

Freudenberger, H. J. (1974). Staff burn-out. *Journal of Social Issues, 30*, 159–165.

Friedman, M. J., Davidson, J. R., Mellman, T. A., & Southwick, S. M. (2000). Pharmacotherapy. In E. B. Foa, T. M. Keane, & M. J. Friedman (Eds.), *Effective treatment for PTSD: Practice guidelines from the International Society for Traumatic Stress Studies* (pp. 326–329). New York: Guilford.

Frizsche, B. A., Finkelstein, M. A., & Penner, L. A. (2000). To help or not to help: Capturing individuals' decision processes. *Social Behavior and Personality, 28,* 561–578.

Fromm, E. (1996). *To have or to be?* New York: Continuum Publishing.

Gerbner, G. (1994). The politics of media violence: Some reflections. In C. Hamelink & O. Linne (Eds.), *Mass communication research: On problems and policies* (pp. 412–418). Norwood, NJ: Ablex.

Gilbar, O., & Eden, A. (2001). Suicide tendency in cancer patients. *Omega Journal of Death and Dying, 42,* 159–170.

Gist, R., & Lubin, B. (1989a). Ecological and community perspectives on disaster. In R. Gist & B. Lubin (Eds.), *Psychosocial aspects of disaster* (pp. 1–8). New York: Wiley.

Gist, R., & Lubin, B. (1989b). Implications for research and practice. In R. Gist & B. Lubin (Eds.), *Psychosocial aspects of disaster* (pp. 341–344). New York: Wiley.

Gist, R., & Woodall, S. J. (2000). There are no simple solutions to complex problems. In J. M. Violanti, D. Paton, & C. Dunning (Eds.), *Posttraumatic stress intervention: Challenges, issues, and perspectives* (pp. 81–95). Springfield, IL: Thomas.

Gleaves, D. H., Hernandez, E., & Warner, M. S. (1999). Corroborating premorbid dissociative symptomatology in dissociative identity disorder. *Professional Psychology: Research and Practice, 30,* 341–345.

Gold, J., & Stricker, G. (2001). A relational psychodynamic perspective on assimilative integration. *Journal of Psychotherapy Integration, 11,* 43–58.

Goldstein, A., & Feske, U. (1994). Eye movement desensitization and reprocessing for panic disorder: A case series. *Journal of Anxiety Disorders, 8,* 351–362.

Goldstein, I. L. (1986). *Training in organizations: Needs assessment, development and evaluation* (2nd ed.). Monterey, CA: Brooks/Cole.

Goldstein, J. (Ed.). (1998) *Why we watch: The attractions of violent entertainment.* New York: Oxford University Press.

Green, A. R., Cross, A. J., & Goodwin, G. M. (1995). Review of the pharmacology and clinical pharmacology of 3,4-methylenedioxymethamphetamine (MDMA or "Ecstasy"). *Psychopharmacology, 119,* 247–260.

Green, J. D., Sommerville, R. B., Mystrom, L. E., Darley, J. M., & Cohen, J. D. (2001). An fMRI investigation of emotional engagement in moral judgment. *Science, 293,* 2105–2108.

Greenwald, R. (2000). Eye movement desensitization and reprocessing. In K. N. Dwivedi (Ed.), *Post-traumatic stress disorder in children and adolescents* (pp. 198–212). London, UK: Whurr.

Guth, A. A., & Pachter, L. (2000). Domestic violence and the trauma surgeon. *American Journal of Surgery, 179,* 134–140.

Guy, J., Brown, C., & Poelstra, P. (1990). Who gets attacked? A national survey of patient violence directed at psychologists in clinical practice. *Professional Psychology: Research and Practice, 21,* 493–495.

Harris, E. A. (1995). The importance of risk management in a managed care environment. In M. B. Sussman (Ed.), *A perilous calling: The hazards of psychotherapy practice* (pp. 247–258). New York: Wiley.

Harris, W. S., Gowda, M., Kolb, J. W., Strychacz, C. P., Vacek, J. L., Jones, P. G., Forker, A., O'Keefe, J. H., & McCallister, B. D. (1999). A randomized, controlled trial of the effects of remote, intercessory prayer on outcomes in patients admitted to the coronary care unit. *Archives of Internal Medicine, 159,* 2273–2278.

Helms, J. M. (1987). Acupuncture for the management of primary dysmenorrhea. *Obstetrics & Gynecology, 69,* 51–56.

Hem, E., Berg, A. M., & Ekeberg, O. (2001). Suicide in police: A critical review. *Suicide and Life Threatening Behavior, 31,* 224–233.

Hendin, H. (1995). *Suicide in America.* New York: Norton.

Henton, J., Cate, R., Koval, J., Lloyd, S., & Christopher, S. (1983). Romance and violence in dating relationships. *Journal of Family Issues, 4,* 467–482.

Herbert, J. D., Lilienfeld, S. L., Lohr, J. M., Montgomery, R. W., O'Donohue, W. T., Rosen, G. M., & Tolin, D. F. (2000). Science and pseudoscience in the development of eye movement desensitization and reprocessing: Implications for clinical practice. *Clinical Psychology Review, 20,* 945–971.

Herman, J. (1997). *Trauma and recovery: The aftermath of violence—from domestic abuse to political terror.* New York: Basic.

Hillhouse, J., & Adler, C. M. (1997). Investigating stress effect patterns in hospital staff nurses: Results of a cluster analysis. *Social Science and Medicine, 45,* 1781–1788.

Hillman, J. (2002). [Differential rates of emergency responding in psychiatrist inpatient units]. Unpublished raw data.

Hillman, J. L. (2000). *Clinical perspectives on elderly sexuality.* New York: Kluwer Academic/Plenum Publishers.

Hillman, J. L. (1998). Health care providers' knowledge of HIV induced dementia among older adults. *Sexuality and Disability, 16,* 181–192.

Hillman, J. L., & Stricker, G. (1998). Some issues in the assessment of HIV among older adults. *Psychotherapy, 35,* 483–489.

Hillman, J., & Stricker, G. (in press). A call for psychotherapy integration in work with older adult patients. *Journal for Psychotherapy Integration.*

Ho, R. T., Jawan, B., Fung, S. T., Cheung, H. K., & Lee, J. H. (1990). Electroacupuncture and postoperative emesis. *Anesthesia, 45,* 327–329.

Ironson, G., Wynings, C., Schneiderman, N., Baum, A., Rodriguez, M., Greenwood, D., Benight, C., Antoni, M., LaPerriere, A., Huang, H., Klimas, N., & Fletcher, M. A. (1997). Posttraumatic stress symptoms, intrusive thoughts, loss, and immune function after Hurricane Andrew. *Psychosomatic Medicine, 59,* 128–141.

Ives, R. (1994). Stop sniffing in the states: Approaches to solvent misuse prevention in the USA. *Drugs: Education, Prevention, and Policy, 1,* 37–48.

Jamison, K. R. (1999). *Night falls fast.* New York: Vintage.

Jansen, P., Richter, L. M., Griesel, R. D., & Joubert, J. (1990). Glue sniffing: A description of social, psychological and neuropsychological factors in a group of South African "street children." *South African Journal of Psychology, 20,* 150–158.

Jenkins, S. R. (1996). Social support and debriefing efficacy among emergency medical workers after a shooting incident. *Journal of Behavior and Personality, 11,* 477–492.

Johnson, D. R., Feldman, S. C., Lubin, H., & Southwick, S. M. (1995). The therapeutic use of ritual and ceremony in the treatment of post-traumatic stress disorder. *Journal of Traumatic Stress, 8,* 283–298.

Jones, E. E., & Nisbett, R. E. (1972). The actor and the observer: Divergent perceptions of the causes of behavior. In E. E. Jones, D. E. Kanouse, H. H. Kelley, R. E. Nisbett, S. Valins, & B. Weiner (Eds.), *Attribution: Perceiving the causes of behavior.* Morristown, NJ: General Learning Press.

Kabat-Zinn, J., Lipworth, L., & Burney, R. (1985). The clinical use of mindfulness meditation for the self-regulation of chronic pain. *Journal of Behavioral Medicine, 8,* 163–191.

Kazarian, S. S., & Evans, D. R. (Eds.). (2001). *Handbook of cultural health psychology.* San Diego, CA: Academic Press.

Kenardy, J. A., & Carr, V. J. (2000). Debriefing post disaster: Follow-up after a major earthquake. In B. Raphael & J. P. Wilson (Eds.), *Psychological debriefing: Theory, practice, and evidence* (pp. 174–181). New York: Cambridge University Press.

Kendall-Tackett, K. A., Williams, L. M., & Finkelhor, D. (1993). Impact of sexual abuse on children: A review and synthesis of recent empirical studies. *Psychological Bulletin, 113,* 164–180.

Kernberg, O. (1984). *Severe personality disorders: Psychotherapeutic strategies.* New Haven, CT: Yale University Press.

Khouzam, H. R., & Kissmeyer, P. (1997). Antidepressant treatment, posttraumatic stress disorder, survivor guilt, and spiritual awakening. *Journal of Traumatic Stress, 10,* 691–696.

Kingsbury, S., Hawton, K., Steinhardt, K., & James, A. (1999). Do adolescents who take overdoses have specific psychological characteristics? *Journal of the American Academy of Child and Adolescent Psychiatry, 38,* 1125–1131.

Kleespies, P. M. (2001). Suicide in the medically ill. *Suicide & Life Threatening Behavior, 31,* 48–59.

Kluft, R. P. (1995). Current controversies surrounding dissociative identity disorder. In L. M. Cohen, J. N. Berzoff, & M. R. Elin (Eds.), *Dissociative identity disorder: Theoretical and treatment controversies* (pp. 347–377). Northvale, NJ: Aronson.

Kluft, R. P. (1999). An overview of the psychotherapy of dissociative identity disorder. *American Journal of Psychotherapy, 53,* 289–319.

Knapp, S., & VandeCreek, L. (1996). Risk management for psychologists: Treating patients who recover lost memories of child abuse. *Professional Psychology: Research and Practice, 27,* 452–459.

Koerner, K., & Linehan, M. M. (1992). Integrative therapy for borderline personality disorder: Dialectical behavior therapy. In J. C. Norcross & M. R. Goldfried (Eds.), *Handbook of psychotherapy integration* (pp. 433–459). New York: Basic Books.

Kroll, J. (1993). *PTSD/borderlines in therapy: Finding the balance.* New York: Norton.

Kubler-Ross, E. (1969) *On death and dying.* New York: MacMillan.

LaGreca, A. M., Silverman, W. K., Vernberg, E. M., & Prinstein, M. J. (1996). Symptoms of posttraumatic stress in children after Hurricane Andrew: A prospective study. *Journal of Consulting and Clinical Psychology, 64,* 712–723.

LaGreca, A. M., Silverman, W. K., & Wasserstein, S. B. (1998). Children's predisaster functioning as a predictor of posttraumatic stress following Hurricane Andrew. *Journal of Consulting and Clinical Psychology, 66,* 883–892.

Lane, P. S. (1993). Critical incident stress debriefing for health care workers. *Omega Journal of Death and Dying, 28,* 301–315.

Labig, C. E. (1995). *Preventing violence in the workplace.* New York: Amacom.

Laitinen, J. (1976). Acupuncutre and transcutaneous electric stimulation in the treatment of chronic sacrolumbalgia and ischialgia. *American Journal of Chinese Medicine, 4,* 169–175.

Lakovics, M. (1983). Classification of countertransference for utilization in supervision. *American Journal of Psychotherapy, 37,* 245–257.

Latane, B., & Darley, J. M. (1970). *The unresponsive bystander: Why doesn't he help?* New York: Appleton-Century-Crofts.

Leippe, M. R., Romanczyk, A., & Manion, A. P. (1991). Eyewitness memory for a touching experience: Accuracy differences between child and adult witnesses. *Journal of Applied Psychology, 76,* 367–379.

Leonard, R., & Alison, L. (1999). Critical incident stress debriefing and its effects on coping strategies and anger in a sample of Australian police officers involved in shooting incidents. *Work and Stress, 13*, 144–161.

Lerner, M. J. (1980). *The belief in a just world: A fundamental delusion.* New York: Plenum.

Lerner, M. J., & Simmons, C. H. (1966). Observer's reaction to the "innocent victim": Compassion or rejection? *Journal of Personality and Social Psychology, 4*, 203–210.

Levine, M. (1999). Rethinking bystander nonintervention: Social categorization and evidence of witnesses at the James Bulger murder trial. *Human Relations, 52*, 1133–1155.

Levine-Perkell, J. (1996). Caregiving issues. In K. M. Nokes (Ed.), *HIV/AIDS and the older adult* (pp. 115–128). New York: Taylor & Francis.

Levy, J. A. (1998). AIDS and injecting drug use in later life. *Research on Aging, 20*, 776–797.

Liberzon, I., & Young, E. A. (1997). Effects of stress and glucocorticoids on CNS oxytocin receptor binding. *Psychoneuroendocrinology, 22*, 411–422.

Lieberman, M. D. (2000). Intuition: A social cognitive neuroscience approach. *Psychological Bulletin, 126*, 109–137.

Lilienfeld, S. O., Kirsch, I., Sarbin, T. R., Lynn, S. J., Chaves, J. F., Ganaway, G. K., & Powell, R. A. (1999). Dissociative identity disorder and the sociocognitive model: Recalling the lessons of the past. *Psychological Bulletin, 125*, 507–523.

Lin, K. M., Poland, R. E., & Nakasaki, G. (Eds.). (1993). *Psychopharmacology and psychobiology of ethnicity.* Washington, DC: American Psychiatric Press.

Lindemann, E. (1944). Symptomatology and management of acute grief. *American Journal of Psychiatry, 101*, 7–21.

Linehan, M. M., Armstrong, H. E., Suarez, A., & Allmon, D. (1991). Cognitive behavioral treatment of chronically parasuicidal borderline patients. *Archives of General Psychiatry, 48*, 1060–1064.

Linehan, M. M., & Kehrer, C. A. (1993). Borderline personality disorder. In D. H. Barlow (Ed.), *Clinical handbook of psychological disorders: A step by step treatment manual* (pp. 396–441). New York: Guilford Press.

Linehan, M. M., Tutek, D. A., Heard, H. L., & Armstrong, H. E. (1994a). Interpersonal outcome of cognitive behavioral treatment for chronically suicidal borderline patients. *American Journal of Psychiatry, 151*, 1771–1776.

Linehan, M. M., Tuteck, D. A., Heard, H. L., & Armstrong, H. E. (1994b). Naturalistic follow-up of a behavioral treatment for chronically parasuicidal borderline patients. *Archives of General Psychiatry, 51*, 422.

Linton, J. C. (1995). Acute stress management with public safety personnel: Opportunities for clinical training and pro bono community service. *Professional Psychology: Research and Practice, 26*, 566–573.

Lipton, D. S., Brewington, V., & Smith, M. (1994). Acupuncture for crack cocaine detoxification: Experimental evaluation of efficacy. *Journal of Substance Abuse Treatment, 11*, 205–215.

Litwack, T. R., Kirschner, S. M., & Wack, R. C. (1993). The assessment of dangerousness and predictions of violence: Recent research and future prospects. *Psychiatric Quarterly, 64*, 245–273.

Lykken, D. (1999). *Happiness: What studies on twins show us about nature, nurture, and the happiness set point.* New York, NY: Golden.

Lkyubomirsky, S. (2001). Why are some people happier than others? The role of cognitive and motivational processes in well-being. *American Psychologist, 56*, 239–249.

Loftus, E. (1993). The reality of repressed memories. *American Psychologist, 48*, 518–537.

Mack, K. A., & Bland, S. D. (1999). HIV testing behaviors and attitudes regarding HIV/AIDS of adults aged 50–64. *The Gerontologist, 39,* 687–694.

Mahl, G. F. (1987). *Explorations in nonverbal and vocal behavior.* Hillsdale, NJ: Lawrence Erlbaum.

Mahler, M. S. (1971). A study of the separation-individuation process: And its possible application to borderline phenomena in the psychoanalytic situation. *Psychoanalytic Study of the Child, 79,* 403–424.

Maltsberger, J. T., & Buie, D. H. (1974). Countertransference hate in the treatment of suicidal patients. *Archives of General Psychiatry, 30,* 625–633.

Mander, J. (1992). *In the absence of the sacred.* San Francisco, CA: Sierra Club Books.

Mann, J. (1973). *Time-limited psychotherapy.* Cambridge: Harvard University Press.

Marshall, S. L. A. (1983). *Island victory: The battle for Kwajalein.* Washington, DC: Zenger Publishing.

Maslow, A. H. (1970). *Motivation and personality* (2nd ed.). New York: Harper.

May, R., Angel, A., & Ellenberger, H. F. (Eds.). (1958). *Existence: A new dimension in psychiatry.* New York: Basic.

McBride, C. A. (1998). The discounting principle and attitudes toward victims of HIV infection. *Journal of Applied Social Psychology, 28,* 595–608.

McDermott, B. M., & Palmer, L. J. (1999). Post-disaster service provision following proactive identification of children with emotional distress and depression. *Australian and New Zealand Journal of Psychiatry, 33,* 855–863.

McDowell, D. M., & Kleber, H. D. (1994). MDMA: Its history and pharmacology. *Psychiatric Annals, 24,* 127–130.

McFarlane, A. C. (1987). Posttraumatic phenomena in a longitudinal study of children following a natural disaster. *Journal of the American Academy of Child and Adolescent Psychiatry, 26,* 764–769.

McFarlane, J., Wiist, W., & Watson, M. (1998). Characteristics of sexual abuse against pregnant Hispanic women by their male intimates. *Journal of Women's Health, 7,* 739–745.

McGarvey, E. L., Clavet, G. J., Mason, W., & Waite, D. (1999). Adolescent inhalant use: Environments of use. *American Journal of Drug and Alcohol Abuse, 25,* 731–741.

McMain, S., Korman, L. M., & Dimeff, L. (2001). Dialectical behavior therapy and the treatment of emotion dysregulation. *Journal of Clinical Psychology, 57,* 183–196.

McNally, V. J. (1999). FBI's Employee Assistance Program: An advanced law enforcement model. *International Journal of Emergency Mental Health, 1,* 109–114.

McNeil, D. E., & Binder, R. L. (1995). Correlates of the accuracy in the assessment of psychiatric inpatients' risk of violence. *American Journal of Psychiatry, 152,* 901–906.

McNeil, D. E., Binder, R. L., & Fulton, F. M. (1998). Management of threats of violence under California's duty-to-protect statute. *American Journal of Psychiatry, 155,* 1097–1101.

Merrill, G. S., & Wolfe, V. A. (2000). Battered gay men: An exploration of abuse, help seeking and why they stay. *Journal-of-Homosexuality, 39,* 1–30.

Miller, L. (1999). Workplace violence: Prevention, response, and recovery. *Psychotherapy, 36,* 160–169.

Mitchell, J. T. (1983). When disaster strikes: The critical incident stress debriefing process. *Journal of Emergency Medical Services, 8,* 36–39.

Mitchell, J. T. (1988). Development and functions of a critical incident stress debriefing team. *Journal of Emergency Medical Services, 13,* 43–46.

Mitchell, J. T., & Everly, G. S. (1996). *Critical Incident Stress Debriefing (CISD): An operations manual for the prevention of traumatic stress among emergency services and disaster workers.* Ellicott City, MD: Chevron Publishing.

Mitchell, J. T., & Everly, G. S. (1998). *Critical Incident Stress Management: The basic course workbook.* Ellicott City, MD: Chevron Publishing.

Mitchell, J. T., Everly, G. S., & Mitchell, D. J. (1999). The hidden victims of disasters and vehicular accidents: The problem and recommended solutions. In E. J. Hicking & E. B. Blanchard (Eds.), *The international handbook of road traffic accidents and psychological trauma: Current understanding, treatment, and law* (pp. 141–153). New York: Elsevier Science Publishing.

Mohandie, K., & Hatcher, C. (1999). Suicide and violence risk in law enforcement. *Behavioral Sciences and the Law, 17,* 357–376.

Moiron, S. (1974). The hell of the inhaler. *CEMEF Informa, 2(4),* 5–8.

Monahan, J. (1993). Limiting exposure to Tarasoff liability: Guidelines for risk containment. *American Psychologist, 48,* 242–250.

Morey, L. C., & Zanarini, M. C. (2000). Borderline personality: Traits and disorder. *Journal of Abnormal Psychology, 109,* 733–737.

Morton, A. J., Hickey, M. A., & Dean, L. C. (2001). Methamphetamine toxicity in mice is potentiated by exposure to loud music. *Neuroreport: For Rapid Communication of Neuroscience Research, 12,* 3277–3281.

Mulvey, E. P., & Cauffman, E. (2001). The inherent limits of predicting school violence. *American Psychologist, 56,* 797–802.

Munroe, J. (1999). Ethical issues associated with secondary trauma in therapist. In B. H. Stamm (Ed.), *Secondary traumatic stress* (pp. 51–64). Lutherville, MD: Sidran.

Myer, R. A., Williams, R. C., Ottens, A. J., & Schmidt, A. E. (1992). A three dimensional model for triage. *Journal of Mental Health Counseling, 14,* 137–148.

Nash, M. (1987). What, if anything, is regressed about hypnotic age regression? A review of the empirical literature. *Psychological Bulletin, 102,* 42–52.

National Institute on Aging. (1998). Impact of aging on the Acquired Immunodeficiency Syndrome. *AIDS, 17,* 5.

Niel, D. E., & Binder, R. L. (1995). Correlates of the accuracy in the assessment of psychiatric inpatients' risk of violence. *American Journal of Psychiatry, 152,* 901–906.

Nisbett, R. E., & Ross, L. (1991). *The person and the situation.* New York: McGraw-Hill.

Nurmi, L. A. (1999). The sinking of the Estonia: The effects of critical incidence stress debriefing (CISD) on rescuers. *International Journal of Emergency Mental Health, 1,* 23–31.

Ory, M. G., & Mack, K. A. (1998). Middle-aged and older people with AIDS: Trends in national surveillance rates, transmission routes, and risk factors. *Research on Aging, 20,* 653–664.

Ory, M. G., Zablotsky, D. L., & Crystal, S. (1998). HIV/AIDS and aging: Identifying a prevention research and care agenda. *Research on Aging, 20,* 637–652.

O'Toole, M. E. (2000). *The school shooter: A threat assessment perspective.* Quantico, VA: Federal Bureau of Investigation.

Paton, D., Violanti, J. M., & Dunning, C. (2000). Posttraumatic stress intervention: Challenges, issues, and perspectives. In J. M. Violanti, D. Paton, & C. Dunning (Eds.), *Posttraumatic stress intervention: Challenges, issues, and perspectives* (pp. 3–9). Springfield, IL: Charles Thomas.

Pelletier, K. R. (2000). *The best alternative medicine: What works and what doesn't.* New York: Simon & Schuster.

Pennebaker, J. W. (2000). The effects of traumatic disclosure on physical and mental health: The values of writing and talking about upsetting events. In J. M. Violanti, D. Paton, & C. Dunning (Eds.), *Posttraumatic stress intervention: Challenges, issues, and perspectives* (pp. 97–114). Springfield, IL: Charles Thomas.

Phelps, E. A., O'Connor, K. J., Cunningham, W. A., Funayama, E. S., Gatenby, J. C., Gore, J. C., & Banaji, M. R. (2000). Performance on indirect measures of race evaluation predicts amygdala activation. *Journal of Cognitive Neuroscience, 12,* 729–738.

Pica, M. (1999). The evolution of alter personality states in dissociative identity disorder. *Psychotherapy, 36,* 404–415.

Pitman, R. K., Van der Kolk, B. A., Orr, S. P., & Greenberg, M. S. (1990). Naloxone-reversible analgesic response to combat-related stimuli in posttraumatic stress disorder: A pilot study. *Archives of General Psychiatry, 47,* 541–544.

Pope, H. G., Oliva, P. S., Hudson, J. K., Bodkin, J., Alexander, B. J., & Gruber, A. J. (1999). Attitudes toward DSM-IV dissociative disorders diagnoses among board certified American psychiatrists. *American Journal of Psychiatry, 145,* 321–323.

Pope, K. S., & Feldman-Summers, S. (1992). National survey of psychologists' sexual and physical abuse history and their evaluation of training and competence in those areas. *Professional Psychology: Research and Practice, 23,* 353–361.

Pope, K. S., & Tabachnick, B. G. (1994). Therapists as patients: A national survey of psychologists' experiences, problems, and beliefs. *Professional Psychology: Research and Practice, 25,* 247–258.

Pope, K. S., & Tabachnick, B. G. (1993). Therapists' anger, hate, fear, and sexual feelings: National survey of therapist responses, client characteristics, critical events, formal complaints, and training. *Professional Psychology: Research and Practice, 24,* 142–152.

Putnam, F. W. (1984). The psychophysiologic investigation of multiple personality disorder: A review. *Psychiatric Clinics of North America, 7,* 31–39.

Putnam, F. W. (2000). Dissociative disorders. In A. J. Sameroff, M. Lewis, & S. M. Miller (Eds.), *Handbook of developmental psychopathology (2nd ed.)* (pp. 739–754). New York: Kluwer Academic/Plenum Publishers.

Ramsey, B. (1993). *Community crisis intervention in Canada.* Paper presented at the Ninth Annual International Congress on Circumpolar Health, Reykjavik, Iceland.

Raphael, B. (1984). Psychiatric consultancy in major disaster. *Australian & New Zealand Journal of Psychiatry, 18,* 303–306.

Raphael, B., Singh, B., Bradbury, L., & Lambert, F. (1983). Who helps the helpers? The effects of a disaster on the rescue workers. *Omega Journal of Death & Dying, 14,* 9–20.

Read, J. (1997). Child abuse and psychosis: A literature review and implications for professional practice. *Professional Psychology: Research and Practice, 28,* 448–456.

Reis, M., & Nahmiash, D. (1998). Validation of the Indicators of Abuse (IOA) screen. *Gerontologist, 38,* 471–480.

Richard, K., & Range, L. M. (2001). Is training in psychology associated with increased responsiveness to suicidality? *Death Studies, 25,* 265–279.

Richman, J. (1999). Similarities and differences between younger and older suicidal people. *Journal of Clinical Geropsychology, 5,* 1–17.

Rieber, R. W. (1999). Hypnosis, false memory and multiple personality: A trinity of affinity. *History of Psychiatry, 10,* 3–11.

Robinson, R. (2000). Debriefing with emergency services: Critical incident stress management. In B. Raphael & J. P. Wilson (Eds.), *Psychological debriefing: Theory, practice, and evidence* (pp. 91–107). New York: Cambridge University Press.

Rose, M. A. (1996). Effect on an AIDS education program for older adults. *Journal of Community Health Nursing, 13,* 141–148.

Rosowsky, E., & Gurian, B. (1991). Borderline personality disorder in late life. *International Psychogeriatrics, 3,* 39–52.

Roth, J., Krishnan, S. P., & Bunch, E. (2001). Barriers to condom use: Results from a study in Mumbai (Bombay), India. *AIDS Education and Prevention, 13,* 65–77.

Ross, L. (1977). The intuitive psychologist and his shortcomings: Distortions in the attribution process. In L. Berkowitz (Ed.), *Advances in experimental social psychology* (Vol. 10, pp. 174–221). New York: Academic Press.

Rudestam, K. E. (1977). Physical and psychological responses to suicide in the family. *Journal of Consulting and Clinical Psychology, 45*, 162–170.

Ruggiero, K. J., Morris, T. L., & Scotti, J. R. (2001). Treatment for children with posttraumatic stress disorder: Current status and future directions. *Clinical Psychology: Science and Practice, 8*, 210–227.

Runyan, C. W., Zakocs, R. C., & Zwerling, C. (2000). Administrative and behavioral interventions for workplace violence prevention. *American Journal of Preventive Medicine, 18*, 116–127.

Rushkoff, D. (2001). Ecstacy: Prescription for cultural renaissance. In J. Holland (Ed.), Ecstacy: The complete guide: A comprehensive look at the risks and benefits of MDMA *(pp. 350–357). Rochester, VT: Park Street Press.*

Ryle, A., & Low, J. (1993). Cognitive analytic therapy. In G. Stricker & J. R. Gold (Eds.), *Comprehensive Handbook of Psychotherapy Integration* (pp. 87–100). New York: Plenum.

Sadavoy, J. (1996). Personality disorder in old age: Symptom expression. *Clinical Gerontologist, 16*, 19–36.

Saigh, P. A. (1998). Effects of flooding on memories of patients with posttraumatic stress disorder. In P. A. Bremner, J. Douglas, & C. R. Marmar (Eds.), *Trauma, memory, and dissociation* (pp. 285–320). Washington, DC: American Psychiatric Press.

Sapolsky, R. M. (1996). Why stress is bad for your brain. *Science, 273*, 749–750.

Sar, V., tutkun, J., Alyanak, B., Bakim, B., & Baral, I. (2000). Frequency of dissociative disorders among psychiatric outpatients in Turkey. *Comprehensive Psychiatry, 41*, 216–222.

Scheflin, A. W. (2000). The evolving standard of care in the practice of trauma and dissociative disorder therapy. *Bulletin of the Menninger Clinic, 64*, 197–234.

Schlitz, M., & Braud, W. (1997). Distant intentionality: Assessing the evidence. *Alternative Therapies, 3*, 62–73.

Schneider, J. (1984). *Stress, loss, and grief: Understanding their origins and growth potential.* Baltimore, MD: University Park Press.

Seligman, M. E. (1995). The effectiveness of psychotherapy: The *Consumer Reports* study. *American Psychologist, 50*, 965–974.

Seligman, M. E., & Csikszentmihalyi, M. (2000). Positive psychology: An introduction. *American Psychologist, 55*, 5–14.

Sells, S. P. (1998). *Treating the tough adolescent: A family-based, step-by-step guide.* New York: Guilford.

Sells, S. P. (2001). *Parenting your out of control teenager.* New York: St. Martin's Press.

Seng, J. S., Oakley, D. J., Sampselle, C. M., Killion, C., Graham-Bermann, S., & Liberzon, I. (2001). Posttraumatic stress disorder and pregnancy complications. *Obstetrics and Gynecology, 97*, 17–22.

Shaffer, D., Fisher, P., Lucas, C. P., & Dulcan, M. K. (2000). NIMH Diagnostic Interview for Children Version IV (NIMH DISC-IV): Description, differences from previous versions, and reliability of some common diagnoses. *Journal of the American Academy of Child and Adolescent Psychiatry, 39*, 28–38.

Shalev, A. Y., Friedman, M. J., Foa, E. B., & Keane, T. M. (2000). Integration and summary. In E. B. Foa, T. M. Keane, & M. J. Friedman (Eds.), *Effective treatment for PTSD: Practice guidelines from the International Society for Traumatic Stress Studies* (pp. 359–379). New York: Guilford.

Shapiro, F. (1989). Efficacy of the eye movement desensitization procedure in the treatment of traumatic memories. *Journal of Traumatic Stress, 2*, 199–223.

Shapiro, F. (1995). *Eye movement desensitization and reprocessing: Basic principles, protocols and procedures.* New York: Guilford.

Shapiro, F. (1996). *Eye Movement Desensitization and Reprocessing: Level I training manual.* Pacific Grove, CA: EMDR Institute.

Shotland, R. L., & Straw, M. K. (1976). Bystander response to an assault: When a man attacks a woman. *Journal of Personality and Social Psychology, 34,* 990–999.

Sicher, F., Targ, E., Moore, D., & Smith, H. S. (1998). A randomized double-blind study of the effect of distant healing in a population with advanced AIDS: A report of a small scale study. *Western Journal of Medicine, 169,* 356–363.

Silberg, J. L. (1998). Dissociative symptomatology in children and adolescents as displayed on psychological testing. *Journal of Personalitiy Assessment, 71,* 421–439.

Silver, S. M., & Wilson, J. P. (1988). Native American healing and purification rituals for war stress. In J. P. Wilson, Z. Harel, & B. Kahana (Eds.), *Human adaptation to extreme stress: From the Holocaust to Vietnam* (pp. 337–355). New York: Plenum.

Simon, L., Greenberg, J., Harmon-Jones, E., Solomon, S., & Pyszczynski, T. (1996). Mild depression, mortality salience, and the defense of the worldview: Evidence of intensified terror management in the mildly depressed. *Personality and Social Psychology Bulletin, 22,* 81–90.

Soisson, E. L., VandeCreek, L., & Knapp, S. (1987). Thorough record keeping: A good defense in a litigious era. *Professional Psychology: Research and Practice, 18,* 498–502.

Solomon, R. M. (1994). *Eye movement desensitization and reprocessing and treatment of grief.* Paper presented at the 4th International Conference on Grief and Bereavement in Contemporary Society, Stockholm, Sweden.

Solomon, R. M., & Shapiro, F. (1997). Eye movement desensitization and reprocessing: A therapeutic tool for trauma and grief. In C. Figley (Ed.), *Death and trauma: The traumatology of grieving* (pp. 231–247). Philadelphia, PA: Taylor & Francis.

Somers, J. U., & Yawkey, T. D. (1984). Imaginary play companions: Contributions of creative and intellectual abilities of young children. *Journal of Creative Behavior, 18,* 77–89.

Southwick, S. M., Krystal, J. H., Morgan, C. A., & Johnson, D. (1993). Abnormal noradrenergic function in posttraumatic stress disorder. *Archives of General Psychiatry, 50,* 266–274.

Spence, K. W. (1956). *Behavior theory and conditioning.* New York: Guilford.

Springer, S. P., & Deutsch, G. (1993). *Left brain, right brain* (4th ed.). New York: Freeman.

Stall, R., & Catania, J. (1994). AIDS risk behaviors among late middle-aged and elderly Americans. *Archives of Internal Medicine, 154,* 57–63.

Stein, D. J., Zungu-Kirwayi, N., van der Linden, G. J. H., & Seedat, S. (2001). Pharmacotherapy for posttraumatic stress disorder (Cochrane review). *The Cochrane Library, 2.* Oxford: Update Software.

Steinberg, M., Rounsaville, B., & Cicchetti, D. (1991). Detection of dissociative disorders in psychiatric patients by a screening instrument and a structured interview. *American Journal of Psychiatry, 148,* 1050–1054.

Sternberg, K. J., Lamb, M. E., Greenbaum, C., Cichetti, D., Dawud, S., Cortes, R. M., Krispin, O., & Lorey, F. (1993). Effects of domestic violence on children's behavior problems and depression. *Developmental Psychology, 29,* 44–52.

Storm, V., McDermott, B., & Finlayson, D. (1994). *The bushfire and me: A story of what happened to me and my family.* Newtown, Australia: New South Wales Department of Health.

Streeck-Fischer, A., & van der Kolk, V. A. (2000). Down will come baby, cradle and all: Diagnostic and therapeutic implications of chronic trauma on child development. *Australian and New Zealand Journal of Psychiatry, 34,* 903–918.

Stricker, G. (1995a). Failures in psychotherapy. *Journal of Psychotherapy Integration, 5,* 91–93.

Stricker, G. (1995b). The lessons of failure. *Journal of Psychotherapy Integration, 5,* 183–188.

Stuhlmiller, C., & Dunning, C. (2000). Challenging the mainstream: From pathogenic to salutogenic models of posttrauma intervention. In J. M. Violanti, D. Paton, & C. Dunning (Eds.), *Posttraumatic stress intervention: Challenges, issues, and perspectives* (pp. 10–42). Springfield, IL: Charles Thomas.

Swann, W. B., Pelham, B. W., & Chidester, T. R. (1988). Change through paradox: Using self-verification to alter beliefs. *Journal of Personality and Social Psychology, 54,* 268–273.

Szostak-Pierce, S. (1999). Even further: The power of subcultural style in techno culture. In K. K. Johnson, & S. J. Lennon (Eds.), *Appearance and power: Dress, body, culture* (pp. 141–151). New York: Berg.

Tarasoff v. Regents of the University of California (1976). 551 P.2d 334.

Tatara, T. (1995). *Elder abuse: Questions and answers.* Washington, DC: National Center on Elder Abuse.

Tatara, T. (Ed). (1999). *Understanding elder abuse in minority populations.* Philadelphia, PA: Brunner/Mazel.

Telch, C. F., Agras, W. S., & Linehan, M. M. (2000). Group dialectical behavior therapy for binge eating disorder: A preliminary, uncontrolled trial. *Behavior Therapy, 31,* 569–582.

Terry, M. J. (1999). Kelengakutelleghpat: An arctic community-based approach to trauma. In B. H. Stamm (Ed.), *Secondary traumatic stress (2nd ed.)* (pp. 149–178). Lutherville, MD: Sidran.

Tolan, P. H., Guerra, N. G., & Kendall, P. C. (1995). A developmental ecological perspective on antisocial behavior in children and adolescents: Toward a unified risk and intervention framework. *Journal of Consulting and Clinical Psychology, 63,* 579–584.

Tsai, G. E., Condie, D., Wu, M., & Chang, I. (1999). Functional magnetic resonance imaging of personality switches in a woman with dissociative identity disorder. *Harvard Review of Psychiatry, 7,* 119–122.

Tseng, W. S., & Hsu, J. (1991). *Culture and family: Problems and therapy.* New York: Haworth.

Tyron, G. (1986). Abuse of therapist by patient: A national survey. *Professional Psychology: Research and Practice, 17,* 357–363.

Van der Hart, L., & Nijenhuis, E. R. (1999). Bearing witness to uncorroborated trauma: The clinician's development of reflective belief. *Professional Psychology: Research and Practice, 30,* 37–44.

Van der Kolk, B. A., Burbridge, J. A., & Suzuki, J. (1997). The psychobiology of traumatic memory. Clinical implications of neuroimaging studies. In R. Yehuda, & A. C. McFarlane (Eds.), *Psychobiology of posttraumatic stress disorder* (pp. 99–113). New York: New York Academy of Sciences.

Van Veldhuizen, P. J. (2000). "Attitudes toward DSM-IV dissociative disorders diagnoses among board-certified American Psychiatrists": Comment. *American Journal of Psychiatry, 157,* 1180–1181.

VandeCreek, L., & Knapp, S. (2000). Risk management and life-threatening patient behaviors. *Journal of Clinical Psychology, 56,* 1335–1351.

Vernberg, E. M., LaGreca, A. M., Silverman, W. K., & Prinstein, M. J. (1996). Prediction of posttraumatic stress symptoms in children after Hurricane Andrew. *Journal of Abnormal Psychology, 105,* 237–248.

Wachtel, P. L. (1977). *Psychoanalysis and behavior therapy: Toward an integration.* New York: Norton.

Walker, L. E. (1979). How battering happens and how to stop it. In D. Moored (Ed.), *Battered women* (pp. 59–78). Newbury Park, CA: Sage.

Walker, L. E. (1984). *The battered woman syndrome.* New York: Springer.

Wee, D. F., Mills, D. M., & Koehler, G. (1999). The effects of critical incidence stress debriefing (CISD) on emergency medical services personnel following the Los Angeles civil disturbance. *International Journal of Emergency Mental Health, 1,* 33–37.

Weed, L. L. (1971). *Medical records, medical education, and patient care: The problem-oriented record as a basic tool.* Chicago: Year Book.

Welfel, E. R., Danzinger, P. R., & Santoro, S. (2000). Mandated reporting of abuse/ maltreatment of older adults: A primer for counselors. *Journal of Counseling and Development, 78,* 284–292.

Wessley, S., Rose, S., & Bisson, J. (1998). A systematic review of brief psychological interventions ("debriefing") for the treatment of immediate trauma related symptoms and the prevention of post traumatic stress disorder (Cochrane review). In *The Cochrane Library, 3.* Oxford: Update Software.

West, C. M. (1998). Leaving a second closet. In J. L. Jasinski & L. M. Williams (Eds.), *Partner violence: A comprehensive review of 20 years of research* (pp. 163–183). Newbury Park, CA: Sage.

Whalen, P. J., Rauch, S. L., Etcoff, N. L., McInerney, S. C., Lee, M. B., & Jenike, M. A. (1998). Masked presentation of emotional facial expressions modulate amygdala activity without explicit knowledge. *Journal of Neuroscience, 18,* 411–418.

Whatley, M. A., & Riggio, R. E. (1993). Gender differences in attributions of blame for male rape victims. *Journal of Interpersonal Violence, 8,* 502–511.

White, M. (2001). House passes FEMA spending measure. *Nation's Cities Weekly, 24,* 2–12.

White, P. A., & Younger, D. P. (1988). Differences in the ascription of transient internal states to self and other. *Journal of Experimental Social Psychology, 24,* 292–309.

Williams, T. M., Zabrack, M. L., & Joy, L. A. (1982). The portrayal of aggression on North American television. *Journal of Applied Social Psychology, 12,* 360–380.

Winnicott, D. W. (1971). *Playing and reality.* Baltimore, MD: Penguin.

Widom, C. S., & Morris, S. (1997). Accuracy of adult recollections of childhood victimization: Part 2. Childhood sexual abuse. *Psychological Assessment, 9.* 34–46.

Wolf, E. S. (1988). *Treating the self: Elements of clinical self psychology.* New York: Guilford.

Yalom, I. (1995). *The theory and practice of group psychotherapy* (4th ed.). New York: Basic.

Young, W. C. (1994). EMDR treatment of phobic symptoms in multiple personality. *Dissociation, 7,* 129–133.

Yufit, R. I. (1991). American Association of Suicidology Presidential Address: Suicide assessment in the 1990's. *Suicide & Life Threatening Behavior, 21,* 152.

Zabukovec, J., Lazrove, S., & Shapiro, F. (2000). Self-healing aspects of EMDR: The therapeutic change process and perspectives of integrated psychotherapies. *Journal of Psychotherapy Integration, 10,* 189–206.

Zeitlin, D., Keller, S. E., Shiflett, S. C., Schleifer, S. J., & Barlett, J. A. (2000). Immunological effects of massage therapy during acute academic stress. *Psychosomatic Medicine, 62,* 83–84.

Zingraff, M., & Randall, T. (1984). Differential sentencing of women and men in the U.S.A. *International Journal of the Sociology of Law, 12,* 401–413.

Zuckerman, M., Miyake, K., & Elkin, C. S. (1995). Effects of attractiveness and maturity of face and voice on interpersonal impressions. *Journal of Research in Personality, 29,* 253–272.

Zweig, R. A., & Hillman, J. (1999). Personality disorders in adults: A review. In E. Rosowsky, R. C. Abrams, & R. A. Zweig (Eds.), *Personality disorders in older adults: Emerging issues in diagnosis and treatment* (pp. 31–54). Mahwah, NJ: Erlbaum.

Index

Printed in the United States
126781LV00007B/36/A

9 780306 473418